Nutrition

7th Edition

by Carol Ann Rinzler

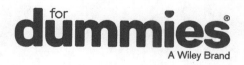

for
dummies®
A Wiley Brand

Nutrition For Dummies®, 7th Edition

Published by: **John Wiley & Sons, Inc.**, 111 River Street, Hoboken, NJ 07030-5774, www.wiley.com

Copyright © 2021 by John Wiley & Sons, Inc., Hoboken, New Jersey

Published simultaneously in Canada

For general information on our other products and services, please contact our Customer Care Department within the U.S. at 877-762-2974, outside the U.S. at 317-572-3993, or fax 317-572-4002. For technical support, please visit https://hub.wiley.com/community/support/dummies.

Wiley publishes in a variety of print and electronic formats and by print-on-demand. Some material included with standard print versions of this book may not be included in e-books or in print-on-demand. If this book refers to media such as a CD or DVD that is not included in the version you purchased, you may download this material at http://booksupport.wiley.com. For more information about Wiley products, visit www.wiley.com.

Library of Congress Control Number: 2021935176

ISBN 978-1-119-72390-5 (pbk); ISBN 978-1-119-72400-1 (ebk); ISBN 978-1-119-72402-5 (ebk)

Manufactured in the United States of America

SKY10029639_091321

Contents at a Glance

Table of Contents

Introduction

The first edition of *Nutrition For Dummies* in 1997 began by noting that once upon a time, people simply sat down to dinner, eating to fill up an empty stomach or just for the pleasure of it. Nobody said, "Wow, that cream soup is loaded with calories," or asked whether the bread was a high-fiber loaf or fretted about the chicken being served with the skin still on. No longer. Today, the dinner table can be a battleground between health and pleasure. You plan your meals with the precision of a major general moving his troops into the front lines, and for most people, the fight to eat what's good for you rather than what tastes good has become a lifelong struggle.

The six editions since then, including this one, have added new information designed to end the war between your need for good nutrition and your equally compelling need for tasty meals, with the facts and figures from nutrition researchers who continue to make it ever more clear that what's good for you can also be good to eat — and vice versa.

About This Book

Nutrition For Dummies, 7th Edition, doesn't aim to send you back to the classroom, sit you down, and make you take notes about what to put on the table every day from now until you're 104 years old. You're reading a reference book, so you don't have to memorize anything — when you want more info, just jump in anywhere to look it up.

Instead, this book means to give you the information you need to make wise food choices — which always means choices that please the palate and soul as well as the body. Some of what you'll read here is really, *really* basic: definitions of vitamins, minerals, proteins, fats, carbohydrates, and, yes, plain (and not so plain) water. You'll also read tips about how to put together a nutritious shopping list and how to use food to make meals so good you can't wait to eat them.

For those who know absolutely nothing about nutrition except that it deals with food, this book is a starting point. For those who know more than a little about nutrition, this book is a refresher course to bring you up to speed on what has happened since the last time you checked out a calorie chart.

For those who want to know *absolutely everything*, this edition of *Nutrition For Dummies* is up to date with hot new info from the 2020 revisions of the *Dietary Guidelines for Americans* and all the twisty "this is good for you" and "this is not" bits and pieces of food info that nutrition scientists have come up with since, well, the last edition.

Wherever you are on your nutrition-information journey, know that some small parts of this book are fun or informative but not necessarily vital to your understanding of nutrition. For example:

» **Text in sidebars:** The sidebars are the shaded boxes that appear here and there. They share personal stories and observations but aren't necessary reading.

» **Anything with a Technical Stuff icon attached:** This information is interesting but not critical to your understanding of nutrition.

Foolish Assumptions

Every book is written with a particular reader in mind, and this one is no different. As I wrote this book, I made the following basic assumptions about who you are and why you plunked down your hard-earned cash for an entire volume about nutrition:

» You didn't study nutrition in high school or college and now you've discovered that you have a better shot at staying healthy if you know how to put together well-balanced, nutritious meals.

» You're confused by conflicting advice on vitamins and minerals, protein, fats, and carbs. In other words, you need a reliable road map through the nutrient maze.

» You want basic information, but you don't want to become an expert in nutrition or spend hours digging your way through medical textbooks and journals.

Icons Used in This Book

Icons are a handy *For Dummies* way to catch your attention as you slide your eyes down the page. The icons come in several varieties, each with its own special meaning.

REMEMBER

The information tagged with this icon is important enough for you to highlight, write down and post it where you'll see it often, or flag for later reference.

TECHNICAL STUFF

This icon points to clear, concise explanations of technical terms and processes — details that are interesting but not necessarily critical to your understanding of a topic. In other words, skip them if you want, but try a few first.

TIP

Bull's-eye! This is time- and stress-saving information that you can use to improve your diet and health.

WARNING

This is a watch-out-for-the-curves icon, alerting you to nutrition pitfalls, such as (oops!) leaving the skin on the chicken — turning a low-fat food into one that is high in fat and cholesterol. This icon also warns you about physical dangers, such as supplements to avoid because they may do more damage than good to your health.

Beyond the Book

In addition to what you're reading right now, this product also comes with a free access-anywhere Cheat Sheet that provides helpful tips on cutting calories, figuring out when you may need extra nutrients, keeping food safe, and understanding nutrition terms and measurements. To get this Cheat Sheet, simply go to www. dummies.com and search for "Nutrition For Dummies Cheat Sheet" in the Search box.

Where to Go from Here

For Dummies books are not linear (proceeding from Chapter 1 to 2 to 3 and so on). In fact, you can choose a subject, such as calories, in Chapter 5, dive right in there, and then skip over to how water works in your body (that's Chapter 12) and still make sense of what you're reading because each chapter delivers a complete message. (Full disclosure: Once in a while there will be a cross reference to a second chapter or even a third, a kind of nutrition fact treasure hunt.)

So, in short, if proteins are your passion, go right to Chapter 6. If you want to know why you absolutely can't resist chocolate-covered pretzels, go to Chapter 15. If you're fascinated by food processing, your choice is Chapter 19. Use the table of contents to find broad categories of information or the index to look up more specific things.

On the other hand, if you're not sure where you want to go, why not just begin at the beginning, Part 1, Chapter 1? It gives you all the basic info you need to understand nutrition and points to places where you can find more detailed information.

1

Nutrition 101: The Basic Facts about Nutrition

Chapter **1**

Nutrition Equals Life: Knowing What to Eat to Get What You Need

Y ou are *what* you eat. You are also *how* you eat. And *when* you eat.

Choosing a varied diet of healthful foods supports any healthy mind and body, but *which* healthful foods you choose says much about your personal tastes as well as the culture from which you come.

How you eat may do the same: Do you use a knife and fork? A pair of sticks? Your hands and a round of bread? Each is a cultural statement. As for *when* you eat (and when you stop), that is a purely personal physiological response to signals from your digestive organs and your brain: "Get food now!" or "Thank you, that's enough."

Understanding more about nutrition means exploring what happens to what you eat and drink as it moves from your plate to your mouth to your digestive tract and into every tissue and cell and discovering how your organs and systems work. You observe firsthand why some foods and beverages are essential to your health. And you find out how to manage your diet so that you can get the biggest bang (nutrients) for your buck (calories).

Discovering the First Principles of Nutrition

Technically speaking, *nutrition* is the science of how the body uses food. In the broader sense, it is nourishment — the process of providing food and the study of what that food offers. In fact, nutrition is life. All living things, including you, need food and water to live. Beyond that, you need good food, meaning food with the proper nutrients, to live well. If you don't eat and drink, you'll die. Period. If you don't eat and drink nutritious food and beverages your body may pay the price:

>> Your bones may bend or break (not enough calcium).

>> Your gums may bleed (not enough vitamin C).

>> Your blood may not carry oxygen to every cell (not enough iron).

And on, and on, and on. Understanding how good nutrition protects you requires a familiarity with the language and concepts of nutrition.

Knowing some basic chemistry is helpful. (Don't panic: Chemistry can be a cinch when you read about it in plain English.) A smattering of sociology and psychology is also useful, because although nutrition is mostly about how food revs up and sustains your body, it's also — as I explain in Chapter 15 — about the cultural traditions and individual differences that explain why you like the food you like.

You've heard "You are what you eat" before. As a matter of fact, it's the first sentence at the top of this chapter. But it bears repeating, because the human body is built with the nutrients it gets from food: water, protein, fat, carbohydrates, vitamins, and minerals.

Nutrition's primary task is to figure out which foods and beverages (in what quantities) are required to construct and maintain every one of your organs and systems. To do this, nutrition concentrates on food's two basic attributes: energy and nutrients.

>> *Energy* is the ability to do work. The amount of energy in food is measured in *calories,* the amount of heat produced when food is burned (metabolized) in your body cells. You can read all about calories in Chapter 5, but for starters, all you need to know is that food is the fuel on which your body runs. Without enough food, you don't have enough energy. No surprise there.

>> *Nutrients* are the natural chemical substances your body uses to build, maintain, and repair tissues. They also make it possible for cells to send messages back and forth to conduct essential chemical reactions such as the ones that make it possible for you to

- Breathe
- Move
- Eliminate waste
- Think
- See
- Hear
- Smell
- Taste

and do everything else common to a healthy living body.

Breaking nutrients into two groups

Each of the nutrients in food fall into one of two distinct groups, macronutrients and micronutrients:

>> **Macronutrients (*macro* = big):** Protein, fat, carbohydrates, and water

>> **Micronutrients (*micro* = small):** Vitamins and minerals and a multitude of other substances

What's the difference between these two groups? The amount you need each day.

Your daily requirements for macronutrients generally exceed 1 gram. An ounce of solid material, such as chicken, has 28 grams, and an ounce of liquid, such as water, has 30 grams. To give you an idea of how that translates into nutrient requirements, the average man needs about 63 grams of protein a day (slightly more than 2 ounces), and the average woman needs about 50 grams (slightly less than 2 ounces).

And remember: That's grams of protein, not grams of a high-protein food such as meat, fish, or poultry.

For example, the USDA National Nutrient Database for Standard Reference (`http://ndb.nal.usda.gov`), one of the ten thoroughly reliable sources listed in Chapter 27, provides the following information for grams of meat versus grams of protein:

>> **Chicken:** 3 ounces/86 grams breast meat (no bones, no skin), roasted, provides 26.7 grams/0.96 ounces protein

>> **Lean ground beef (7% fat):** 4 ounces/113 grams provides 23.6 grams/0.86 ounces protein

>> **Canned salmon:** 3.5 ounces/100 grams provides 19.68 grams/0.70 ounces protein

Your daily requirements for micronutrients are much smaller. Consider vitamins. The Recommended Dietary Allowance (RDA) for vitamin C is measured in milligrams (1/1,000 of a gram), while the RDAs for vitamin D, vitamin B12, and folate are even smaller, measured in micrograms (1/1,000,000 of a gram). For more about the RDAs, including how they vary for people of different ages, check out Chapter 3.

Looking at essential nutrients

A reasonable person may assume that an essential nutrient is one you need to sustain a healthy body. But who says a reasonable person thinks like a nutritionist? In nutrition speak, an *essential nutrient* is a very special thing:

>> **An essential nutrient can't be manufactured in the body.** You have to get essential nutrients from food or from a nutritional supplement.

>> **An essential nutrient is linked to a specific deficiency disease,** such as scurvy, the deficiency disease that may afflict people who go without sufficient vitamin C for extended periods of time, or kwashiorkor, the protein deficiency disease. A diet rich in the essential nutrient prevents or cures the deficiency disease, but you need the proper nutrient. In other words, you can't cure a vitamin C deficiency with extra amounts of protein.

TECHNICAL STUFF

Not all nutrients are essential for all species of animals. Take vitamin C (and you should, every day). It's an essential nutrient for human beings but not for dogs because a dog's body manufactures the vitamin C it needs. Check out the list of nutrients on a can or bag of dog food. See? No vitamin C. The dog already has the vitamin C it — sorry, he or she — requires.

WHAT'S A BODY MADE OF?

Sugar and spice and everything nice well, more precisely water and fat and protein and carbohydrates (the simple and complex sugars described in Chapter 8) and vitamins and minerals.

On average, when you step on the scale, approximately 60 percent of your weight is water, 20 percent is body fat (slightly less for a man), and 20 percent is a combination of mostly protein, plus carbohydrates, minerals, vitamins, and other naturally occurring biochemicals.

Based on these percentages, you can reasonably expect that an average 140-pound person's body weight consists of about

- 84 pounds of water

- 28 pounds of body fat

- 28 pounds of a combination of protein (up to 25 pounds), minerals (up to 7 pounds), carbohydrates (up to 1.4 pounds), and vitamins (a trace)

You're right: Those last figures do total more than 28 pounds. That's because "up to" (as in "up to 25 pounds of protein") means that the amounts may vary from person to person. Ditto for minerals and carbohydrates.

Why? And how? Because a young person's body has proportionately more muscle and less fat than an older person's, and a woman's body has proportionately less muscle and more fat than a man's. As a result, more of a man's weight comes from protein and muscle and bone mass, while more of a woman's weight comes from fat. Protein-packed muscles and mineral-packed bones are denser tissue than fat.

Weigh a man and a woman of roughly the same height and size, and his greater bone and muscle mass means he's likely to tip the scale higher every time.

Here are three other examples of nutrients that are essential for some pets and plants but not necessarily for humans:

>> **Myo-inositol:** Myo-inositol, an organic compound similar to glucose — the fuel we get from carbohydrates — is an essential nutrient for gerbils and rats who can't make it in their own bodies and thus must get what they need from food. It's nonessential for human beings who can synthesize myo-inositol and then use it in dozens of important body processes, such as transmitting signals between cells.

>> **Taurine:** The amino acid taurine is essential for cats, but *conditionally essential for humans*, which means essential for some people but not all. All human bodies except newborns synthesize taurine from the amino acids methionine and cysteine (see Chapter 6), so although adults can make their own taurine, newborns need to get theirs from food, either breast milk or formula. That's why its essential nature is conditional.

>> **Boron:** Several minerals, such as boron, are essential for plants but haven't been proven essential for either microorganisms, such as bacteria, or for animals, including people.

For more on the vitamins and minerals, *amino acids* (the so-called building blocks of proteins), and fatty acids that are considered essential for your human body, check out Chapters 6, 7, 10, and 11.

Protecting the Nutrients in Your Food

Identifying nutrients is one thing. Making sure you get them into your body is another. What's essential is keeping nutritious food nutritious by preserving and protecting its components.

Some people see the term *food processing* as a nutritional dirty word, or two words. They're wrong. Without food processing and preservatives, you and I would still be forced to gather or kill our food each morning and down it fast before it spoiled. For more about which processing and preservative techniques produce the safest, most nutritious — and yes, delicious — dinners, check out Part 4.

Considering how vital food preservation can be, you may want to think about when you last heard a rousing cheer for the anonymous cook who first noticed that salting or pickling food could extend food's shelf life. Or for the guys who invented the refrigeration and freezing techniques that slow food's natural tendency to spoil.

Or for Louis Pasteur, the man who made it absolutely clear that heating food to boiling kills bugs (microorganisms) that might otherwise cause food poisoning. So give them a hand, right here.

Knowing Your Nutritional Status

Nutritional status is a phrase that describes the state of your health as related to your diet. *Malnutrition* is what happens when the diet goes wrong. Most people think of malnutrition as the result of diet too low in calories and essential nutrients, such as vitamins, but a diet that delivers too much food leads to malnutrition in the form of obesity. The latter is more common in developed countries with an abundant food supply and a relatively sedentary population. The former may arise from

>> **A diet that simply doesn't provide enough food:** This situation can occur in times of famine or through voluntary starvation due to an eating disorder or because something in your life disturbs your appetite. Among older people, malnutrition may follow tooth loss or age-related loss of appetite or because they live alone and sometimes just forget to eat.

>> **A diet that, while otherwise adequate, is deficient in a specific nutrient:** This kind of nutritional inadequacy can lead to a deficiency disease, such as beriberi — the disease caused by a lack of vitamin B1 (thiamine).

>> **A metabolic disorder or medical condition that prevents your body from absorbing specific nutrients, such as carbohydrates or protein:** One common example is diabetes, the inability to produce enough insulin, the hormone your body uses to metabolize (digest) carbohydrates. Another is celiac disease, a condition that makes it impossible for the body to digest gluten, a protein in wheat. Need more info on either diabetes or celiac disease? Check out *Diabetes For Dummies,* by Alan L. Rubin; *Diabetes Meal Planning & Nutrition For Dummies,* by Toby Smithson and Alan L. Rubin; and *Gluten-Free All-in-One For Dummies,* a five-books-in-one bargain on living with celiac disease (all books published by Wiley).

Doctors and registered dietitians have many tools with which to rate your nutritional status. They can

>> Review your medical history to see whether you have any conditions (such as dentures) that may make eating certain foods difficult or that interfere with your ability to absorb nutrients.

>> Perform a physical examination to look for obvious signs of nutritional deficiency, such as dull hair and eyes (a lack of vitamins?), poor posture (not enough calcium to protect the spinal bones?), or extreme thinness (not enough food? an underlying disease?).

>> Order laboratory blood and urine tests that may identify early signs of malnutrition, such as the lack of red blood cells that characterizes anemia caused by an iron deficiency.

At every stage of life, the aim of a good diet is to maintain a healthy nutritional status.

Fitting Food into the Medicine Chest

Food is medicine for the body and the soul. Good meals make good friends, and modern research validates the virtues not only of Granny's chicken soup but also of heart-healthy sulfur compounds in garlic and onions, anticholesterol dietary fiber in grains and beans, bone-building calcium in milk and greens, and mood elevators in coffee, tea, and chocolate.

Of course, foods pose some risks as well: food allergies, food intolerances, food and drug interactions, and the occasional harmful substances, such as the dreaded *saturated fats* and *trans fats* (see Chapter 7). In other words, constructing a healthful diet can mean tailoring food choices to your own special body, which is the subject of Part 5.

Finding Nutrition Facts

Getting reliable information about nutrition can be a challenge. For the most part, you're likely to get your nutrition information from TV and radio talk shows or news, your daily newspaper, your favorite magazine, a variety of nutrition-oriented books, and the Internet.

If you're not a nutrition expert, how can you tell whether what you hear or read is really right? By looking for the validation from people who are, of course, and by knowing what questions to ask.

Nutrition people

Not every piece of nutrition news is nutritious. The person who makes the news may simply have wandered in with a new theory — "Artichokes cure cancer!" "Never eat cherries and cheese at the same meal!" "Women who take vitamin C are more likely to give birth to twins!" The more bizarre, the better.

Those most likely to give you news you can use with confidence are

>> **Nutrition scientists and researchers:** These are people with undergraduate or graduate degrees in science subjects, such as chemistry, biology, biochemistry, or physics, and are engaged in research dealing primarily with the biological effects of food on animals and human beings. Some nutrition investigators come from other fields entirely, such as a historian or sociologist, whose research concentrates on food history and habits.

>> **Dietitians and nutritionists:** These people have undergraduate degrees in food and nutrition science or the management of food programs. A person with the letters RD *(registered dietitian)* after his name has completed a dietetic internship and passed an American Dietetic Association licensing exam. In some states, a person who claims the title "nutritionist" must have a graduate degree in basic science courses related to nutrition.

>> **Nutrition reporters and writers:** These are people who specialize in giving you information about the medical and/or scientific aspects of food. Most have the science background required to translate technical information into language nonscientists can understand. Some have been trained as dietitians, nutritionists, or nutrition scientists; others gain their expertise through years of covering their beat.

REMEMBER

Regardless of the source, nutrition news should always pass what you might call *The Reasonableness Test.* In other words, if a story or report or study or theory sounds ridiculous, as in the earlier examples, it probably is.

Questions to ask about any study

You open your morning newspaper or turn on the evening news and read or hear that a group of researchers at an impeccably prestigious scientific organization has published a study showing that yet another thing you've always taken for granted is hazardous to your health. So you throw out the offending food or drink or rearrange your daily routine to avoid the once-acceptable, now-dangerous food, beverage, or additive. And then what happens? Two weeks, two months, or two years down the road, a second, equally prestigious group of scientists publishes a study conclusively proving that the first group got it wrong.

Consider the saga of dietary fiber and colon cancer. In the early 1990s, based on a respectably large number of studies including a 1992 meta-analysis of 13 case-control efforts in nine different nations, all kinds of health experts urged everyone to increase his or her consumption of high-fiber foods to reduce the risk of colon cancer. Then in 1999, data from the long-running Nurses' Health Study at the Harvard School of Public Health showed absolutely no difference in the risk of colon and rectal cancer between women who ate lots of high-fiber foods and those who didn't.

Imagine the confusion. Imagine the number of boxes of high-fiber cereal tossed in favor of scrambled eggs, once considered a cholesterol risk, now regarded as perfectly healthful, for breakfast. Imagine the reaction to a report in the *Journal of the National Cancer Institute* two years later saying that while cereal high in dietary fiber may not be protective, people whose diets are low in fruit and vegetables have the greatest risk of colorectal cancer. What to do? Toss the cereal? Keep the banana?

Nobody seems to know. That leaves you, a layperson, on your own to come up with the answer. Never fear — you may not be a nutritionist, but that doesn't mean you can't ask five common-sense questions about any study to arrive at a sensible conclusion that says, "Yes, this may be true," or "No, this may not be."

Does this study include human beings?

True, animal studies can alert researchers to potential problems, but working with animals alone can't give you conclusive proof of the effect in human beings because different species react differently to various foods and chemicals and diseases. Cows and horses can digest grass and hay; humans can't. Mouse and rat embryos suffer no ill effects when their mothers are given thalidomide, the sedative that's known to cause deformed fetal limbs when given to pregnant monkeys — and human beings — at the point in pregnancy when limbs are developing.

Are there enough people in this study?

No, a researcher's saying, "Well, I did give this to a couple of people," is not enough. To provide a reliable conclusion, a study must include sufficient numbers of people to establish a pattern. Otherwise, there's always the possibility that an effect occurred by chance.

Equally important, the study needs people of different ages, races, ethnicity, and, yes, gender. Without them, the results may not apply across the board. One good example can be found in the original studies linking high blood cholesterol levels to an increased risk of heart disease and linking small doses of aspirin to a reduced risk of a second heart attack involved only men. It wasn't until follow-up studies were conducted with women that researchers were able to say with any certainty that high cholesterol may be hazardous for men and women and that aspirin is protective for women as well as men — but not in quite the same way. As cardiovascular researchers eventually learned, men taking low-dose aspirin tend to lower their risk of heart attack. For women, the aspirin reduces the risk of stroke. *Vive la difference!*

Is there anything in the design or method of this study that may affect the accuracy of its conclusions?

Some testing methods are more likely than others to lead to biased or inaccurate conclusions. A *retrospective study* (which asks people to tell what they did in the past) is always considered less accurate than a *prospective study* (one that follows people while they're actually doing what the researchers are studying), because memory isn't always reliable. People tend to forget details or, without meaning to, alter them to fit the researchers' questions.

Was this study reviewed by the author's peers?

Serious researchers subject their studies to peer review, which means they have others working in the same field read the data and approve the conclusions. All reliable scientific journals require peer review before publishing a study.

Are the study's conclusions reasonable?

If you find a study's conclusions illogical, chances are the researchers feel the same way. In 1990, the Nurses' Health Study reported that a high-fat diet raised the risk of colon cancer. But the data showed a link only to diets high in beef. No link was found to diets high in dairy fat. In short, this study was begging for a second study to confirm (or deny) its results, and in 2005, a large study of more than 60,000 Swedish women, reported in the *American Journal of Clinical Nutrition*, showed that eating lots of high-fat dairy foods actually reduced the risk of colorectal cancer.

EXTREME NUTRITION: CANNIBALISM

Cannibalism, from *Canibales*, the name early Spanish explorers pinned on a tribe in the West Indies, is one of civilized mankind's strongest taboos, but anthropologists know that men and women have been tossing their friends and neighbors and relatives and defeated enemies onto the fire or into the stew pot ever since there was a written or drawn record of human activity.

The heyday of cannibalism reports was the Age of Exploration when stories of man-eating savages went along with virtually every voyage to the New World. Clearly, many of the terrifying tales were true, but the cannibal label was also used to belittle or demonize unknown or resistant peoples.

In fact, cannibalism has crept into virtually every society, civilized and not, driven by religious or cultural ritual such as the idea that devouring the heart of a brave man confers bravery upon the diner, but more commonly by simple necessity of survival during famine. In 1609, for example, George Percy, an original member of the Jamestown Colony in Virginia, wrote: *" now famin beginneinge to Looke gastely and pale in every face, thatt notheinge was Spared to mainteyne Lyfe and to doe those things which seame incredible, as to digge upp deade corpes outt of graves and to eate them. And some have Licked upp the Bloode which hathe fallen from their weake fellowes."*

Although they did not reach into graves, members of the Donner Party, caught in winter storms and starving as they tried to cross the Rockies (1846–1847), were also driven to cannibalism, as were those caught in the dreadful 842-day Siege of Leningrad (1941–1944) when more than 800,000 people starved to death; in China during the Great Leap Forward (1958–1961); and high in the Andes among the young athletes stranded after the crash of Uruguayan Air Force Flight 571 (1972).

But this is *Nutrition For Dummies,* not *History For Dummies,* so what you want to know is this: How nutritious is human flesh? According to James Cole, Senior Lecturer in Archaeology a lecturer on human origins at the University of Brighton in England: Very.

Human bodies, like other animal carcasses are red meat, fat, and offal. Based on data from four (dead) male adults, Cole estimates that a whole, cooked human body serves up about 82,000 calories. At a recommended 2,500 calories a day for an average adult male and 2,000 for an average adult woman, that's about 34 days' worth of sustenance for the former and 43 for the latter. A piece at a time, Cole rates a human arm at about 1,800 calories; a leg at 7,150; the lungs, liver, and alimentary canal about 1,500 calories each; the bundle of brain, spinal cord, and nerve and trunk about 2,700 calories. The brave heart? A mere 122.

Of course, while law-abiding folks are unlikely to slice, dice, and serve other folks anytime soon, other species are doing in their fellows day after day. The list of cannibalistic creatures who eat their enemies, their lovers, or their offspring includes fish such as the tiger shark and walleye, cute and cuddly prairie dogs, hamsters, hedgehogs, some snakes, caterpillars, ladybugs, spiders, some toads and tadpoles, hermit crabs, ducklings, cats, dogs, and polar bears (the last three often kill and sometimes consume sickly newborns). Chickens also make the list — but their cannibal dish is eggs not chicks.

And by the way, cannibalism is a species-neutral term. The word for people eating people is *anthropophagy* from the Greek words *anthropos* meaning "human being" and *phagein* meaning "to eat."

Chapter **2**

Digestion: The 24/7 Food Factory

When you see (or smell) something appetizing, your digestive organs leap into action. Your mouth waters. Your stomach contracts. Intestinal glands begin to secrete the chemicals that turn food into the nutrients that build new tissues and provide the energy you need for work, pleasure, and everyday life. This chapter provides a basic primer on the digestive system from start to finish with a few stops along the way to explain how you metabolize everything from apples to zucchini.

Introducing the Digestive System

Your *digestive system* is a collection of organs specifically designed to turn complex substances (food) into basic components (nutrients). These organs form one long, exceedingly well-organized tube that starts at your mouth, continues down through your throat to your stomach, and then goes on to your small and large intestines to end at your anus.

In between, with the help of the liver, pancreas, and gallbladder, the usable (digestible) parts of everything that you eat are converted to simple compounds that your body can easily absorb to burn for energy or to build new tissue. The indigestible residue is bundled off and eliminated as waste.

Figure 2-1 shows the body parts and organs that comprise your digestive system.

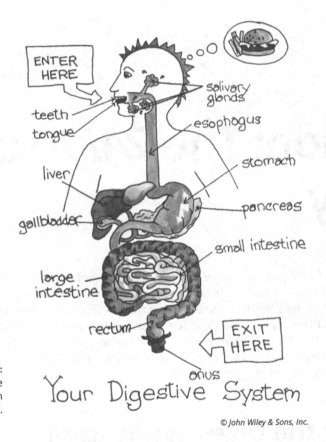

FIGURE 2-1:
Your digestive system in all its glory.

© John Wiley & Sons, Inc.

The digestive process run by these organs works in two simple ways, one mechanical and one chemical.

>> *Mechanical digestion* takes place in your mouth and your stomach. First, your teeth break food into small, easy-to-swallow pieces that slide quickly from your mouth down through your esophagus (throat) to your stomach. Here, a churning action called *peristalsis* continues to break food into smaller particles and then moves the particles along to your small intestine, where the churning and breaking continues.

>> *Chemical digestion* occurs at every point in the digestive tract where enzymes and other substances, such as *hydrochloric acid* (from stomach glands) and *bile* (from the liver), dissolve food, releasing the nutrients inside.

The rest of this chapter explains exactly what occurs and where along the digestive tract.

Digestion: One Step at a Time

Each organ in the digestive system plays a specific role in the digestive drama. But the first act occurs in three places rarely listed as part of the digestive tract: your brain, your eyes, and your nose.

The next acts take place in your mouth, your stomach, and your small and large intestines.

Your brain, eyes, and nose

When you see appetizing food, you experience a conditioned response. (For the lowdown on how your digestive system can be conditioned to respond to food, see Chapter 14; for information on your food preferences, see Chapter 15.) In other words, your thoughts — "Wow! That looks good!" — stimulate your brain to tell your digestive organs to get ready for action.

What happens in your nose is purely physical. The tantalizing aroma of good food is transmitted by molecules that fly from the surface of the food to settle on the membrane lining of your nostrils; these molecules stimulate the receptor cells on the olfactory nerve fibers that stretch from your nose back to your brain. When the receptor cells communicate with your brain, your brain sends encouraging messages to your mouth and digestive tract as the sight and scent of food make your mouth water and your stomach contract in anticipatory hunger pangs.

What if you hate what you see or smell? For some people, even the thought of liver is enough to make them want to leave the room. At that point, your body takes up arms to protect you: You experience a *rejection reaction*. Your mouth purses, and your nose wrinkles as if to keep the food (and its odor) as far away as possible. Your throat tightens, and your stomach *turns* as muscles contract, not in anticipatory pangs but in movements preparatory for vomiting up the unwanted food. Not a pleasant moment.

But assume that you like what's on your plate. Go ahead. Take a bite.

Your mouth

Lift your fork to your mouth, and your teeth and salivary glands swing into action. Your teeth chew, grinding and breaking food into small, manageable pieces. As a result,

>> You can swallow easily.

>> You break down the indigestible wrapper of fibers surrounding the edible parts of some foods (fruits, vegetables, whole grains) so that your digestive enzymes can get to the nutrients inside.

At the same time, salivary glands under your tongue and in the back of your mouth secrete the watery liquid called *saliva*, which performs two important functions:

>> It moistens and compacts food so your tongue can push it to the back of your mouth and you can swallow, sending the food down your esophagus into your stomach.

>> It provides *amylases,* enzymes that start the digestion of complex carbohydrates (starches), breaking the starch molecules into simple sugars. (Check out Chapter 8 for more on carbs.)

TURNING STARCHES INTO SUGARS

Salivary enzymes (like amylases) don't lay a finger on proteins and leave fats pretty much alone, but they do begin to digest complex carbohydrates, breaking the long, chainlike molecules of starches into individual units of sugars. The following simple experiment enables you to taste firsthand the effects of amylases on carbohydrates.

1. **Put a small piece of plain, unsalted cracker on your tongue.**

   No cheese, no chopped liver — just the cracker, please.

2. **Close your mouth and let the cracker sit on your tongue for a few minutes.**

   Do you taste a sudden, slight sweetness? That's the salivary enzymes breaking a long, complex starch molecule into its component parts (sugars).

3. **Now swallow.**

   The rest of the digestion of the starch takes place farther down, in your small intestine.

No protein digestion occurs in your mouth, and although saliva does contain very small amounts of *lingual lipases* — fat-busting enzymes secreted by cells at the base of the tongue — the amount is so small that the fat digestion here is insignificant.

Your stomach

If you were to lay your digestive tract out on a table, most of it would look like a simple, rather narrow, tube. The exception is your stomach, a pouchlike structure just below your esophagus, which few non-physicians have ever seen except for those TV viewers addicted to the show *My 600-lb. Life.*

Like most of the digestive tube, your stomach is circled with strong muscles whose rhythmic peristaltic contractions turn your stomach into a sort of food processor that mechanically breaks pieces of food into ever smaller particles. While this is going on, glands in the stomach wall are secreting *stomach juices* — a potent blend of enzymes, hydrochloric acid, and mucus.

One stomach enzyme — *gastric alcohol dehydrogenase* — digests small amounts of alcohol, an unusual nutrient that can be absorbed directly into your bloodstream even before it's been digested. Other enzymes, plus stomach juices, begin the digestion of proteins and fats, separating them into their basic components, amino acids and fatty acids.

If the words *amino acids* and *fatty acids* are completely new to you and if you're suddenly consumed by the desire to know more about them this instant, stick a pencil in the book to hold your place and flip to Chapters 6 and 7 for the details.

For the most part, digestion of carbohydrates comes to a temporary halt in the stomach. Stomach acids can break some carb bonds, but overall, the liquids here are so acidic that they deactivate *amylases,* the enzymes that break complex carbohydrates apart into simple sugars. Eventually, your churning stomach blends its contents into a thick soupy mass called *chyme* (from *cheymos,* the Greek word for "juice"). When a small amount of chyme spills past the stomach into the small intestine, the digestion of carbohydrates resumes in earnest, and your body begins to extract nutrients from food.

Your small intestine

Open your hand and put it flat against your belly button, with your thumb pointing up to your waist and your little finger pointing down.

Your hand is now covering most of the relatively small space into which your 20-foot-long small intestine is neatly coiled. When the partially digested chyme spills from your stomach into this part of the digestive tube, a whole new set of gastric juices are released:

>> *Pancreatic and intestinal enzymes* finish the digestion of proteins into amino acids.

>> *Bile,* a greenish liquid (made in the liver and stored in the gallbladder), enables fats to mix with water (emulsification like an oil and vinegar dressing).

>> *Alkaline pancreatic juices* make the chyme less acidic so that amylases can go back to work separating complex carbohydrates into simple sugars.

>> *Intestinal alcohol dehydrogenase* digests alcohol not previously absorbed into your bloodstream.

While these chemicals work, contractions of the small intestine continue to move the food mass down through the tube so your body can absorb sugars, amino acids, fatty acids, vitamins, and minerals into cells in the intestinal wall.

TECHNICAL STUFF

The lining of the small intestine is a series of folds covered with projections that have been described as "fingerlike" or "small nipples." The scientific name for these small structures is *villus* (singular) and *villi* (plural). Each villus is covered with smaller projections called *microvilli*, and every villus and microvillus is programmed to accept a specific nutrient — and no other.

Nutrients are absorbed not in their order of arrival in the intestine but according to how fast they're broken down into their basic parts, as follows:

>> Carbohydrates — which separate quickly into single sugar units — are absorbed first.

>> Proteins (as amino acids) go next.

>> Fats — which take the longest to break apart into their constituent fatty acids — are last. That's why a high-fat meal keeps you feeling fuller longer than a meal such as chow mein or plain tossed salad, which are mostly low-fat carbohydrates.

>> Vitamins that dissolve in water are absorbed earlier than vitamins that dissolve in fat.

After you've digested your food and absorbed its nutrients through your small intestine, this is what happens:

» Amino acids, sugars, vitamin C, the B vitamins, iron, calcium, and magnesium are carried through the bloodstream to your liver, where they're processed and sent out to the rest of the body.

» Fatty acids, cholesterol, and vitamins A, D, E, and K go into the lymphatic system and then into the blood. They, too, end up in the liver, are processed, and are shipped out to other body cells.

Inside the cells, nutrients are *metabolized* — burned for heat and energy or used to build new tissues. The metabolic process that gives you energy is called *catabolism* (from *katabole*, the Greek word for casting down). The metabolic process that uses nutrients to build new tissues is called *anabolism* (from *anabole*, the Greek word for raising up).

How the body uses nutrients for energy and new tissues is, alas, a subject for another chapter. In fact, this subject is enough to fill seven different chapters, each devoted to a specific kind of nutrient. For information about metabolizing proteins, turn to Chapter 6; for fats, Chapter 7; for carbohydrates, Chapter 8; for alcohol, Chapter 9; for vitamins, Chapter 10; for minerals, Chapter 11; and for water, Chapter 12.

Your large intestine

When every useful, digestible ingredient other than water has been wrung out of your food, the rest — indigestible waste such as fiber — moves into the top of your large intestine, the area known as your *colon*. The colon's primary job is to absorb water from this mixture and then to squeeze the remaining matter into the compact bundle known as feces.

Feces (whose brown color comes from leftover bile pigments) are made of indigestible material from food, plus cells that have sloughed off the intestinal lining and the bodies of bacteria, members of the microbiome (see the nearby sidebar "Prebiotics and probiotics: The good gut twins"). In fact, about 30 percent of the entire weight of the feces comprises the bodies of these microorganisms, which live in permanent colonies in your colon, where they

» Manufacture vitamin B12, which is absorbed through the colon wall

» Produce vitamin K, also absorbed through the colon wall

» Break down amino acids and produce nitrogen (which gives feces a characteristic odor)

» Feast on indigestible complex carbohydrates (fiber), excreting the gas that sometimes makes you physically uncomfortable — or a social pariah

When the bacteria have finished and their bodies have been incorporated into the waste, the feces — small remains of yesterday's copious feast — pass down through your rectum and out through your anus. But not necessarily right away: Digestion of any one meal may take longer than a day to complete.

PREBIOTICS AND PROBIOTICS: THE GOOD GUT TWINS

A little more than 100 years ago, Ilya Ilyich (Elie) Metchnikoff, a Russian scientist, decided that humans who died young had succumbed to the effects of "putrefying bacteria" in their intestines. Searching for a remedy, Metchnikoff ended up with Bulgarian peasants, a significant number of whom lived well into their late 80s. Historians may argue that the only way to have lived long in Bulgaria was to avoid Bulgarian politics, but Metchnikoff credited the national longevity to yogurt, the first time someone recognized the benefits of probiotics, a discovery that won him the Nobel Prize in physiology and medicine in 1908.

The National Institutes of Health (NIH) defines probiotics as "live microorganisms that are similar to the beneficial microorganisms found in the human gut." The most common probiotics in our food are members of the *Lactobacilli* family, such as the ones in Metchnikoff's magic Bulgarian yogurt. Probiotic microbes are also active in other fermented food, including kefir, tempeh, some pickles, sauerkraut, and kimchi. (***Note:*** Heat kills these microbes, so to be useful they must be live as noted on the labels for many yogurts.) Recently, a new term has entered the conversation: prebiotics. As you can assume, the "pre" means something that comes before probiotics — in this case, dietary fiber your body cannot absorb but which serves as food for those protective probiotic microbes. (See Chapter 8 for more on dietary fiber.)

While food is your best natural source of prebiotics and probiotics, the hot market right now is in supplements: probiotic tablets, capsules, powders, lozenges, and gums whose worldwide sales are expected to rise from $2.5 billion in 2018 to an astronomical $74.69 billion by 2025. And no wonder. Healthwise, proponents claim a slew of benefits for probiotics, including the prosaic but highly welcome ability to prevent or ease diarrhea due to an infection or treatment with antibiotics that wipes out normal bacterial colonies in the intestines. In 2014, a metanalysis for 24 different trials showed that probiotics also helped prevent a life-threatening intestinal inflammation in newborn premature infants.

Some studies also suggest that probiotics may alleviate symptoms of digestive disorders such as irritable bowel syndrome (IBS) and improve and perhaps relieve depression, but no evidence supports claims that they strengthen your immune system or make it easier for you to lose weight. And there's this: Probiotic products are supplements, which means the Food and Drug Administration (FDA) regulates them as food, not drugs, so they don't have to prove that they're safe or effective. (See Chapter 13 for more on supplement safety.) That matters because with all the hoopla surrounding a "natural" product, there is a clear lack of data regarding the possible risks of long-term use of these supplements.

The bottom line: Probiotics are a promising field of research, and one day they may be used to treat or help prevent many disorders. But right now, not enough evidence exists to recommend their widespread use.

Chapter **3**

How Much Nutrition Do You Need?

A healthful diet provides sufficient amounts of all the nutrients that your body needs. The question is, how much is enough?

Today, three sets of recommendations provide the answers, and each one comes with its own virtues and deficiencies. The first, and most familiar, is the *RDA* (short for *Recommended Dietary Allowance*). The second, originally known as the *Estimated Safe and Adequate Daily Dietary Intakes (ESADDI)*, now shortened to *Adequate Intake* or simply *AI*, describes recommended amounts of nutrients for which no RDAs exist. The third is the *DRI (Dietary Reference Intake)*, an umbrella term that includes RDAs plus several innovative categories of nutrient recommendations: EAR (Estimated Average Requirement), AI (Adequate Intake), and UL (Tolerable Upper Intake Level).

Confused? Not to worry. This chapter spells it all out.

RDAs: Guidelines for Good Nutrition

The Recommended Dietary Allowances (RDAs) were created in 1941 by the Food and Nutrition Board, a subsidiary of the National Research Council, which is part of the National Academy of Sciences in Washington, D.C., in order to investigate issues of nutrition that might "affect national defense." The committee was renamed the Food and Nutrition Board in 1941, after which they began to deliberate on a set of recommendations of a standard daily allowance for each type of nutrient. The standards would be used for nutrition recommendations for the armed forces, for civilians, and for overseas populations who might need food relief.

RDAs originally were designed to make planning several days' meals in advance easy for you. The *D* in RDA stands for *dietary*, not daily, because the RDAs are an average. You may get more of a nutrient one day and less the next, but the idea is to hit an average over several days.

For example, the current RDA for vitamin C is 75 milligrams for a woman and 90 milligrams for a man (age 18 and older). One 8-ounce glass of fresh orange juice has 120 milligrams of vitamin C, so a woman can have an 8-ounce glass of orange juice on Monday and Tuesday, skip Wednesday, and still meet the RDA for the three days. A man may have to toss in something else — maybe a stalk of broccoli — to be able to do the same thing. No big deal.

The amounts recommended by the RDAs provide a margin of safety for healthy people, but they're not therapeutic. In other words, RDA servings won't cure a nutrient deficiency, but they can prevent one from occurring.

Proteins, vitamins, and minerals: The essentials

RDAs offer recommendations for protein and 18 essential vitamins and minerals. For the specific amounts, check out Chapter 6 (protein), Chapter 10 (vitamins), and Chapter 11 (minerals).

Recommendations for carbohydrates, fats, dietary fiber, and alcohol

What nutrients are missing from the RDA list of essentials? Carbohydrates, fiber, fat, and alcohol. The reason is simple: If your diet provides enough protein, vitamins, and minerals, it's almost certain to provide enough carbohydrates and probably more than enough fat. Although no specific RDAs exist for carbohydrates and fat, guidelines definitely exist for them and for dietary fiber and alcohol.

In 1980, the U.S. Public Health Service and the U.S. Department of Agriculture joined forces to produce the first edition of *Dietary Guidelines for Americans* (see Chapter 16). A new edition of the Dietary Guidelines has been issued every five years since then to set parameters for what you can consider reasonable amounts of calories, carbohydrates, dietary fiber, fats, protein, and alcohol. According to these guidelines, several general rules advise you to

>> **Balance your calorie intake with energy output in the form of regular exercise.** Check out Chapter 5 for specifics on how many calories a person of your weight, height, and level of activity (couch potato? marathon runner?) needs to consume each day.

>> **Make foods with complex carbohydrates and dietary fiber (defined in Chapter 8) the base of your total daily calories.** These should make up to 900 to 1,300 calories and up to 25 grams dietary fiber on a 2,000 calorie per day diet.

>> **Concentrate on unsaturated fats.** For more specific guidelines, check out Chapters 16 and 17 and Chapter 7 for everything you need to know about the individual dietary fats.

>> **Drink alcohol only in moderation.** That means one drink a day for a woman and two for a man. As the *Guidelines* note, neither is a component of the USDA Dietary Patterns.

Different people, different needs

Because different bodies require different amounts of nutrients, RDAs currently address as many as 22 specific categories of human beings: boys and girls, men and women, from infancy through middle age. In 2006, the RDAs were expanded to include recommendations for groups of people age 50 to 70 and 71 and older.

REMEMBER These expanded groupings are a *really* good idea. In 1990, the U.S. Census counted 31.1 million Americans older than 65. By 2050, the U.S. government expects more than 60 million mostly active older citizens.

If age is important, so is gender. For example, because women of child-bearing age lose iron when they menstruate, their RDA for iron is higher than the RDA for men. On the other hand, because men who are sexually active lose zinc through their ejaculations, the zinc RDA for men is higher than the zinc RDA for women.

REMEMBER And gender affects body composition, which influences other RDAs, such as protein: The RDA for protein is set in terms of grams of protein per kilogram (2.2 pounds) of body weight. Because the average man weighs more than the average woman, his RDA for protein is higher than hers. The RDA for an adult male, age 19 or older, is 56 grams; for a woman, it's 46 grams.

SEVEN RULES FOR LADIES-IN-WAITING

The 2020 edition of the *Dietary Guidelines for Americans* is the first one in which the scientific advisory committees chose to focus on how what a pregnant woman eats affects the health of her developing baby. Here's their advice based on what they found:

1. Women of child-bearing age should be encouraged to achieve and maintain a healthy weight before becoming pregnant and during pregnancy itself. (For more on healthful weight, check out Chapter 4.)

2. When picking a dietary pattern, aim for one rich in fruits and veggies, whole grains, seafood, and vegetable oils while cutting back on added sugars, refined grains, and red and processed meats. (More on that in Chapter 17.)

3. Choose plant foods that are good sources of important vitamins such as folate and minerals such as calcium.

4. Don't worry about allergens unless it's the mother's allergy. What a pregnant woman eats does not appear to create allergies in the baby.

5. Include at least 8 ounces and as much as 12 ounces of seafood once a week. Aim for seafood low in mercury and high in protective omega-3 fatty acids.

6. No alcohol. Period.

7. Stay away from chancy, possibly contaminated foods such as unpasteurized milk and undercooked meats.

AIs: The Nutritional Numbers Formerly Known as ESADDIs

In addition to the RDAs, the Food and Nutrition Board has created an *Adequate Intake* (AI) for eight nutrients considered necessary for good health, even though nobody really knows exactly how much your body needs. Not to worry: Sooner or later, some smart nutrition researcher will come up with a hard number and move the nutrient to the RDA list.

You can find the AIs for biotin, choline, and pantothenic acid in Chapter 10, along with the requirements for other vitamins. The AIs for the minerals calcium, chromium, molybdenum, and manganese are in Chapter 11 with the other dietary minerals.

DRI: The Totally Complete Nutrition Guide

In 1993, the Food and Nutrition Board's Dietary Reference Intakes committee set up several panels of experts to review the RDAs and other recommendations for major nutrients (vitamins, minerals, and other food components) in light of new research and nutrition information. The first order of business was to establish a new standard for nutrient recommendations called the *Dietary Reference Intake* (DRI). DRI is an umbrella term that embraces several categories of nutritional measurements for vitamins, minerals, and other nutrients. It includes

>> **Estimated Average Requirement (EAR):** The amount that meets the nutritional needs of half the people in any one group (such as teenage girls or people older than 70). Nutritionists use the EAR to figure out whether an entire population's normal diet provides adequate amounts of nutrients.

>> **Recommended Dietary Allowance (RDA):** The RDA, now based on information provided by the EAR, is still a daily average that meets the needs of 97 percent of a specific population, such as women age 18 to 50 or men age 70 and older.

>> **Adequate Intake (AI):** The AI is a new measurement, providing recommendations for nutrients for which no RDA is set. (***Note:*** AI replaces ESADDI.)

>> **Tolerable Upper Intake Level (UL):** The UL is the highest amount of a nutrient you can consume each day without risking an adverse effect.

The DRI panel's first report, listing new recommendations for calcium, phosphorus, magnesium, and fluoride, appeared in 1997. Its most notable change was upping the recommended amount of calcium from 800 milligrams to 1,000 milligrams for adults age 31 to 50 as well as postmenopausal women taking estrogen supplements; for postmenopausal women not taking estrogen, the recommendation is 1,500 milligrams.

The DRI panel's second report appeared in 1998. The report included new recommendations for thiamin, riboflavin, niacin, vitamin B6, folate, vitamin B12, pantothenic acid, biotin, and choline. The most important revision was increasing the folate recommendation to 400 micrograms a day based on evidence showing that folate reduces a woman's risk of giving birth to a baby with spinal cord defects and lowers the risk of heart disease for men and women. (See the sidebar "Reviewing terms used to describe nutrient recommendations" in this chapter to brush up on your metric abbreviations.)

As a result of the 1998 DRI panel's report, the FDA ordered food manufacturers to add folate to flour, rice, and other grain products. (Multivitamin products already contain 400 micrograms of folate.) In May 1999, data released by the Framingham Heart Study, which has followed heart health among residents of a Boston suburb for nearly half a century, showed a dramatic increase in blood levels of folate. Before the fortification of foods, 22 percent of the study participants had folate deficiencies; after the fortification, the number fell to 2 percent.

A DRI report with revised recommendations for vitamin C, vitamin E, the mineral selenium, beta carotene, and other antioxidant vitamins was published in 2000. In 2001, new DRIs were released for vitamin A, vitamin K, arsenic, boron, chromium, copper, iodine, iron, manganese, molybdenum, nickel, silicon, vanadium, and zinc. In 2004, the Institute of Medicine (IOM) released new recommendations for sodium, potassium, chloride, and water, plus a special report on recommendations for two groups of older adults (age 50 to 70 and 71 and over). By 2005, the Food and Nutrition Board had established an AI of 600 IU (international units) vitamin D for men and women older than 71. Put all these findings together, and they spell out the recommendations you find in this chapter.

Table 3-1 shows the most recent RDAs for vitamins for healthy adults; Table 3-2 shows RDAs for minerals for healthy adults. Where no RDA is given, an AI is indicated by an asterisk (*) by the column heading.

REVIEWING TERMS USED TO DESCRIBE NUTRIENT RECOMMENDATIONS

Nutrient listings use the metric system. RDAs for protein are listed in grams. The RDA and AIs for vitamins and minerals are shown in milligrams (mg) and micrograms (mcg). A milligram is 1/1000 of a gram; a microgram is 1/1000 of a milligram.

Vitamin A, vitamin D, and vitamin E are special cases. For instance, one form of vitamin A is *preformed vitamin A,* a form of the nutrient that your body can use right away. Preformed vitamin A, known as *retinol,* is found in food from animals — liver, milk, and eggs. Carotenoids (red or yellow pigments in plants) also provide vitamin A. But to get vitamin A from carotenoids, your body has to convert the pigments to chemicals similar to retinol. Because retinol is a ready-made nutrient, the RDA for vitamin A is listed in units called retinol equivalents (RE). One microgram (mcg) RE is approximately equal to 3.33 international units (IU, the former unit of measurement for vitamin A).

Vitamin D consists of three compounds: vitamin D1, vitamin D2, and vitamin D3. Cholecalciferol, the chemical name for vitamin D3, is the most active of the three, so the RDA for vitamin D is measured in equivalents of cholecalciferol.

Your body gets vitamin E from two classes of chemicals in food: tocopherols and tocotrienols. The compound with the greatest vitamin E activity is a tocopherol: *alpha*-tocopherol. The RDA for vitamin E is measured in milligrams of alpha-tocopherol equivalents (a-TE).

HOW MUCH IS THAT?

Nutrient amounts are measured in various units:

- g = gram

- mg = milligram = 1 / 1,000 of a gram

- mcg = microgram = 1 / 1,000,000 of a gram

- IU = international unit

- RE = retinol equivalent = the amount of "true" vitamin A in an IU

- a-TE = alpha-tocopherol equivalent = the amount of alpha-tocopherol in a unit of vitamin E

TABLE 3-1 ## Vitamin RDAs for Healthy Adults

Age (Years)	Vitamin A (RE/IU)[†]	Vitamin D (mcg/IU)[‡*]	Vitamin E (a-TE)	Vitamin K (mcg)[*]	Vitamin C (mg)
Males					
19–30	900/2,970	15/600	15	120	90
31–50	900/2,970	15/600	15	120	90
51–70	900/2,970	15/600	15	120	90
71 and older	900/2,970	20/800	15	120	90
Females					
19–30	700/2,310	15/600	15	90	75
31–50	700/2,310	15/600	15	90	75
51–70	700/2,310	15/600	15	90	75
71 and older	700/2,310	20/900	15	90	75

*Adequate Intake (AI)

†The "official" RDA for vitamin A is still 1,000 RE/5,000 IU for a male, 800 RE/4,000 IU for a female who isn't pregnant or nursing; the lower numbers listed on this chart are the currently recommended levels for adults.

‡The current recommendations are the amounts required to prevent vitamin D deficiency disease; recent studies suggest that the optimal levels for overall health may actually be higher, in the range of 800–1,000 IU a day.

Age (years)	Thiamin (Vitamin B1) (mg)	Riboflavin (Vitamin B2) (mg)	Niacin (NE)	Pantothenic acid (mg)*	Vitamin B6 (mg)	Folate (mcg)	Vitamin B12 (mcg)	Biotin (mcg)*
Males								
19–30	1.2	1.3	16	5	1.3	400	2.4	30
31–50	1.2	1.3	16	5	1.3	400	2.4	30
50–70	1.2	1.3	16	5	1.7	400	2.4	30
71 and older	1.2	1.1	16	5	1.7	400	2.4	30
Females								
19–30	1.1	1.1	14	5	1.3	400	2.4	30
31–50	1.1	1.1	14	5	1.3	400	2.4	30
51–70	1.1	1.1	14	5	1.5	400	2.4	30
71 and older	1.1	1.1	14	5	1.5	400	2.4	30
Pregnant	1.4	1.1	18	6	1.9	600	2.6	30
Nursing	1.4	1.1	17	7	2.0	500	2.8	35

Adequate Intake (AI)

TABLE 3-2   ## Mineral RDAs for Healthy Adults

Age (years)	Calcium (mg)*	Phosphorus (mg)	Magnesium (mg)	Iron (mg)	Zinc (mg)	Copper (mcg)
Males						
19–30	1,000	700	400	8	11	900
31–50	1,000	700	420	8	11	900
51–70	1,200	700	420	8	11	900
71 and older	1,200	700	420	8	11	900
Females						
19–30	1,000	700	310	18	8	900
31–50	1,000	700	320	18	8	900
51–70	1,000/1,500**	700	320	8	8	900
71 and older	1,000/1,500**	700	320	8	8	900

Age (years)	Calcium (mg)*	Phosphorus (mg)	Magnesium (mg)	Iron (mg)	Zinc (mg)	Copper (mcg)
Pregnant	1,000–1,300	700–1,250	350–400	27	11–12	1,000
Nursing	1,000–1,300	700–1,250	310–350	9–10	12–13	1,300

*Adequate Intake (AI)

**The lower recommendation is for postmenopausal women taking estrogen supplements; the higher figure is for postmenopausal women not taking estrogen supplements.

Age (years)	Iodine (mcg)	Selenium (mcg)	Molybdenum (mcg)	Manganese (mg)*	Fluoride (mg)*	Chromium (mcg)*	Choline (mg)*
Males							
19–30	150	55	45	2.3	4	36	550
31–50	150	55	45	2.3	4	36	550
51–70	150	55	45	2.3	4	30	550
71 and older	150	55	45	2.3	4	30	550
Females							
19–30	150	55	45	1.8	3	25	425
31–50	150	55	45	1.8	3	25	425
51–70	150	55	45	1.8	3	20	425
71 and older	150	55	45	1.8	3	20	425
Pregnant	220	60	50	2.0	1.5–4.0	29–30	450
Nursing	290	70	50	2.6	1.5–4.0	44–45	550

*Adequate Intake (AI)

Adapted with permission from Recommended Dietary Allowances (Washington D.C.: National Academy Press, 1989), and DRI panel reports, 1997–2004

Hankering for more details? Notice something missing? Right — no recommended allowances for fat, carbohydrates, and, of course, water. You can find those (respectively) in Chapters 7, 8, and 12.

REMEMBER

The slogan "No Sale Ever Is Final," printed on the sales slips at one of my favorite clothing stores, definitely applies to nutritional numbers. RDAs, AIs, and DRIs should always be regarded as works in progress, subject to revision at the first sign of a new study. In other words, in an ever-changing world, here's one thing of which you can be *absolutely* certain: The numbers in this chapter will change. Sorry about that.

IN THIS CHAPTER

» Defining obesity

» Listing the fattest and fittest states

» Figuring out how much you should weigh

» Understanding how you fit into the equation

Chapter **4**

Bigger But Not Better

According to the Federal Centers for Disease Control (CDC), in 2016, nearly seven of every ten American adults was either *overweight* or *obese*, two terms this chapter defines. And movie titles aside, the kids are *not* all right. Overall, the 2013 National Survey of Children's Health reported that more than one in every five American children age 12 to 19 weigh too much. This excess poundage isn't pretty, and it comes at a cost to our health. One 2019 study that followed more than 1,000,000 American women showed a link between obesity in middle age and dementia later in life. Another suggested that childhood obesity may affect the accuracy of routine blood tests. There's also a cost in dollars and cents. The CDC puts the price of treating obesity-related illnesses at nearly $200 billion each year, an amount equal to about 6 percent of all medical spending in the United States.

If these trends continue, researchers at the Johns Hopkins Bloomberg School of Public Health, the Agency for Healthcare Research and Quality, and the University of Pennsylvania School of Medicine predict that by the year 2030, nearly 90 percent of American adults will be overweight, at which point the cost of treating their obesity-related health problems will approach $1 trillion a year. No wonder the American Heart Association says we're in the grip of an obesity epidemic. And that is only one of the topics I cover in this chapter. Add on how much your own body should weigh, the methods by which to judge your obesity or lack thereof (and how to evaluate the accuracy of the numbers), plus the conditions that make obesity more hazardous to your health, and you have a lot to put on your plate about weight.

The Obesity Epidemic

The word *epidemic* conjures up images of polio, plague, flu, measles — a host of contagious illnesses that pass more or less easily from one person to another. But does obesity qualify? Believe it or not, maybe.

In 2007, Harvard sociologist Nicholas Christakis and James Fowler, a political scientist at the University of California, San Diego, suggested in *The New England Journal of Medicine* that gaining weight may be a "socially contagious" event. In other words, people in groups tend to adopt similar behavior, and gaining or losing weight right along with friends and relatives may be one of those activities.

To reach this conclusion, Christakis and Fowler analyzed more than 30 years' worth of information for more than 12,000 volunteers in the famed Framingham Heart Study, the project that has tracked the incidence and causes of heart disease in a Massachusetts city since 1948.

The Framingham people were weighed during checkups every two to four years. When Christakis and Fowler toted up the results, they discovered that the risk of becoming obese rose nearly 60 percent for someone with an obese friend, 40 percent for someone with an obese brother or sister, and 37 percent for someone whose husband or wife is obese. And these people didn't even have to live close to each other for the risk to rise: The coincidence of obesity existed even when the subjects lived in different cities, which leads right to the next section, stats showing the cities and states where overweight Americans are most likely to be found.

Observing the Obesity Map

How many people are fat and how many leans varies from state to state and city to city depending on a whole list of variables ranging from genetics to physical activity and, of course, the local diet. Table 4-1 shows the ten leanest and fattest states. Table 4-2 does the same for the top ten fattest and leanest cities. In both cases, the information is solidly reliable drawn from such eminent statistics sources as the Centers for Disease Control and Prevention, the U.S. Census, and the U.S. Department of Agriculture.

What do the fattest cities and states have in common? According to Michael Wimberly of the Geographic Information Science Center of Excellence at South Dakota State University, the people living there are

>> Less likely to engage in physical activity

>> Less likely to eat five servings of fruits and vegetables a day

>> More likely to eat the "wrong" foods

>> More likely to be living somewhere pretty far away from a really good supermarket

TABLE 4-1

The Ten Fattest and Leanest U.S. States

Fattest States (Fattest First)	Leanest States (Leanest First)
Mississippi	Utah
Kentucky	Colorado
Oklahoma	Connecticut
West Virginia	Idaho
Tennessee	Oregon
Alabama	Minnesota
Arkansas	Montana
Louisiana	Massachusetts
Michigan	Alaska
Ohio	Washington

From "Fattest States in the U.S." https://wallethub.com/edu/fattest-states/16585/

TABLE 4-2

The Ten Fattest and Leanest American Cities

Fattest Cities (Fattest First)	Leanest Cities (Leanest First)
McAllen-Edinburg-Mission, TX	San Francisco-Oakland, CA
Shreveport-Bossier City, LA	Honolulu, HI
Memphis, TN	Minneapolis-St Paul, MN
Jackson, MS	Seattle-Tacoma-Belleville, WA
Knoxville, TN	Portland, OR
Tulsa, OK	Boston, MA
Mobile, AL	Denver, CO
Nashville, TN	Alexandria-D.C., VA
Columbia, SC	Colorado Springs, CO
Lafayette, LA	Salt Lake City, UT

From https://walletyhub.com/edu/fattest-cities-in-america/10532

Wimberly calls this an *obesogenic environment,* a situation that encourages weight gain.

Determining How Much You Should Weigh

Over the years, many health organizations ranging from insurance companies to the U.S. federal government have created charts and tables purporting to establish *healthy weight* standards for adult Americans. Some of these efforts set the figures so low that you can hardly get there without severely restricting your diet — or being born again with a different body, preferably with light bones and no curves. Others are more reasonable.

Weight charts and tables

In 1959, the Metropolitan Life Insurance Company published the first set of standard weight charts. The weights were drawn from insurance statistics showing what the healthiest, longest-living people weighed — with clothes on and (for the women) wearing shoes with one-inch heels. The problem? At the time, the class of people with insurance was so small and so narrow that it was hard to say with certainty that their weight could predict healthy poundage for the rest of the population.

Thirty-one years later, the government published the weight chart shown in Table 4-3. This moderate, eminently usable set appeared in the 1990 edition of *Dietary Guidelines for Americans* (more about the *Dietary Guidelines* in Chapter 16). The weights in this table are listed in ranges for both men and women of specific heights. Height is measured without shoes, and weight is measured without clothes. Because most people gain some weight as they grow older, the people who compiled these recommendations did a really sensible thing: They divided the ranges into two broad categories, one for people age 19 to 34, the other for those age 35 and older.

Muscle is heavier than fat, so individuals with a small frame and proportionately more fat tissue than muscle tissue are likely to weigh in at the low end. People with a large frame and proportionately more muscle than fat are likely to weigh in at the high end. As a general but by no means invariable rule, that means that women — who have smaller frames and less muscle — weigh less than men of the same height and age.

TABLE 4-3

How Much Should You Weigh?

Height	Weight (Pounds) for 19- to 34-Year-Olds	Weight (Pounds) for 35-Year-Olds and Older
5′	97–128	108–138
5′1″	101–132	111–143
5′2″	104–137	115–148
5′3″	107–141	119–152
5′4″	111–146	122–157
5′5″	114–150	126–162
5′6″	118–155	130–167
5′7″	121–160	134–172
5′8″	125–164	138–178
5′9″	129–169	142–183
5′10″	132–174	146–188
5′11″	136–179	151–194
6′	140–184	155–199
6′1″	144–189	159–205
6′2″	148–195	164–210
6′3″	152–200	168–216
6′4″	156–205	173–222
6′5″	160–211	177–228
6′6″	164–216	182–234

From Nutrition and Your Health: Dietary Guidelines for Americans, 3rd ed. (Washington D.C.: U.S. Department of Agriculture, U.S. Department of Health and Human Services, 1990)

Later editions of the Dietary Guidelines omitted the higher weight allowances for older people so that the "healthy" weights for everyone, young or old, became the ones listed in 1990 in the column for 19- to 34-year-olds. I'm going to go out on a limb here to say that I prefer the 1990 recommendations because they are

>> Achievable without constant dieting

>> Realistic about how your body changes as you get older

>> Less likely to make you totally crazy about your weight

AGE IS NOT JUST A WEIGHT NUMBER

Losing weight to stay healthily slim is generally regarded as a positive thing, but in 2019, a study published in the *British Medical Journal* showed that there could be problems associated with losing weight later in life. Based on data gathered from 36,000 subjects in the U.S. National Health & Examination Survey, it turns out taking off pounds in middle age and late adulthood may actually raise your risk of dying prematurely, especially if you have an underlying medical condition such as diabetes, cancer, or heart disease. The important message from the researchers: "Try not to gain weight while you're young and when you're older focus on maintaining a healthy lifestyle."

These are a pretty good description of how nutritional guidelines need to work, don't you think?

The BMI: Another way to rate your weight

The *body mass index* (BMI) is a number that measures the relationship between your weight and your height. Currently in the United States, a BMI below 18.5 is considered underweight, 18.5 to 24.9 is normal, 25.0 to 29.9 is overweight, 30.0 to 39.9 is obese, and 40.00 or greater is severely obese. Previously, other countries were slightly more lenient in their estimate of normal and overweight; for example, in Australia, a BMI of less than 20 was considered underweight. Today, the American standards are generally accepted around the world.

The equation used to calculate your BMI is called the *Quetelet Index*, named after the 19th-century Belgian mathematician and astronomer who invented the concept of "the average man" (see the nearby sidebar "The man who invented the average man"). The equation is W/H^2, which originally meant weight (in kilograms) divided by height (in meters, squared). The American equation, however, divides your weight in pounds by your height in inches, squared. So if you are five foot three inches tall and weigh 138 pounds, the U.S. equation looks like this:

$$BMI = W/H^2 \times 705$$

$$= (138 \text{ pounds}/63 \times 63 \text{ inches}) \times 705$$

$$= (138/3{,}969) \times 705$$

$$= 24.5 \text{ BMI}$$

THE MAN WHO INVENTED THE AVERAGE MAN

Lambert Adolphe Jacques Quetelet (1795–1874) was a Belgian mathematician, astronomer, statistician, and sociologist who invented the concept of the *homme moyen* (middle man), the average Joe who stands at the center of any bell curve.

Quetelet's main concern was predicting criminal behavior. To this end, he hoped to develop statistical patterns based on a person's deviation from average (read: normal) social behavior that could be used to predict his actions, including moral (good) and criminal (bad) behavior. Although this idea provoked many lively discussions among 19th-century social scientists, it never really worked as a crime-fighting tool. But it is extremely useful in estimating health risks.

(Figure adapted from Clinical Guidelines on the Identification, Evaluation, and Treatment of Overweight and Obesity in Adults: The Evidence Report.)

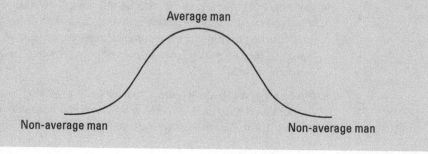

For a simpler solution, go to www.nhlbi.nih.gov/health/educational/lose_wt/BMI/bmicalc.htm, fill in the numbers, and bingo! The Baylor College of Medicine has an even niftier calculator site that gives you BMI plus the daily calorie intake that keeps you where you are or what you need to lose a few pounds. Check it out at www.bcm.edu/cnrc-apps/caloriesneed.cfm/TheBaylorCollegeof Medicine%20Calorie%20Needs%20and%20BMI%20calculator.

Or you could just run your finger down the screen showing the National Institute of Health's BMI chart for men and women from four feet ten inches to six feet four inches tall, weighing 91 to 443 pounds with "normal" being within a pound or two of the healthful weights proposed for younger people in the 1990 *Dietary Guidelines for Americans.* You can find the chart at https://www.nhlbi.nih.gov/health/educational/lose_wt/BMI/bmi_tbl.pdf.

HIGH-TECH FAT FINDING

A tape measure or a weight chart is a low-tech tool anyone can handle. But science loves complexity, so weight experts have several complicated ways to figure out if you're fat. Here are three of the most interesting. *Warning*: These are not your handy home tests — they're performed in some doctor's office but more likely in a research hospital or bariatric clinic.

- **Bioelectric impedance:** Your body is full of fluids packed with *electrolytes*, such as sodium and potassium, ions that conduct the electrical impulses that send messages back and forth among your cells. Muscle tissue contains more fluid than fat tissue, so a body with more muscle than fat is less resistant to an outside electrical current. To measure your body's resistance to electrical current (a phenomenon known as *impedance*), the technician conducting the test places electrodes at your wrists and ankles and zaps a harmless low-intensity electrical current through your body. Then she calculates how resistant your tissues were to the current. The final number indicates how much body fat you have.

- **The BOD POD:** This egg-shape chamber measures how much air you displace when you step in. Because muscle is denser tissue than body fat and displaces more air, the tech running the test can calculate the amount of fat in your body by looking at your weight and then at the amount of air you push aside when you enter the chamber.

- **Dual-energy X-ray absorptiometry (DEXA):** This test uses X-rays to measure muscle, bone, and body fat. The test — which takes about ten minutes — produces an image of the tissues that allows the tech to estimate the amount of body fat.

Understanding What the Numbers Really Mean

Weight charts, tables, numbers, and stats are so plentiful that you may think they're totally reliable in predicting who's healthy and who's not. They aren't. Real people and their real differences keep sneaking into the equation.

For example, BMI is not a reliable guide for

>> Women who are pregnant or nursing

>> People who are very tall or very short

>> Professional athletes or weight trainers with very well-developed muscle tissue. *Remember:* Muscle weighs more than fat, so a person with lots of muscle tissue may have a higher BMI and still be really healthy.

In addition, the value of the BMI in predicting your risk of illness appears to be tied to your age. If you're in your 30s, a lower BMI is clearly linked to better health. If you're in your 70s or older, no convincing evidence points to your weight playing a significant role in determining how healthy you are or how much longer you'll live. In between, from age 30 to age 74, the relationship between your BMI and your health is, well, in between — more important early on, less important later in life.

Increasing the odds of accuracy

To make the BMI a more accurate tool for predicting the health risks of carrying extra weight, the National Institutes of Health suggests adding a second measurement, the waist circumference — in other words, the apple/pear test.

An apple is a body with lots of fat around the middle: your waist. A pear has fat around the hips and thighs. Apples have a higher risk of diabetes, high blood pressure, and heart disease.

To identify your body type, wrap a measuring tape around your middle, just above your hip bones. Take a deep breath. Let it out. See what the tape says. That's your waist.

Table 4-4 shows the relative risks of Type 2 diabetes, hypertension, and heart disease associated with different waist measurements.

Seeing red flags on weight and health

No one factor, such as weight, gives a complete picture of how healthy — or unhealthy — you are. Regardless of your BMI or any other measurement, the risk of health problems rises if you have more than one other common problem. Here is a sample list:

>> High blood pressure

>> High levels of LDL ("bad") cholesterol

>> Low levels of HDL ("good") cholesterol

>> High levels of triglycerides (a kind of fat found in blood)

TABLE 4-4 **Estimated Risk Linked to BMI and Waist Size**

	BMI category	Risk at Waist size <40 Inches (Men), <35 Inches (Women)	Risk at Waist Size >40 Inches (Men), >35 Inches (Women)
Underweight	<18.5	—	—
Normal	19–24.9	—	—
Overweight	25–29.9	Increased	High
Obese	30–34.9	High	Very high
	35–39.9	Very high	Very high
	>40	Extremely high	Extremely high

National Heart, Lung and Blood Institute, National Institutes of Health, www.nhlbi.nih.gov/health/public/ heart/obesity/lose_wt/bmi_dis.htm

>> A family history of premature heart disease, meaning one or more close relatives who suffered a heart attack before age 50 for a man or age 60 for a woman

>> Not being physically active or being a smoker

If the profile fits, check with your doctor about a sensible wellness plan.

Facing the Numbers When They Don't Fit Your Body

Right about here, you probably feel the strong need for a really big chocolate bar — not such a bad idea now that nutritionists have discovered that dark chocolate is rich in disease-fighting antioxidants that benefit your various organs (as long as you stick to a 1-ounce, high cocoa content daily "dose").

REMEMBER

But it makes sense to consider the alternative — realistic rules that enable you to control your weight safely and effectively.

>> **Not everybody starts out with the same set of genes — or fits into the same pair of jeans.** Some people are naturally larger and heavier than others. If that's you, and all your vital stats satisfy your doctor, don't waste time trying to fit someone else's idea of perfection. Relax and enjoy your own body.

>> **If you're overweight and your doctor agrees with your decision to diet, you don't have to set world records to improve your health.** Even a moderate drop in poundage can be highly beneficial. According to the CDC, losing just 5 to 10 percent of your body weight can lower high blood sugar, high cholesterol, and high blood pressure, reducing your risks of diabetes, heart disease, and stroke.

>> **The number you really need to remember is 3,500, the number of calories it takes to gain or lose one pound of body fat.** In other words, 3,500 food calories equal one pound of body weight. So if you simply

- Cut your calorie consumption from 2,000 calories a day to 1,700 and continue to do the same amount of physical work, you'll lose one pound of fat in approximately just 12 days (*approximately* because different bodies burn calories/energy at different rates).

- Go the other way and increase calories from 1,700 to 2,000 a day without increasing the amount of work you do, approximately 12 days later, you'll be one pound heavier.

>> **Moderation is the best path to weight control.** Moderate calorie deprivation on a sensible diet produces healthful, moderate weight loss; this diet includes a wide variety of different foods containing sufficient amounts of essential nutrients. Abusing this rule and cutting calories to the bone can turn you literally into skin and bones, depriving you of the nutrients you need to live a normal healthy life. For more on the potentially devastating effects of starvation, voluntary and otherwise, check out Chapter 14.

>> **Be more active.** Exercise allows you to take in more calories and still lose weight. In addition, exercise reduces the risk of many health problems, such as heart disease. Sounds like a recipe for success.

Although many Americans should work at losing weight, the fact is that many larger people, even people who are clearly obese, do live long, happy, and healthy lives.

To figure out why some overweight people's health status doesn't follow the "rules," many nutrition scientists now focus on the importance of *confounding variables* — science speak for "something else is going on here."

Here are three potential confounding variables in the obesity/health equation:

>> Maybe people who are overweight are more prone to illness because they exercise less, in which case stepping up the workouts may reduce the perceived risk of being overweight.

SNOOZE TO LOSE

In 2010, two separate studies, one at the University of Chicago Medical Center and the other at the Division of Sleep Medicine at Brigham and Women's Hospital and Beth Israel Deaconess Medical Center in Boston, linked lack of several good nights' sleep to weight gain. Naturally, that called for follow-up studies, and sure enough, in 2012, researchers at Columbia University College of Physicians and Surgeons discovered that sleep deprivation appears to impact the "fullness" hormones ghrelin (which says, "I need food") and leptin (which says "Enough!"), producing more ghrelin, less leptin, and thus eventually more pounds on your body. In plain speak, a sleepy brain makes bad decisions whether for late-night snacking or reaching for a candy bar rather than an apple the following day.

>> People who are overweight may be more likely to be sick because they eat lots of foods containing high-calorie ingredients, such as saturated fat, that can trigger adverse health effects; in this case, the remedy may simply be a change in diet and a healthier lifestyle including, yes, exercise.

Chapter 5

Calories: Powering Up the Body

A utomobiles burn gasoline to get the energy they need to move. Your body burns (*metabolizes*) food to produce energy in the form of heat that keeps you warm and (as energy) powers your every move and thought.

The amount of heat produced by metabolizing food is measured in a unit called the *kilocalorie* — the amount of energy it takes to raise the temperature of 1 kilogram of water 1 degree on a Centigrade (Celsius) thermometer at sea level.

TECHNICAL STUFF

For the non-chemists in the room, 1 kilogram = 1 liter = 1/4 U.S. gallon. As for temperature, 1 degree on the Celsius thermometer = 33.8 degrees on a Fahrenheit thermometer. To convert any temperature from Celsius to Fahrenheit or vice versa, use the following equations, which illustrate a 0 degree temperature, the simplest example:

$$°F = °C × 9/5 + 32$$

$$32°F = 0°C × 9/5 = 0 + 32 = 32°F$$

$$°C = (°F - 32) × 5/9$$

$$0°C = (32°F - 32) = 0 × 5/9 = 0°C$$

Nutritionists commonly substitute the word *calorie* for *kilocalorie*. Strictly speaking, a true calorie is just 1/1,000 of a kilocalorie, but the word *calorie* is easier to say and easier to remember, so that's what you see when you read about the energy in food.

Counting the Calories in Food

When someone says that a serving of food — say, one banana — has 105 calories, that means your metabolizing the banana produces 105 calories of energy your body can use for work.

Different foods have different amounts of calories depending on their nutritional components. For example, high-fat foods have more calories than low-fat foods because a gram of fat has more calories than a gram of carbs or protein or alcohol:

>> Protein has 4 calories per gram.

>> Carbohydrates have 4 calories per gram.

>> Fat has 9 calories per gram.

>> Alcohol has 7 calories per gram.

In other words, ounce for ounce, proteins and carbohydrates give you fewer than half as many calories as fat. That's why — again, ounce for ounce — high-fat foods, such as cream cheese, are calorie-rich, while low-fat foods, such as fruits and vegetables, are not.

MEASURING THE NUMBER OF CALORIES

Nutrition scientists measure the number of calories in food by actually burning the food in a *bomb calorimeter,* which is a box with two chambers, one inside the other. The researchers weigh a sample of the food, put the sample in a dish, and put the dish into the inner chamber of the calorimeter. They fill the inner chamber with oxygen and then seal it so the oxygen can't escape. The outer chamber is filled with a measured amount of cold water, and the oxygen in the first chamber (inside the chamber with the water) is ignited with an electric spark. When the food burns, an observer records the rise in the temperature of the water in the outer chamber. If the temperature of the water goes up 1 degree per kilogram, the food has 1 calorie; if it goes up 2 degrees, it has 2 calories; 235 degrees, 235 calories — or one 8-ounce chocolate malt made with powder mix and whole milk.

Sometimes foods that seem to be equally low calorie really aren't. You have to watch all the angles, paying attention to fat in addition to protein and carbohydrates. Here's a good example: A chicken breast and a hamburger are both high-protein foods. Both should have the same number of calories per ounce. But if you serve the chicken without its skin, it contains very little fat, while the hamburger has a lot. So a 3-ounce serving of skinless chicken gives you 140 calories, while a 3-ounce burger yields 230 to 245 calories, depending on the cut of the meat and its fat content.

Empty calories

All food provides calories. All calories provide energy. But some foods are said to give you *empty calories.* This term has nothing to do with the energy the calorie provides. It simply describes a food whose protein, fat, and carb calories come "naked" without the additional nutrients such, as dietary fiber, vitamins, and minerals, that improve the nutrition value of the foods on your plate.

The best-known empty-calorie foods are table sugar and *ethanol* (the kind of alcohol found in beer, wine, and spirits). On their own, sugar and ethanol give you energy — but no nutrients. (See Chapter 8 for more about sugar and Chapter 9 for more about alcohol.)

Of course, sugar and alcohol are often found in foods that do provide other nutrients. For example, sugar is found in bread, and alcohol is found in beer — two very different foods that both provide calcium, phosphorus, iron, potassium, sodium, and B vitamins.

In the United States, some people are malnourished because they can't afford enough food to get the nutrients they need. The school lunch program started by President Franklin Delano Roosevelt in 1935 and expanded by almost every president, Republican and Democrat, since then has been a largely successful attempt to prevent malnutrition among poor schoolchildren.

Some Americans live in "food deserts," places where fresh produce and healthier options are just not available — or available but at really high prices.

Many other Americans who can afford enough food are malnourished because they simply don't know how to choose a diet that gives them nutrients as well as calories. For these people, eating too many foods with empty calories may cause significant health problems, such as weak bones, bleeding gums, skin rashes, mental depression, and preventable birth defects. Too many empty calories may also lead to obesity, an epidemic in current American society and, increasingly, around the world, which I outline in Chapter 4.

KEEPING UP WITH KETO

Choose a basic balanced healthy diet, and your body runs on glycogen, the sugar produced when you digest carbohydrates. A ketogenic diet changes that by restricting carbs so that you burn fats instead. That leads to your liver's creating ketones, alternate chemicals your cells can use for fuel, a situation called *ketosis*.

The original ketogenic ("ketone-making") diet, created in the 1920s as a treatment for epileptic children who did not respond to anti-seizure meds, drew 90 percent of daily calories from fat, 6 percent from protein, and just 4 percent form carbs. After a year on this regimen, nearly half the children experienced fewer seizures, and 12 percent were actually seizure free, a result confirmed today by the Epilepsy Foundation.

The strictest modern medical keto diet is more flexible, reducing calories from fat to 75 percent of the daily total, raising calories from protein to 20 percent, and adding one percent point to carbs. Non-medical versions such as the multiple varieties of the Atkins diet promoted as a fast way to peel off the pounds, are even more relaxed. *Caution:* To date, there are no serious long-term studies that show that keto diets produce anything more than a temporary weight loss.

None of the keto diets are risk free. The most common side effects among children who followed the original ketogenic plan were constipation, weight loss, and growth problems thought to be due to limiting proteins. Today, obesity experts know that the keto diet may trigger high calcium levels in urine (hypercalciuria), kidney stones, temporarily high cholesterol, bad breath, dizziness, and, in the first few weeks, low energy levels commonly called *the keto flu*. This list of potential problems suggests that pregnant women, diabetics, and those with a history of kidney stones should not try keto without a doctor's approval.

Every calorie counts

Although your body burns some calories faster than others — your first source of energy is carbohydrates, which you metabolize before fats — people who say that "calories don't count" or that "some calories count less than others" are usually trying to convince you to follow a diet that concentrates on one kind of food to the exclusion of most others. One common example that arises like a phoenix in every generation of dieters is the *high-protein diet.*

WARNING

The high-protein diet, most commonly known today as the Atkins or ketogenic/keto diet, tells you to cut back or even entirely eliminate carbohydrate foods on the assumption that because your muscle tissue is mostly protein, the protein foods you eat will go straight from your stomach to your muscles, while everything else turns to fat. In other words, this diet says that you can stuff yourself with protein foods because no matter how many calories you get, they'll all be protein calories, and they'll all end up in your muscles, not on your hips. Wouldn't it be nice if that were true? The problem is, it isn't. All calories, regardless of where they come from, give you energy. If you take in more energy (calories) than you spend each day, you'll gain weight. If you take in fewer calories than you use up, you'll lose weight. This nutrition rule is an equal opportunity, one-size-fits-all proposition that generally applies to everyone and everybody.

Determining How Many Calories You Need

Think of your energy requirements as a bank account. You make deposits when you consume calories. You make withdrawals when your body spends energy on work. Nutritionists divide the amount of energy you withdraw each day into two parts:

>> The energy you need when your body is at rest

>> The energy you need to do your daily "work"

To keep your energy account in balance, you need to take in enough each day to cover your withdrawals. As a general rule, infants and adolescents burn more energy per pound than adults do, because they're continually making large amounts of new tissue. Similarly, an average man burns more energy than an average woman because his body is larger and has more muscle (see the upcoming section "Sex, glands, and chocolate cake"), thus leading to the totally unfair but totally true proposition that a man who weighs, say, 150 pounds can consume about 10 percent more calories than a woman who weighs 150 pounds and still not gain weight. For the numbers, check out the next section and Table 5-1.

Resting energy expenditure (REE)

Even when you're at rest, your body is busy. Your heart beats. Your lungs expand and contract. Your intestines digest food. Your liver processes nutrients. Your glands secrete hormones. Your muscles flex, usually gently. Cells send electrical impulses back and forth among themselves, and your brain continually sends messages to every tissue and organ.

TABLE 5-1
How Many Calories Do You Need When You're Resting?

Gender and Age	Equation to Figure Out Your REE
Males	
18–30	(15.3 x weight in kg) + 679
31–60	(11.6 x weight in kg) + 879
61 and older	(13.5 x weight in kg) + 487
Females	
18–30	(14.7 x weight in kg) + 496
31–60	(8.7 x weight in kg) + 829
61 and older	(10.5 x weight in kg) + 596

The National Research Council, Recommended Dietary Allowances (Washington, D.C.: National Academy Press, 1989)

The energy that your resting body uses to do all of this is called *resting energy expenditure*, abbreviated REE. The REE, also known as the *basal metabolism*, accounts for 60 to 70 percent of all the energy you need each day.

To find your resting energy expenditure (REE), you must first figure out your weight in kilograms (kg). One kilogram equals 2.2 pounds. So to get your weight in kilograms, divide your weight in pounds by 2.2. For example, if you weigh 150 pounds, that's equal to 68.2 kilograms (150 ÷ 2.2). Plug that into the appropriate equation in Table 5-1, and there's your REE.

What do you do with this information? First, simply appreciate its scientific value in describing the most basic fact about how many calories you need to survive. Second, and more pragmatically, regard it as a base on which to build a nutritional, real-life daily menu.

Sex, glands, and chocolate cake

A *gland* is an organ that secretes *hormones* — chemical substances that can change the function and sometimes the structure of other body parts. Hormones secreted by three glands — the pituitary, the thyroid, and the adrenals — influence how much energy you use when your body's at rest.

Your pituitary gland, a small structure in the center of your brain, stimulates your thyroid gland (which sits at the front of your throat) to secrete hormones that impact the rate at which your tissues burn nutrients to produce energy.

When your thyroid gland doesn't secrete enough hormones (a condition known as *hypothyroidism*), you burn food more slowly, and your REE drops. When your thyroid secretes excess amounts of hormones (a condition known as *hyperthyroidism*), you burn food faster, and your REE is higher.

When you're frightened or excited, your adrenal glands (two small glands, one on top of each kidney) release *adrenaline*, the hormone that serves as your body's wake-up call. When you release adrenaline, your heartbeat increases. You breathe faster. Your muscles clench. And you burn food faster, converting it as fast as possible to the energy you need for the reaction commonly known as *fight or flight*. But these effects are temporary. The effects of your sex glands, on the other hand, last as long as you live.

If you're a woman, you know that your appetite may rise and fall in tune with your menstrual cycle. In fact, this fluctuation parallels what's happening to your REE, which goes up just before or at the time of ovulation. Your appetite is highest when menstrual bleeding starts and then falls sharply. Being a man (and making lots of testosterone) makes satisfying your nutritional needs on a normal American diet easier. Your male bones are naturally denser, so you're less dependent on dietary or supplemental calcium to prevent *osteoporosis* (severe loss of bone tissue) later in life. You don't lose blood through menstruation, so you need only less than half as much iron (8 milligrams for an adult male; 18 milligrams for a premenopausal woman who is neither pregnant nor nursing). Best of all, you can consume about 10 percent more calories than a woman of the same weight without adding pounds.

It is no accident that while teenage boys are developing wide shoulders and biceps, teenage girls are getting hips. Testosterone, the male hormone, promotes the growth of muscle and bone. Estrogen gives you fatty tissue. As a result, the average male body has proportionally more muscle; the average female body, proportionally more fat.

Muscle is active tissue. It expands and contracts. It works. And when a muscle works, it uses more energy than fat (which insulates the body and provides a source of stored energy but does not move an inch on its own). What this muscle versus fat battle means is that the average man's REE is about 10 percent higher than the average woman's. In practical terms, that means a 140-pound man can hold his weight steady while eating about 10 percent more than a 140-pound woman who is the same age and performs the same amount of physical work.

WARNING

No amount of dieting changes this unfair situation. A woman who exercises strenuously may reduce her body fat so dramatically that she no longer menstruates, an occupational hazard for some professional athletes. But she'll still have proportionately more body fat than an adult man of the same weight. If she eats what he does, and they perform the same amount of physical work, she still must take in fewer calories than he to hold her weight steady.

MUSCLE VERSUS FAT VERSUS WEIGHT LOSS

Muscle weighs more than fat. This is why many people who take up exercise to lose weight discover, one month or so into the barbells and step-up-step-down routine, their clothes fit better, but the scale points slightly higher. They've traded lightweight fat for heavier muscle, a case where less is more that can be momentarily confusing but definitely healthier in the long term.

Energy for work

Your second largest chunk of energy after the REE is the energy you spend on physical work, everything from brushing your teeth in the morning to planting a row of petunias in the garden or working out in the gym.

Your total energy requirement (the number of calories you need each day) is your REE plus enough calories to cover the amount of work you do.

Does thinking about this use up energy? Yes, but not as much as you'd like to imagine. To solve a crossword puzzle, or write a chapter of this book, the average brain uses about 1 calorie every four minutes. That's only one-third the amount needed to keep a 60-watt bulb burning for the same length of time.

Table 5-2 defines the energy level of various activities ranging from the least energetic (sleep) to the most (playing football, digging ditches). Table 5-3 shows how to make these numbers personal.

TABLE 5-2   **How Active Are You When You're Active?**

Activity Level	Activity
Resting	Sleeping, reclining
Very light	Seated and standing activities, painting, driving, laboratory work, typing, sewing, ironing, cooking, playing cards, and playing a musical instrument
Light	Walking on a level surface at 2.5 to 3 mph, garage work, electrical trades, carpentry, restaurant trades, housecleaning, child-care, golfing, sailing, and table tennis
Moderate	Walking 3.5 to 4 mph, weeding and hoeing, carrying a load, cycling, skiing, tennis, and dancing
Heavy	Walking with a load uphill, tree felling, heavy manual digging, basketball, climbing, football, and soccer
Exceptionally heavy	Professional athletic training

The National Research Council, Recommended Dietary Allowances (Washington, D.C.: National Academy Press, 1989)

TABLE 5-3

How Many Calories Do You Need to Do the Work You Do?

Activity Level	Calories Needed for This Work for One Hour
Very light	80–100
Light	110–160
Moderate	170–240
Heavy	250–350
Exceptionally heavy	350+

"Food and Your Weight," House and Garden Bulletin, No. 74 (Washington, D.C.: U.S. Department of Agriculture)

Calculating Your Daily Calorie Needs

Figuring out exactly how many calories to consume each day can be a consuming task. Luckily, the Institute of Medicine, the group whose Food and Nutrition Board determines the RDAs for vitamins, minerals, and other nutrients, has created a list of the average daily calorie allowance for healthy people from infants to senior citizens who maintain a healthful weight (see Chapter 4) based on the amount of activity a person performs each day.

Table 5-4 shows the calorie recommendations as estimated by the U.S. Department of Agriculture and Health and Human Services. Note that in this context, *sedentary* means a lifestyle with only the light physical activity associated with daily living; *moderately active* means a lifestyle that adds physical activity equal to a daily 1.5-to-3-mile walk at a speed of 3 to 4 miles per hour; *active* means adding physical activity equal to walking 3 miles a day at the 3 to 4 miles per hour clip.

TABLE 5-4

Estimated Daily Calorie Requirements for Healthy Adults Based on Activity Level

Gender	Age (years)	Sedentary	Moderately Active	Active
Child	2–3	1,000	1,000-1,400	1,000-1,400
Female	4–8	1,200	1,400–1,600	1,400–1,600
	9–13	1,600	1,600–2,000	1,800–2,200
	14–18	1,800	2,000	2,400
	19–30	2,000	2,000–2,200	2,400
	31–50	1,800	2,000	2,200

(continued)

TABLE 5-4 *(continued)*

Gender	Age (years)	Sedentary	Moderately Active	Active
	51–60	1,600	1,800	
Male	4–8	1,400	1,400–1,600	1,600–2,000
	9–13	1,800	1,800–2,200	2,000–2,600
	14–18	2,200	2,400–2,800	2,800–3,200
	19–30	2,400	2,600–2,800	3,000
	31–50	2,200	2,400–2,600	2,800–3,000
	51–60	2,200	2,200–2,400	2,400–2,800
	61–65	2,000	2,400	2,800
	66–75	2,000	2,200	2,600
	76+	2,000	2,200	2,400

Note: "Sedentary" means lifestyle with only light physical activity such as that associated with typical day-to-day life. "Moderately active" means adding physical activity equal to walking 1.5 to 3 miles a day at about 3 to 4 miles per hour. "Active" means adding a walk longer than 3 miles per day at the same clip of 3 to 4 miles per hour.

Source https://www.webmd.com/diet/features/estimated-calorie-requirement *based on* https://fns-prod.azureedge.net/sites/default/files/usda_food_patterns/EstimatedCalorieNeedsPerDayTable.pdf

REMEMBER

Calories are not your enemy. On the contrary, they give you the energy you need to live a healthy life. The trick is to manage your calories and not let them manage you. When you know which foods provide what energy, you can strategize your energy intake to match your energy expenditure, and vice versa. When you do, your body will say, "Thank you," every day.

2

The Good Stuff in Your Food

Chapter **6**

Protein Power

rotein is an essential nutrient whose name comes from the Greek word *protos*, which means "first." To visualize a molecule of protein, close your eyes and see a very long chain, rather like a chain of sausage links. The links in the chains are *amino acids*, commonly known as the building blocks of protein. In addition to carbon, hydrogen, and oxygen atoms, amino acids contain a nitrogen (amino) group. The *amino group* is essential for synthesizing (assembling) specialized proteins in your body.

In this chapter, you discover how your body uses the proteins you get from food and, equally important, how your body manufactures some special proteins you need for a healthy life.

Understanding How Your Body Uses Proteins

The human body is chock-full of proteins used to build new cells and to maintain tissues. To make that possible, proteins are present in the outer and inner membranes of every living cell as well as

» **Your hair, your nails, and the outer layers of your skin:** All three are made of keratin, a *scleroprotein,* from the Greek word *skleros* meaning "hard."

Scleroproteins are impervious to digestive enzymes. In other words, if you bite your nails, you can't digest the pieces.

>> **Muscle tissue:** The special proteins in muscle are *myosin, actin,* and *myoglobin.*

>> **Bone marrow:** The outer layer of your bones is hardened with minerals, such as calcium, but the rubbery inner structure is protein; and bone marrow, the soft material inside the bone, is also protein-rich.

>> **Red blood cells:** This is where you find *hemoglobin,* a protein compound that carries oxygen throughout the body. *Plasma,* the clear fluid in blood, contains fat and protein particles known as *lipoproteins,* which ferry cholesterol around and out of the body (more on the various lipoproteins in Chapter 7).

About half the dietary protein that you consume each day is used to make *enzymes,* the specialized worker proteins that do specific jobs, such as digesting food and assembling or dividing molecules to make new cells and chemical substances. To perform these functions, enzymes often need specific vitamins and minerals.

DNA/RNA

Nucleoproteins are chemicals in the nucleus of every living cell. They're made of proteins linked to *nucleic acids* — complex compounds that contain phosphoric acid, a sugar molecule, and nitrogen-containing molecules made from amino acids.

Nucleic acids (molecules found in the chromosomes and other structures in the center of your cells) carry the genetic codes, the genes that help determine what you look like, your general intelligence, and who you are. They also contain one of two sugars, either *ribose* or *deoxyribose.* The nucleic acid containing ribose is called *ribonucleic acid* (RNA). The nucleic acid containing deoxyribose is called *deoxyribonucleic acid* (DNA).

DNA, which carries and transmits the genetic inheritance in your chromosomes, is a very long molecule with two strands twisting about each other (the *double helix*). DNA's job is to provide instructions that determine how your body cells are formed and how they behave. RNA, a single-strand molecule, is created in the cell nucleus according to the pattern determined by the DNA. Then RNA carries the DNA's instructions to the rest of the cell.

DNA is the most distinctly "you" thing about your body. The possibility that another person on Earth has exactly the same DNA as you is infinitesimal. That's why DNA analysis is so valuable in identifying individuals in various situations. Most commonly, this means criminal behavior, but some now propose that parents store a sample of their children's DNA to have a conclusive way of identifying a missing child, even years later.

Although many enzymes such as pepsin (the enzyme that breaks down proteins) have unique names, many more end in the three letters *-ase*. For example, the enzyme that acts on fat *(lip-)* is called lipase, and the enzyme that breaks down starches is called amylase from *amyl-*, the biochemist's term for "pertaining to starch."

Your ability to see, think, hear, and move — in fact, to do just about everything that you consider part of a healthy life — requires your nerve cells to send messages back and forth to each other and to other specialized kinds of cells, such as muscle cells. Sending these messages requires chemicals called *neurotransmitters*. Making neurotransmitters requires proteins.

Finally, proteins play an important part in the creation of every new cell and every new individual. Your chromosomes, after all, consist of *nucleoproteins*, substances made of amino acids and nucleic acids. (See the nearby "DNA/RNA" sidebar for more information about nucleoproteins.)

Moving Proteins from Your Dinner Plate to Your Cells

The cells in your digestive tract can absorb only single amino acids or very small chains of two or three amino acids called *peptides*. So proteins from food are broken into their component amino acids by digestive enzymes, which are, of course, specialized proteins. Then other enzymes in your body cells build new proteins by reassembling the amino acids into specific compounds that your body needs to function. This process is called *protein synthesis*. During protein synthesis

» Amino acids hook up with fats to form *lipoproteins,* the molecules that ferry cholesterol around and out of the body. Or amino acids may join up with carbohydrates to form the *glycoproteins* found in the mucus secreted by the digestive tract.

» Proteins combine with phosphoric acid to produce *phosphoproteins,* such as casein, a protein in milk.

» While most of us think "muscle" when we hear "protein," in fact nucleic acids combine with proteins to create *nucleoproteins,* essential components of every cell nucleus and of cytoplasm, the living material inside each cell.

The carbon, hydrogen, and oxygen that are left over after protein synthesis is complete are converted to glucose and used for energy. The nitrogen residue (ammonia) is processed by the liver, which converts the ammonia to urea. Most of the urea produced in the liver is excreted through the kidneys in urine; very small amounts are sloughed off in skin, hair, and nails.

Every day, you *turn over* (reuse) more proteins than you get from the food you eat, so you need a continuous supply to maintain your protein status. If your diet doesn't contain sufficient amounts of proteins, you start digesting the proteins in your body, including the proteins in your muscles and — in extreme cases, which is to say starvation — your heart muscle (see the section "Dodging protein deficiency," later in this chapter).

Differentiating Dietary Proteins

All the proteins in your food are made of amino acids, but not all proteins contain all the amino acids you require to maintain a healthy body. Some proteins are essential, others not so much. Some are high quality, others not so much again. This section explains it all.

Essential and nonessential proteins

For optimal health, human beings require 22 different amino acids. Ten are considered *essential*, which means you can't synthesize them in your body and must get them from food. (Two of these, arginine and histidine, are essential only for children.) Several more are *nonessential*: If you don't get them in food, you can manufacture them yourself from fats, carbohydrates, and other amino acids. Three — glutamine, ornithine, and taurine — are somewhere in between essential and nonessential for humans, essential only under certain conditions, such as with injury or disease. See the following for a list of the essential and nonessential amino acids for humans.

Essential Amino Acids	Nonessential Amino Acids
Arginine*	Alanine
Histidine*	Asparagine
Isoleucine	Aspartic acid
Leucine	Citrulline
Lysine	Cysteine
Methionine	Glutamic acid

Essential Amino Acids	Nonessential Amino Acids
Phenylalanine	Glycine
Threonine	Norleucine
Tryptophan	Proline
Valine	Serine
	Taurine
	Tyrosine

*Essential for children; nonessential for adults — but essential for healthy cats and dogs.

#Found in breast milk and considered possibly essential for newborns; nonessential for adult humans; essential for cats and songbirds.

Evaluating proteins

There are two basic ways to describe the value of proteins. The first is *high quality versus low quality*. The second is *complete versus limited or incomplete*.

High-quality versus low-quality proteins

Because an animal's body is similar to yours, its proteins contain similar combinations of amino acids. That's why nutritionists call proteins from foods of animal origin — meat, fish, poultry, eggs, and dairy products — *high-quality proteins.* Your body absorbs these proteins more efficiently and uses them with very little waste to synthesize other proteins. The proteins from plants — grains, fruits, vegetables, legumes (beans), nuts, and seeds — often have limited amounts of some essential amino acids.

The basic standard against which you measure the value of proteins in food is the egg, which nutrition scientists have arbitrarily given a *biological value* of 100 percent, meaning that, gram for gram, it's the food with the best supply of complete proteins. Other foods that have proportionately more protein may not be as valuable as the egg because they lack sufficient amounts of one or more essential amino acids.

For example, eggs are 11 percent protein, and dry beans are 22 percent protein. However, the proteins in beans don't provide sufficient amounts of *all* the essential amino acids. The prime exception is the soybean, a legume that's packed with abundant amounts of all the amino acids essential for human adults. Obviously, soybeans are an excellent source of proteins for vegetarians, especially *vegans* — those vegetarians who avoid all products of animal origin, including milk and eggs.

SUPER SOY: THE SPECIAL PROTEIN FOOD

Nutrition fact number 1: Food from animals has complete proteins. Nutrition fact number 2: Vegetables, fruits, and grains have incomplete proteins. Nutrition fact number 3: Nobody told the soybean.

Unlike other vegetables, including other beans, soybeans have complete proteins with sufficient amounts of all the amino acids essential for human health. In fact, food experts rank soy proteins on par with egg whites and casein (the protein in milk), the two proteins easiest for your body to absorb and use (see Table 6-1).

One-half cup (4 ounces) of cooked soybeans has 14 grams of protein; 4 ounces of tofu has 13. Either serving gives you approximately twice the protein you get from one large egg or one 8-ounce glass of skim milk, or two-thirds the protein in 3 ounces of lean ground beef. Eight ounces of fat-free soy milk has 7 grams of protein — a mere 1 gram less than a similar serving of skim milk — and no cholesterol. Soybeans are also jam-packed with dietary fiber, which helps move food through your digestive tract.

So what could go wrong? A whole lot.

Soybeans contain phytoestrogens, plant compounds such as isoflavone, that mimic the effects of natural mammalian estrogen. Once promoted as an alternative to estrogen products for women at and after menopause, soybeans and soy supplements may be problematic in specific situations. For example, according to WebMD, one of the reliable food and medicine websites listed in Chapter 27, even short-term use (up to six months) may cause gastric upset such as constipation, bloating, and nausea. Long-term use may possibly be unsafe. Although some studies suggest that soy products protect against reproductive cancers, others imply that they may actually stimulate breast and endometrial tumors. During pregnancy, soy estrogens may be hazardous for the fetus. Soy "milks" are considered safe for infants and young children who are sensitive to cow's milk, but supplements or other products containing larger amounts of phytoestrogens than found in these formulas may not be safe.

Conclusion? As with everything else in life from food to whatever, balance matters. Some soy: Good. Too much: Not so much.

The term used to describe the value of the proteins in any one food is *amino acid score*. Because the egg contains ample amounts of all the essential amino acids, it scores 100. Table 6-1 shows the protein quality of representative foods relative to the egg.

In 1993, the FDA and FAO/WHO adopted the Protein Digestibility Corrected Amino Acid Score as the preferred method for determining protein quality.

TABLE 6-1

Scoring the Amino Acids in Food

Food	Protein Content (Grams)	Amino Acid Score (Compared to the Egg)
Egg	33	100
Fish	61	100
Beef	29	100
Milk (cow's whole)	23	100
Soybeans	29	100
Dry beans	22	75
Rice	7	62–66
Corn	7	47
Wheat	13	50
Wheat (white flour)	12	36

Nutritive Value of Foods (Washington, D.C.: U.S. Department of Agriculture, 1991); George M. Briggs and Doris Howes Calloway, Nutrition and Physical Fitness, 11th ed. (New York: Holt, Rinehart and Winston, 1984)

Complete proteins and incomplete proteins

Another way to describe the quality of proteins is to say that they're either complete or incomplete. A *complete protein* is one that contains ample amounts of all essential amino acids; an *incomplete protein* does not. A protein low in one specific amino acid is called a *limiting protein* because it can build only as much tissue as the smallest amount of the necessary amino acid. You can improve the protein quality in a food containing incomplete/limiting proteins by eating it along with one that contains sufficient amounts of the limited amino acids.

Matching foods to create complete proteins is called *complementarity*, a concept first popularized by Frances Moore Lappe in her bestselling book, *Diet for a Small Planet* (Ballantine Books). Moore's intent was to convince people to become vegetarians or at least to increase the amount of plant foods in their diets while decreasing the amount of foods from animals so as to conserve energy and reduce the overall cost of producing food.

One example of complementarity is rice and beans. The rice is low in the essential amino acid lysine, and beans are low in the essential amino acid methionine. By eating rice with beans, you improve (or complete) the proteins in both. Another example is pasta and cheese. Pasta is low in the essential amino acids lysine and isoleucine; milk products have abundant amounts of these two amino acids. Shaking Parmesan cheese onto pasta creates a higher-quality protein dish. In each case, the foods have complementary amino acids. Other examples of complementary protein dishes are peanut butter with bread, and milk with cereal. Many such combinations are a natural and customary part of the diet in parts of the world where animal proteins are scarce or very expensive.

Table 6-2 shows how to combine foods to improve the quality of their proteins. Once upon a time, nutritionists insisted that you had to consume these combinations in rigorous combination — that is, in the same dish or the same meal. But time moves on, and so does nutrition knowledge. Today, those same nutritionists accept the idea that when you eat a food with incomplete proteins, the proteins hang around in your body several hours, long enough to hook up with incomplete proteins in other foods in your next meal, which certainly makes meal planning ever so much easier.

TABLE 6-2   **Combining Foods to Complement Proteins**

This Food	Complements This Food	Examples
Whole grains	Legumes (beans)	Rice and beans
Dairy products	Whole grains	Cheese sandwich, pasta with cheese, pancakes (wheat and milk/egg batter)
Legumes (beans)	Nuts and/or seeds	Chili soup (beans) with caraway seeds
Dairy products	Legumes (beans)	Chili beans with cheese
Dairy products	Nuts and seeds	Yogurt with chopped nut garnish

THE LOWDOWN ON GELATIN AND YOUR FINGERNAILS

Everyone knows that gelatin is a protein that strengthens fingernails. Too bad *everyone's* half-wrong.

Yes, gelatin is protein, and yes, protein makes nails strong. But the protein in gelatin, a food made by treating animal bones with acid, thus destroying the essential amino acid tryptophan, is incomplete. Luckily, you can improve the protein value of gelatin by slicing a banana onto the dish (bananas are tryptophan-rich) and pouring on some milk (also a good source of tryptophan).

Figuring Out How Much Protein You Need

The National Academy of Sciences Food and Nutrition Board, which sets the requirements for vitamins and minerals, such as the Recommended Dietary Allowances, or RDAs, and the Dietary Reference Intakes, or DRIs, described in Chapter 3, also sets goals for daily protein consumption. As with other nutrients, the board has different recommendations for different groups of people: young, old, male, and female.

Calculating the correct amount

In 2005, the Academy set a DRI of 46 grams of protein per day for a healthy adult woman and 56 grams per day for a healthy adult man. You can easily meet these amounts by having two to three 3-ounce servings of lean meat, fish, or poultry (21 grams each). Vegetarians can get their protein from 2 eggs (12 to 16 grams), 2 slices of packaged fat-free cheese (10 grams), 4 slices of bread (3 grams each), and 1 cup of yogurt (10 grams). Vegans (those who don't eat any foods from animals, including dairy products) can get the protein they need from a cup of oatmeal (6 grams) with a cup of soymilk (7 grams), 2 tablespoons peanut butter (8 grams) sandwiched on one large pita (5 to 6 grams), 6 ounces soy milk yogurt (6 grams), 6 ounces tofu (13 grams) with 1 cup cooked brown rice (5 grams), and 1 cup steamed broccoli (5 grams).

For the protein values in literally thousands of servings of literally thousands of foods, check out the USDA National Nutrient Database for Standard Reference at http://ndb.nal.usda.gov/.

MUSCLE TURNS INTO FAT? NO WAY

An older body synthesizes new proteins less efficiently than a younger one, so muscle mass (protein tissue) diminishes while fat content stays the same or rises. This change is often erroneously described as muscle "turning to fat." In fact, an older body still uses protein to build new tissue, including hair, skin, and nails, which continue to grow until death. By the way, the idea that nails continue to grow after death — a staple of shock movies and horror comics — arises from the fact that tissue around the corpse's nails shrinks, making the nails look longer.

Dodging protein deficiency

The first sign of protein deficiency is likely to be weak muscles — the body tissue most reliant on protein. For example, children who don't get enough protein have shrunken weak muscles. They may also have thin hair, their skin may be covered with sores, and blood tests may show abnormally low blood levels of *albumin*, a protein that helps maintain the body's fluid balance, keeping a proper amount of liquid in and around body cells.

A protein deficiency may also affect red blood cells. The cells live for only 120 days, so the body needs a regular supply of protein to make new ones. People who don't get enough protein may become *anemic*, having fewer red blood cells than they need. Other signs of protein deficiency are fluid retention (the big belly on a starving child), hair loss, and muscle wasting caused by the body's attempt to protect itself by digesting the proteins in its own muscle tissue, a phenomenon that explains why victims of starvation are, literally, skin and bones.

Given the high-protein content of a normal American diet (which generally provides far more protein than you actually require), protein deficiency is rare in the United States except as a consequence of eating disorders such as *anorexia nervosa* (refusal to eat) and *bulimia* (regurgitation after meals), both discussed in Chapter 14.

Boosting your protein intake: Special considerations

Anyone who's building new tissue quickly needs extra protein. For example, the DRI for protein for women who are pregnant or nursing is 71 grams per day, 25 grams higher than the RDA for an adult woman who is not pregnant.

Injuries also raise your protein requirements because an injured body releases above-normal amounts of protein-destroying hormones from the pituitary and adrenal glands. As a result, you need extra protein to protect existing tissues, and after severe blood loss, you need extra protein to make new hemoglobin for red blood cells. Cuts, burns, or surgical procedures mean that you need extra protein to make new skin and muscle cells, and fractures mean extra protein is needed to make new bone. The need for extra protein is so important if you've been badly injured and are in the hospital and can't take protein by mouth, and you'll be given an intravenous solution of amino acids with glucose (sugar) or emulsified fat.

TECHNICAL STUFF

Do athletes need more proteins than the rest of us? Recent research suggests that the answer may be yes, but athletes easily meet their requirements simply by eating more food, not by increasing the amount of any specific food.

Avoiding protein overload

Yes, you can get too much protein. Several medical conditions make it difficult for people to digest and process proteins properly. As a result, waste products build up in different parts of the body.

People with liver disease or kidney disease either don't process protein efficiently into urea or don't excrete it efficiently through urine. The result may be uric acid kidney stones or *uremic poisoning* (an excess amount of uric acid in the blood). The pain associated with *gout* (a form of arthritis that affects nine men for every one woman) is caused by uric acid crystals collecting in the spaces around joints. Doctors may recommend a low-protein diet as part of the treatment in these situations.

Nutrition experts also draw a distinction between proteins from plants and dairy products versus protein from animal foods, primarily red meat, which has been linked to an increased risk of coronary artery disease, as well as some cancers. (More about a similar difference between fats in Chapter 7.)

Chapter 7

Facing Facts on Fat and Cholesterol

The chemical family name for fats and related compounds, such as cholesterol, is *lipids*, from *lipos*, the Greek word for "fat." Liquid fats are called *oils*; solid fats are called, well, *fat*, and the fat in food is called *dietary fat*.

With the exception of *cholesterol* and other *sterols* (a fatty substance that has no calories and provides no energy), dietary fats are high-energy nutrients. Gram for gram, fats have more than twice as much energy potential (calories) as protein and carbohydrates: 9 calories per fat gram versus 4 calories per gram for the other two. (For more calorie information, see Chapters 3 and 5.)

This chapter cuts the fat away from the subject of fats and zeroes in on what you really need to know.

Discovering How Your Body Uses Fats

Dietary fats are sources of energy that add flavor to food — the characteristic sizzle on the steak, so to speak. Unfortunately, some forms of this tasty nutrient may also be hazardous to your health. The trick is to separate the good from the bad.

Understanding what fats do for you

A healthy body needs fats to build body tissues and manufacture biochemicals such as hormones. Some of the *adipose* (fatty) tissue in your body is plain to see. For example, even though your skin covers it, you can *see* the fat deposits in female breasts, hips, thighs, buttocks, and belly or on the male abdomen and shoulders.

This relatively visible body fat

>> Provides a source of stored energy

>> Gives shape to your body

>> Cushions your skin (imagine sitting in a chair without your buttocks to pillow your bones)

>> Acts as an insulation blanket that reduces heat loss

Other body fat is tucked away in and around your internal organs. This hidden fat is

>> Part of every cell membrane (the outer skin that holds each cell together).

>> A component of *myelin,* the fatty material that sheathes nerve cells and makes it possible for them to send the electrical messages that enable you to think, see, speak, move, and perform the multitude of tasks natural to a living body. Your brain is about 60 percent fat, giving a whole new meaning to the term "fat head."

>> A constituent of hormones and other biochemicals such as vitamin D and bile.

>> A shock absorber that protects your organs (as much as possible) if you fall or are injured.

Pulling energy from fat

Although dietary fat has more energy (calories) per gram than protein and carbohydrates, your body has a more difficult time pulling the energy out of fatty foods than out of foods high in protein and carbs.

Imagine a chain of long balloons — the kind people twist into shapes that resemble dachshunds, flowers, and other amusing things. When you drop one of these balloons into water, it floats. That's exactly what happens when you swallow fat-rich foods. The fat floats on top of the watery food-and-liquid mixture in your stomach, which limits the effects of *lipases,* the enzymes that break fats apart so you can digest them. As a result, fat is digested more slowly than proteins and carbohydrates, so you feel fuller, a condition called *satiety* (pronounced say-*ty*-eh-tee) longer after eating high-fat food.

Into the intestines

When the fat moves down your digestive tract into your small intestine, an intestinal hormone called *cholecystokinin* alerts your gallbladder to release *bile.* Bile is an emulsifier, a substance that enables fat to mix with water so that lipases can start breaking the fat into *glycerol* and *fatty acids.* These smaller fragments may be stored in special cells (fat cells) in adipose tissue, or they may be absorbed into cells in the intestinal wall, where one of the following happens:

» They're combined with oxygen (or burned) to produce heat/energy, water, and the waste product carbon dioxide.

» They're used to make lipoproteins that haul fats, including cholesterol, through your bloodstream.

Into the body

Glucose, the molecule you produce by digesting carbohydrates, is the body's basic source of energy. Burning glucose is easier and more efficient than burning fat, so your body always goes for carbohydrates first. But if you've used up all your available glucose — maybe you're stranded in a cabin in the Arctic, you haven't eaten for a week, a blizzard's howling outside, and the corner deli 500 miles down the road doesn't deliver — then it's time to start in on your body fat.

The first step is for an enzyme in your fat cells to break up stored *triglycerides* (the form of fat in adipose tissue). The enzyme action releases glycerol and fatty acids, which travel through your blood to body cells, where they combine with oxygen to produce heat/energy, plus water — lots of water — and the waste product carbon dioxide.

As anyone who has used a high-protein/high-fat/low-carb weight-loss diet such as the Atkins regimen or a keto diet (more about them in Chapter 5) can tell you, in addition to all that water, burning fat for energy produces *ketones.* For people on a low-carb diet, the more likely sign of all those ketones, a condition known as *ketosis,* is stinky urine or breath that smells like acetone (nail polish remover).

Defining Fatty Acids and Their Relationship to Dietary Fat

Like amino acids, which are the building blocks of protein (explained in Chapter 6), fatty acids are the building blocks of fats. Chemically speaking, a *fatty acid* is a chain of carbon atoms with hydrogen atoms attached and a *carbon-oxygen-oxygen-hydrogen group* (the unit that makes it an acid) at one end.

An *essential fatty acid* is one that your body needs but can't assemble from other fats. You have to get it whole, from food. Linoleic acid, found in vegetable oils, is an essential fatty acid. Two others — linolenic acid and arachidonic acid — occupy a somewhat ambiguous position. You can't make them from scratch, but you can make them if you have enough linoleic acid on hand, so food scientists often argue about whether linolenic and arachidonic acids are actually "essential."

In practical terms, who cares? Linoleic acid is so widely available in food, you're unlikely to experience a deficiency of any of the three — linoleic, linolenic, or arachidonic acids — as long as a measly 2 percent of the calories you get each day come from fat.

EXPLORING THE CHEMICAL STRUCTURE OF FATTY ACIDS

Molecules are groups of atoms hooked together by chemical bonds. Different atoms form different numbers of bonds with other atoms. For example, a hydrogen atom can form one bond with one other atom; an oxygen atom can form two bonds with other atoms; and a carbon atom can form four bonds to other atoms.

To actually see how this bonding works, visualize a carbon atom as one of those round pieces in a child's Erector set or Tinker toy kit. Your carbon atom (C) has — figuratively speaking, of course — four holes: one on top, one on the bottom, and one on each side. If you stick a peg into each hole and attach a small piece of wood representing a hydrogen atom (H) to the pegs on the top, the bottom, and the left, you have a structure that looks like this:

Methyl group

This unit, called a *methyl group,* is the first piece in any fatty acid. To build the rest of the fatty acid, you add carbon atoms and hydrogen atoms to form a chain. At the end, you tack on a group with one carbon atom, two oxygen atoms, and a hydrogen atom. This group is called an *acid group,* the part that makes the chain of carbon and hydrogen atoms a fatty acid.

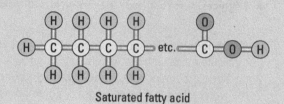

Saturated fatty acid

The preceding molecule is a *saturated fatty acid* because it has a hydrogen atom at every available carbon link in the chain. A *monounsaturated fatty acid* drops two hydrogen atoms and forms one double bond (two lines instead of one) between two carbon atoms. A *polyunsaturated fatty acid* drops more hydrogen atoms and forms several (poly) double bonds between several carbon atoms. Every hydrogen atom still forms one bond, and every carbon atom still forms four bonds, but they do so in a slightly different way. These sketches are not pictures of real fatty acids, which have many more carbons in the chain and have their double bonds in different places, but they can give you an idea of what fatty acids look like up close.

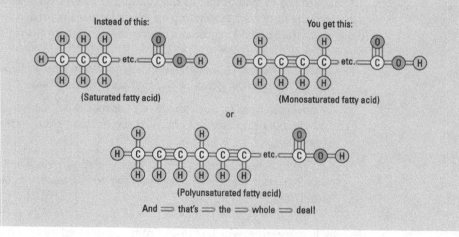

Focusing on the Fats in Food

Food contains three kinds of fats: triglycerides, phospholipids, and sterols. Here's how they differ:

>> **Triglycerides:** Your body uses these fats to make adipose tissue and burns for energy.

>> **Phospholipids:** Phospholipids are hybrids — part lipid, part phosphate (a molecule made with the mineral phosphorus) — that ferry hormones and the fat-soluble vitamins A, D, E, and K through your blood and back and forth in the watery fluid that flows across cell membranes.

>> **Sterols (steroid alcohols):** These are fat and alcohol compounds with no calories. Vitamin D is a sterol. So is the sex hormone testosterone. And so is cholesterol, the base on which your body builds hormones and vitamins.

Looking at the fatty acids in food

All the fats in food are combinations of fatty acids. Nutritionists characterize fatty acids as saturated fatty acids (SFA), monounsaturated fatty acids (MUFA), or polyunsaturated fatty acids (PUFA), depending on how many hydrogen atoms are attached to the carbon atoms in the chain. The more hydrogen atoms, the more saturated the fatty acid. Depending on which fatty acids predominate, a food fat is likewise characterized as saturated, monounsaturated, or polyunsaturated.

>> A *saturated fat,* such as butter, has mostly saturated fatty acids. Saturated fats are solid at room temperature and get harder when chilled.

>> A *monounsaturated fat,* such as olive oil, has mostly monounsaturated fatty acids. Monounsaturated fats are liquid at room temperature; they get thicker when chilled.

>> A *polyunsaturated fat,* such as corn oil, has mostly polyunsaturated fatty acids. Polyunsaturated fats are liquid at room temperature; they stay liquid when chilled.

So why is margarine, which is made from unsaturated fats such as corn and soybean oil, a solid? Because it's been artificially saturated by food chemists who add hydrogen atoms to some of its unsaturated fatty acids. This process, known as *hydrogenation,* turns an oil, such as corn oil, into a solid fat that can be used in products such as margarines without leaking out all over the table. A fatty acid with extra hydrogen atoms is called a *hydrogenated fatty acid.* (*Trans fatty acids* are hydrogenated fatty acids.) Because of those extra hydrogen atoms, hydrogenated fatty acids behave like saturated fats, clogging arteries and raising the levels of cholesterol in your blood.

One answer to the problem of hydrogenated fatty acids is plant *sterols* and *stanols*. Plant sterols are natural compounds in the oils in grains, fruits, and vegetables, including soybeans. *Stanols* are compounds created by adding hydrogen atoms to sterols from wood pulp and other plant sources; the first commercial stanol food was Benecol (bene = good, col = cholesterol) spread.

Sterols and stanols work like little sponges, sopping up cholesterol in your intestines before it can make its way into your bloodstream. As a result, your total cholesterol levels and your levels of low-density lipoproteins (LDLs or "bad" cholesterol) go down. In some studies, one to two 1-tablespoon servings a day of sterols and stanols can lower levels of bad cholesterol by 10 to 17 percent, with results showing up in as little as two weeks.

Table 7-1 shows the kinds of fatty acids found in some common dietary fats and oils. Fats are characterized according to their predominant fatty acids. For example, as you can plainly see in the table, nearly 25 percent of the fatty acids in corn oil are monounsaturated fatty acids. Nevertheless, because corn oil has more polyunsaturated fatty acid, corn oil is considered a polyunsaturated fat. Note for math majors: Some totals in Table 7-1 don't add up to 100 percent because these fats and oils also contain other kinds of fatty acids in amounts so small that they don't affect the basic character of the fat.

TABLE 7-1   ## What Fatty Acids Are in That Fat or Oil?

Fat or Oil	Saturated Fatty Acid (%)	Monounsaturated Fatty Acid (%)	Polyunsaturated Fatty Acid (%)	Kind of Fat or Oil
Canola oil	7	53	22	Monounsaturated
Corn oil	13	24	59	Polyunsaturated
Olive oil	14	74	9	Monounsaturated
Palm oil	52	38	10	Saturated
Peanut oil	17	46	32	Monounsaturated
Safflower oil	9	12	74	Polyunsaturated
Soybean oil	15	23	51	Polyunsaturated
Soybean-cottonseed oil	18	29	48	Polyunsaturated
Butter	62	30	5	Saturated
Lard	39	45	11	Saturated*

Because more than one-third of its fats are saturated, nutritionists label lard a saturated fat.

Nutritive Value of Foods (Washington, D.C.: U.S. Department of Agriculture); Food and Life (New York: American Council on Science and Health)

Identifying the foods with fats

Not all foods have fats. True, all animal foods, such as milk, meat, fish, and poultry, have naturally occurring fats. Some grains and some grain products do as well, naturally or from added ingredients such as the butter or margarine and eggs used to make cake and cookie batter. But fruits and vegetables are a whole different story. A very short list that includes olives and avocados does contain natural fats, but most foods in these categories are fat free. In short, as a general rule:

>> Fruits and vegetables have only traces of fat, primarily unsaturated fatty acids.

>> Grains have small amounts of fat, up to 3 percent of their total weight.

>> Dairy products vary. Cream is a high-fat food. Regular milks and cheeses are moderately high in fat. Skim milk and skim milk products are low-fat foods. Most of the fat in any dairy product is saturated fatty acids.

>> Meat is moderately high in fat, and most of its fats are saturated fatty acids.

>> Poultry (chicken and turkey), without the skin, is relatively low in fat.

>> Fish may be high or low in fat, primarily unsaturated fatty acids that — lucky for the fish — remain liquid even when the fish is swimming in cold water. (Remember, saturated fats harden when cooled.)

>> Vegetable oils, butter, and lard are high-fat foods. Most of the fatty acids in vegetable oils are unsaturated; most of the fatty acids in lard and butter are saturated.

>> Processed foods, such as cakes, breads, canned or frozen meat, and vegetable dishes, are generally higher in fat than plain grains, meats, fresh fruits, and fresh vegetables.

TIP

Here's a simple guide to finding which foods are high (or low) in fat. Oils are virtually 100 percent fat. Butter and lard are close behind. After that, the fat level drops, from 70 percent for some nuts down to 2 percent for most bread. The rule to take away from these numbers? A diet high in grains and plants always is lower in fat than a diet high in meat and oils.

Getting the right amount of fat

Getting the right amount of fat in your diet is a delicate balancing act. Too much, and you increase your risk of obesity, diabetes, heart disease, and some forms of cancer. Too little fat, and infants don't thrive, children don't grow, and everyone, regardless of age, is unable to absorb and use fat-soluble vitamins that smooth the skin, protect vision, bolster the immune system, and keep reproductive organs functioning.

So, exactly how much dietary fat is safe to consume each day? Nutrition experts have laid out general suggestions for specific kinds of fat like the infamous saturated sort believed to clog your arteries. As a result, you can find their recommendations right there on the Nutrition Facts Label for every packaged food. But overall, every day? Your guess is as good as theirs. For several years, *The Dietary Guidelines for Americans* had proposed exactly what percentage of your daily calories should come from fats, but that changed in 2015 when the specific numbers were eliminated, aiming instead for quality over quantity limits. This position, which relies on Patterns, the stratagem described in Chapter 17, makes food plans such as the Mediterranean Diet, with its emphasis on fats from plants, an attractive, protective and pragmatic scheme.

With exceptions, naturally.

WARNING

Sometimes, dietary recommendations come with surprises. For many years, the best advice on dietary fats was to take in less than you might actually enjoy. But then, in January 2020, an article in the *Journal of the American Urological Association* reported that, for men, a low-fat diet might be linked to a "small but significant" reduction in testosterone. There are also cautions regarding dietary fats and children. Although many organizations, such as the American Academy of Pediatrics, the American Heart Association, and the National Heart, Lung, and Blood Institute, recommend restricting fat intake for older children, they stress that infants and toddlers require fatty acids for proper physical growth and mental development. Never limit the fat in your baby's diet without checking first with your pediatrician.

REELING IN FACTS ON A FISH STORY

When Sir William Gilbert, lyricist to songsmith Sir Arthur Sullivan, wrote, "Here's a pretty kettle of fish!" in *Iolanthe*, he may well have been talking about the latest skinny on seafood.

The good news from a 2002 Harvard survey of more than 43,000 male health professionals was that those who ate 3 to 5 ounces of fish just once a month have a 40 percent lower risk of *ischemic stroke,* a stroke caused by a blood clot in a cranial artery. The Harvard study didn't include women, but a report on women and stroke published in the *Journal of the American Medical Association* in 2000 showed that women who consume about 4 ounces of fish — think one small can of tuna — two to four times a week appear to cut their risk of stroke by a similar 40 percent.

(continued)

(continued)

From the 1970s through the 1990s, these benefits were thought to be due to the presence of *omega-3 fatty acids* — unsaturated fatty acids found most commonly in fatty fish such as salmon and sardines. The primary omega-3 is *alpha*-linolenic acid, which your body converts to hormonelike substances called *eicosanoids*. The eicosanoids — eicosapentaenoic acid (EPA) and docosahexaenoic acid (DHA) — reduce inflammation, perhaps by inhibiting an enzyme called COX-2, which is linked to inflammatory diseases such as rheumatoid arthritis (RA).

So it makes sense to think that omega-3s are heart-friendly and that taking fish oil supplements would offer protection against heart attack and stroke. Alas, to date, most clinical trials show no such results. In 2013, data from a study of 12,000 people known to have atherosclerosis (plaque deposits in their arteries) published in *The New England Journal of Medicine* showed that daily doses of fish oil had no effect on the incidence of death from heart attack or stroke. Seven years later, pharmaceutical giant Astra-Zeneca stopped testing its own fish oil pill, Epanova, because it showed no benefit when combined with a statin for patients at risk of heart disease due to high levels if LDLs. On the other hand, eating fatty fish itself seems to be beneficial in many ways, not the least of which, according to a 2014 study at Ronald Reagan UCLA Medical Center, is bigger brain area where memory and cognition live.

Fish also is a good source of *taurine,* an amino acid the journal *Circulation* notes helps maintain the elasticity of blood vessels. Finally, omega-3s are bone builders. Fish oils enable your body to create *calciferol,* a naturally occurring form of vitamin D, the nutrient that enables your body to absorb bone-building calcium — which may be why omega-3s appear to help hold minerals in bone — and increase the formation of new bone.

A pretty kettle of fish, indeed.

Consumer Alert: Despite all the benefits fish bring to a healthful diet, it's also true that some fish, particularly those caught in the wild (rather than raised on a fish farm), may be contaminated with metals such as methyl mercury, a metal that makes its way into the water as industrial pollution and may be hazardous for children as well as women who are or may be pregnant, because mercury targets the developing fetal and child's brain and spinal cord. To keep methyl mercury ingestion as low as possible, experts recommend these people avoid all king mackerel, swordfish, and tile fish, species most likely to be contaminated.

Considering Cholesterol and You

Surprise: Every healthy body *needs* cholesterol. Look carefully, and you will find cholesterol in and around your cells, in your fatty tissue, in your organs, in your brain, and in your glands. What's it doing there? Plenty. Cholesterol

» Protects the integrity of cell membranes

» Helps nerve cells to send messages back and forth

» Is a building block for vitamin D (a sterol), made when sunlight hits the fat just under your skin (for more about vitamin D, see Chapter 11)

» Enables your gallbladder to make *bile acids,* digestive chemicals that, in turn, enable you to absorb fats and fat-soluble nutrients, such as vitamin A, vitamin D, vitamin E, and vitamin K

» Is a base on which you build steroid hormones, such as estrogen and testosterone

Cholesterol and heart disease

Doctors measure your cholesterol level by taking a sample of blood and counting the milligrams of cholesterol in 1 deciliter (1/10 liter) of blood. When you get your annual report from the doctor, your total cholesterol level looks something like this: 225 mg/dL. In other words, you have 225 milligrams of cholesterol in every tenth of a liter of blood. The more cholesterol you have floating in your blood, the more cholesterol is likely to cross into your arteries, where it may stick to the walls, form deposits that eventually block the flow of blood, and thus increase your risk of heart attack or stroke.

Blood tests aren't the only way to measure cholesterol risk. The next time you go for your annual eye exam and your doctor takes a picture of the back of your eyes, she can give you a good estimate of the health of your coronary arteries based on the diameter of the small ocular arteries (arterioles) and veins (venules) she sees there. A report in the *British Medical Journal* based on the measurement of these vessels in the eyes of 3,600 men and women age 49 to 75 found that wider venules and narrower arterioles were linked to a higher risk of dying from coronary artery disease.

CHOLESTEROL SEASON

Even if you allow yourself to indulge in (a few) high-cholesterol ice-cream cones and burgers every day of the year, your cholesterol level may still be naturally lower in the summer than in winter.

The basis for this intriguing culinary conclusion is the 2004 University of Massachusetts SEASONS (Seasonal Variation in Blood Lipids) Study of 517 healthy men and women age 20 to 70. The volunteers started out with an average cholesterol level of 213 milligrams per deciliter (women) to 222 milligrams per deciliter (men). A series of five blood tests during the one-year study showed an average drop of 4 points in the summer for men and 5.4 points for women. People with high cholesterol (above 240 milligrams per deciliter) did better, dropping as much as 18 points in the summer.

U. Mass cardiologists say one explanation for the summer downswing may be the normal increase in human blood volume in hot weather. Cholesterol levels reflect the total amount of cholesterol in your bloodstream. With more blood in the stream, the amount of cholesterol per deciliter declines, producing a lower total cholesterol reading. A second possibility is that people tend to eat less and be more active in summer. They lose weight, and weight loss equals lower cholesterol.

The first bit of wisdom from this study is obvious: Being physically active reduces your cholesterol level. The second is that environment matters. In other words, if you're planning to start a new cholesterol-buster diet, you may just do better to start during the cool weather, when your efforts may lower your total cholesterol as much as 12 points over a reasonable period of time, say, six months. Then when your doctor runs a follow-up test the following summer, you'll get the added benefit of the seasonal slip to make you feel really, really good about how well you're doing. For more on controlling your cholesterol, check out *Controlling Cholesterol For Dummies,* 2nd Edition, which I wrote with Martin W. Graf, MD (published by Wiley).

Lipoproteins

A *lipoprotein* is a fat and protein particle that carries cholesterol through your blood. Your body makes four types of lipoproteins: chylomicrons, very low-density lipoproteins (VLDLs), low-density lipoproteins (LDLs), and high-density lipoproteins (HDLs). As a general rule, LDLs take cholesterol into blood vessels; HDLs carry it out of the body.

A lipoprotein is born as a *chylomicron*, made in your intestinal cells from protein and triglycerides (fats). After 12 hours of traveling through your blood and around your body, a chylomicron has lost virtually all its fats. By the time the chylomicron makes its way to your liver, the only thing left is protein.

The liver, a veritable fat and cholesterol factory, collects fatty acid fragments from your blood and uses them to make cholesterol and new fatty acids. Time out! How much cholesterol you get from food may affect your liver's daily output: Eat more cholesterol, and your liver may make less. If you eat less cholesterol, your liver may make more. And so it goes.

Churning out harmful lipoproteins

After your liver has made cholesterol and fatty acids, it packages them with protein as very low-density lipoproteins (VLDLs), which have more protein and are denser than their precursors, the chylomicrons. As VLDLs travel through your bloodstream, they lose triglycerides, pick up cholesterol, and turn into low-density lipoproteins (LDLs). LDLs supply cholesterol to your body cells, which use it to make new cell membranes and manufacture sterol compounds such as hormones. That's the good news.

The bad news is that both VLDLs and LDLs are soft and squishy enough to pass through blood vessel walls. The larger and squishier they are, the more likely they are to slide into your arteries, which means that VLDLs are more hazardous to your health than LDLs, although elevated levels of all LDLs are regarded as being strongly linked to an increased risk of cardiovascular disease, such as a blocked blood vessel leading to a heart attack.

REMEMBER

VLDLs and LDLs are sometimes called "bad cholesterol," but this characterization is a misnomer. They aren't cholesterol; they're just the rafts on which cholesterol sails into your arteries. Traveling through the body, LDLs continue to lose cholesterol. In the end, they lose so much fat that they become mostly protein — turning them into high-density lipoproteins, the particles sometimes called "good cholesterol." Once again, this label is inaccurate. HDLs aren't cholesterol: They're simply protein and fat particles too dense and compact to pass through blood vessel walls, so they carry cholesterol out of the body rather than into arteries.

That's why a high level of HDLs may reduce your risk of heart attack regardless of your total cholesterol levels. Conversely, a high level of LDLs may increase your risk of heart attack, even if your overall cholesterol level is low.

Setting limits on the bad guys

At one point, back in the Dawn of the Cholesterol Age, the "safe" upper limit for LDLs was assumed to be around 160 milligrams per deciliter. Now, the National Heart, Lung, and Blood Institute, American College of Cardiology, and the American Heart Association have all put their stamps of approval on the National Cholesterol Education Program's (NCEP) recommendations for new, lower levels of LDLs.

Table 7-2 lays out the specifics on the National Cholesterol Education Program (NCEP) and the National Heart, Lung, and Blood Institute descriptions of and recommendations for total cholesterol levels, levels of high-density lipoproteins (HDLs), the so-called "good cholesterol," and low-density lipoproteins, the so-called "bad cholesterol" that invades and may clog blood vessels.

TABLE 7-2 **Recommended Optimal Cholesterol Levels By Age and Gender**

Anyone age 19 and younger	Men age 20 or older	Women age 20 or older
Total cholesterol*		
Less than 170	125-200	125-200
Non-HDL cholesterol		
Less than 120	less than 130	less than 130
LDL cholesterol		
less than 100	less than 100	less than 100
HDL cholesterol		
More than 45	40 or higher	50 or higher

*All levels listed in mg/dc (milligrams per deciliter), the number of milligrams (1000th of a gram) in one-tenth of a liter
Source: U.S. National Library of Medicine (20-19) "Cholesterol Levels: What You Need To Know"

TIP

But total cholesterol levels alone aren't the entire story. Many people with high cholesterol levels live to a ripe old age, while others with low total cholesterol levels develop heart disease because cholesterol is only one of several risk factors for heart disease. Here are some more:

>> An unfavorable ratio of lipoproteins (see the next section)

>> Smoking

>> Obesity

>> Age (being older is riskier)

>> Sex (being male is riskier)

>> A family history of heart disease

Diet and cholesterol

Most of the cholesterol you need is made right in your own liver, which churns out about 1 gram (1,000 milligrams) a day from the raw materials in the proteins, fats, and carbohydrates that you consume. But you also get cholesterol from food of animal origin: meat, poultry, fish, eggs, and dairy products. Although some plant foods, such as coconuts and cocoa beans, are high in saturated fats, no plants produce cholesterol.

TECHNICAL STUFF

For the past several years, there has been an ongoing debate about whether the cholesterol in your food is as important in determining the levels of cholesterol in your blood as is the cholesterol you produce in your liver. In other words, for some people, it is possible that even a diet very low in cholesterol and saturated fats may not lower their own cholesterol levels. Chapter 16 gives you the lowdown on the conclusions drawn in the *Dietary Guidelines for Americans 2015*. Meanwhile, for those of you who prefer to track your dietary cholesterol, Table 7-3 lists the amount of cholesterol in normal servings of some representative foods.

TABLE 7-3   ## How Much Cholesterol Is on That Plate?

Food	Serving Size	Cholesterol (mg)
Meat		
Beef (stewed) lean and fat	3 ounces	87
Beef (stewed) lean	2.2 ounces	66
Beef (ground) lean	3 ounces	74
Beef (ground) regular	3 ounces	76
Beef steak (sirloin)	3 ounces	77
Bacon	3 strips	16
Pork chop, lean	2.5 ounces	71
Poultry		
Chicken (roast) breast	3 ounces	73
Chicken (roast) leg	3 ounces	78
Turkey (roast) breast	3 ounces	59
Fish		
Clams	3 ounces	43
Flounder	3 ounces	59
Oysters (raw)	1 cup	120
Salmon (canned)	3 ounces	34
Salmon (baked)	3 ounces	60

(continued)

TABLE 7-3 *(continued)*

Food	Serving Size	Cholesterol (mg)
Tuna (water canned)	3 ounces	48
Tuna (oil canned)	3 ounces	55
Cheese		
American	1 ounce	27
Cheddar	1 ounce	30
Cream	1 ounce	31
Mozzarella (whole milk)	1 ounce	22
Mozzarella (part skim)	1 ounce	15
Swiss	1 ounce	26
Milk		
Whole	8 ounces	33
2%	8 ounces	18
1%	8 ounces	18
Skim	8 ounces	10
Other dairy products		
Butter	Pat	11
Other		
Eggs, large	1	213
Lard	1 tbsp.	12

Nutritive Value of Foods (Washington, D.C.: U.S. Department of Agriculture)

RED VERSUS WHITE

For years, dietary recommendations regarding cholesterol have said that "white meat" (chicken) is more healthful than "red meat" (beef). Maybe no longer. In June 2019 researchers from the Children's Hospital Oakland Research Institute reported that while a chicken breast sounds more healthful than a steak, in fact their effects on your cholesterol levels are pretty much the same. Both raise your cholesterol levels. The conclusion? Although the chicken was marginally better than the beef, the best advice is to replace animal protein with plant protein. Think beans. Think chili. Think lower cholesterol.

IN THIS CHAPTER

» Identifying the different kinds of carbohydrates

» Understanding how your body uses carbohydrates

» Choosing the foods with the best carbs

» Deciphering dietary fiber

Chapter **8**

Carbohydrates: A Complex Story

C arbohydrates are sugar compounds that plants make when they're exposed to light. (The name means "carbon plus water.") This process of making sugar compounds is called *photosynthesis*, from the Latin *photo-*, meaning "light," and *synthese*, meaning "put together."

This chapter shines a bright light on the different kinds of carbohydrates, illuminating all the nutritional nooks and crannies to explain how each contributes to your vim and vigor — not to mention a tasty daily menu.

Checking Out Carbohydrates

Carbohydrates come in three varieties: simple carbohydrates, complex carbohydrates, and dietary fiber. All are composed of units of sugar. What makes one carbohydrate different from another is the number of sugar units it contains and how the units are linked together.

Simple carbohydrates

What makes simple carbs simple is, well, *simple*. These relatively small molecules have only one or two units of sugar, which makes them easy to digest — which is why they provide a fast energy lifter.

>> A carbohydrate with one unit of sugar is called a *simple sugar* or a *monosaccharide* (*mono* = one; *saccharide* = sugar). Fructose (fruit sugar) is a monosaccharide, and so are glucose (blood sugar), the sugar produced when you digest carbohydrates, and galactose, the sugar derived from digesting lactose (milk sugar).

>> A carbohydrate with two units of sugar is considered pretty simple but its real name is *double sugar* or a *disaccharide* (*di* = two). Sucrose (table sugar), which is made of one unit of fructose and one unit of glucose, is a disaccharide.

Complex carbohydrates

Complex carbohydrates, which are also known as *polysaccharides* (*poly* = many), have more than two units of sugar linked together. Carbs with three to ten units of sugar are sometimes called *oligosaccharides* (*oligo* = few).

>> Raffinose is a *trisaccharide* (*tri* = three) that's found in potatoes, beans, and beets. It has one unit each of galactose, glucose, and fructose.

>> Stachyose is a *tetrasaccharide* (*tetra* = four) found in the same vegetables mentioned in the previous item. It has one fructose unit, one glucose unit, and two galactose units.

>> Starch, a complex carbohydrate in potatoes, pasta, and rice, is a definite polysaccharide. In fact, it's an *oligosaccharide (with more than 10 glucose units)* built of many units of glucose.

Because complex carbohydrates may have anywhere from three to several thousand units of sugars, your body takes longer to digest them than it takes to digest simple carbohydrates. As a result, digesting complex carbohydrates releases glucose into your bloodstream more slowly and evenly than digesting simple carbs. (For more about digesting carbs, see the section "Carbohydrates and Energy: A Biochemical Love Story," later in this chapter.)

Dietary fiber

Dietary fiber is a term used to distinguish the fiber in food from the natural and synthetic fibers (silk, cotton, wool, and nylon) used in fabrics. Dietary fiber is a third kind of carbohydrate. Like the complex carbohydrates, dietary fiber (cellulose, hemicellulose, pectin, beta-glucans, and gum) is a polysaccharide. Lignin, a different kind of chemical, is also called a dietary fiber.

Some kinds of dietary fiber also contain units of soluble or insoluble uronic acids, compounds derived from the sugars fructose, glucose, and galactose. For example, *pectin* — a soluble fiber in apples — contains soluble galacturonic acid.

TIP

Dietary fiber isn't like other carbohydrates. The bonds that hold its sugar units together can't be broken by human digestive enzymes. Although the bacteria living naturally in your intestines convert very small amounts of dietary fiber to fatty acids, dietary fiber isn't considered a source of energy. (For more about fatty acids, see Chapter 7.)

Carbohydrates and Energy: A Biochemical Love Story

Your body runs on glucose, the molecules your cells burn for energy. (For more information on how you get energy from food, check out Chapter 3.)

Proteins, fats, and alcohol (as in beer, wine, and spirits) also provide energy in the form of calories. And protein does give you glucose, but it takes a long time, relatively speaking, for your body to get it.

TECHNICAL STUFF

When you eat carbohydrates, your pancreas secretes insulin, the hormone that enables you to digest starches and sugars. This release of insulin is sometimes called an *insulin spike*, also known as "insulin secretion."

Eating simple carbohydrates such as sucrose (table sugar) provokes higher insulin secretion than eating complex carbohydrates such as starch. If you have a metabolic disorder such as diabetes that keeps you from producing enough insulin, you must be careful not to take in more carbs than you can digest. (See the section "Some people have problems with carbohydrates," later in this chapter.)

Most healthy people can metabolize even very large amounts of carbohydrate foods easily. Their insulin secretion rises to meet the demand and then quickly settles back to normal. In other words, the fact remains that for most people, a carb is a carb is a carb, regardless of how quickly the sugar enters the bloodstream. You can find the complete story in *Diabetes For Dummies*, by Alan L. Rubin, MD (Wiley).

GLIDING THROUGH THE GLYCEMIC INDEX

Some perfectly healthful foods, such as carrots and potatoes, contain a larger amount of easily digestible and absorbed carbs than do others. Early on, the *Glycemic Index (GI)*, a carbohydrate measurement scheme developed at the University of Toronto in 1981, offered a way to gauge the simple carb content by ranking foods according to how quickly the food affected blood sugar levels when compared to glucose (the form of sugar your body uses as energy).

Some foods contain such small amounts of carbs that the GI may not be a useful guide. As Meri Raffetto explains in *The Glycemic Index Diet For Dummies* (Wiley), a second measurement, the Glycemic Load (GL), developed at the Harvard School of Public Health in 1997, is a more accurate guide. For example, the (primarily) simple sugars in an apple may rate a GI from 28 to 44, but the amount is so small that the GL is only 4.

For more examples, go straight to www.health.harvard.edu and type "glycemic index" into the Search box.

For info on why the difference between simple and complex carbs can matter for athletes, see the later section "Some people need extra carbohydrates."

How glucose becomes energy

Inside your cells, glucose is burned to produce heat and *adenosine triphosphate*, a molecule that stores and releases energy as required by the cell. By the way, nutrition scientists, who have as much trouble pronouncing polysyllabic words as you probably do, usually refer to adenosine triphosphate by its initials: ATP.

The transformation of glucose into energy occurs in one of two ways: with oxygen or without it. Glucose is converted to energy with oxygen in the *mitochondria* — tiny bodies in the jellylike substance inside every cell. This conversion yields energy (ATP, heat) plus water and carbon dioxide, a waste product.

Red blood cells don't have mitochondria, so they change glucose into energy without oxygen. This yields energy (ATP, heat) and lactic acid.

Glucose is also converted to energy in muscle cells. When it comes to producing energy from glucose, muscle cells are, well, double-jointed. They have mitochondria, so they can process glucose with oxygen. But if the level of oxygen in the muscle cell falls very low, the cells can just go ahead and change glucose into energy without it. This is most likely to happen when you've been exercising so strenuously that you (and your muscles) are, literally, out of breath.

Being able to turn glucose into energy without oxygen is a handy trick, but here's the downside: One byproduct is lactic acid. Why is that a big deal? Because too much lactic acid makes your muscles ache.

How pasta ends up on your hips when too many carbs pass your lips

Your cells budget energy very carefully. They don't store more than they need right now. Any glucose the cell doesn't need for its daily work is converted to glycogen (animal starch) and tucked away as stored energy in your liver and muscles.

Your body can pack about 400 grams (14 ounces) of glycogen into liver and muscle cells. A gram of carbohydrates — including glucose — has 4 calories. If you add up all the glucose stored in glycogen to the small amount of glucose in your cells and blood, it equals about 1,800 calories of energy.

If your diet provides more carbohydrates than you need to produce this amount of stored calories in the form of glucose and glycogen in your cells, blood, muscles, and liver, the excess will be converted to fat. And that's how your pasta ends up on your hips.

Other ways your body uses carbohydrates

Providing energy is an important job, but it isn't the only thing carbohydrates do for you. Carbohydrates also protect your muscles. When you need energy, your body looks for glucose from carbohydrates first. If none is available, because you're on a carbohydrate-restricted diet or have a medical condition that prevents you from using the carbohydrate foods you consume, your body begins to pull energy out of fatty tissue and then moves on to burning its own protein tissue (muscles). If this use of proteins for energy continues long enough, you run out of fuel and die.

REMEMBER

A diet that provides sufficient amounts of carbohydrates keeps your body from eating its own muscles. That's why a carbohydrate-rich diet is sometimes described as *protein sparing*.

Carbohydrates also

>> Regulate the amount of sugar circulating in your blood so all your cells get the energy they need

>> Provide nutrients for the friendly bacteria in your intestinal tract that help digest food

>> Assist in your body's absorption of calcium

>> May help lower cholesterol levels and regulate blood pressure, the special benefits of dietary fiber (see the section "Dietary Fiber: The Non-Nutrient in Carbohydrate Foods," later in this chapter)

Finding the Carbohydrates You Need

The most important sources of carbohydrates are plant foods — fruits, vegetables, and grains. Milk and milk products contain the carbohydrate lactose (milk sugar), but meat, fish, and poultry have no carbohydrates at all.

The National Academy of Sciences Institute of Medicine (IOM) recommends that 45 to 65 percent of your daily calories come from carbohydrate foods, such as grains (bread, cereals, pasta, and rice), fruit, and vegetables, foods that provide simple carbohydrates, complex carbohydrates, and the natural bonus of dietary fiber. Table sugar, honey, and sweets — which provide simple carbohydrates — are recommended only on a once-in-a-while basis.

TECHNICAL STUFF

One gram of carbohydrates has 4 calories. To find the number of calories from the carbohydrates in one food serving, multiply the number of grams of carbohydrates by 4. For example, one whole bagel has about 38 grams of carbohydrates, equal to about 152 calories (38×4). (You have to say "about" because the dietary fiber in the bagel provides no calories, because the body can't metabolize it.) Wait — that number doesn't account for all the calories in the serving. Remember, the foods listed here may also contain at least some protein and fat, and these two nutrients add calories.

Some people have problems with carbohydrates

Some people have a hard time handling carbohydrates. For example, people with Type 1 ("insulin dependent") diabetes don't produce sufficient amounts of insulin, the hormone needed to carry all the glucose produced from carbohydrates into body cells. As a result, the glucose continues to circulate in the blood until it's excreted through the kidneys. That's why one way to tell whether someone has diabetes is to test the level of sugar in that person's urine.

Other people can't digest carbohydrates because their bodies lack the specific enzymes needed to break the bonds that hold a carbohydrate's sugar units together. For example, many (some say most) Asians, Africans, Middle Easterners, South Americans, and Eastern, Central, or Southern Europeans are deficient in lactase, the enzyme that splits lactose (milk sugar) into glucose and galactose. If these people drink milk or eat milk products, they end up with a lot of undigested lactose in their intestinal tracts. This undigested lactose makes the bacteria living there happy as clams — but not the person who owns the intestines: As bacteria feast on the undigested sugar, they excrete waste products that give their host gas and cramps.

To avoid this anomaly, many national cuisines purposely avoid milk as an ingredient. (Quick! Name one native Asian dish that's made with milk. No, coconut milk doesn't count.) To get the calcium their bodies need, these people simply substitute high-calcium foods such as greens or calcium-enriched soy products for milk.

TIP

A second solution for people who don't make enough lactase is to use a *predigested milk product*, such as yogurt or buttermilk or sour cream, all of which are created by adding friendly bacteria that digest the milk (that is, break the lactose apart) without spoiling it. Other solutions include lactose-free cheeses and enzyme-treated milk.

Some people need extra carbohydrates

The small amount of glucose in your blood and cells provides the energy you need for your body's daily activities. The 400 grams of glycogen stored in your liver and muscles provides enough energy for ordinary bursts of extra activity.

But what happens when you have to work harder or longer than that? For example, what if you're a long-distance athlete, which means that you use up your available supply of glucose before you finish your competition? (That's why marathoners often run out of gas — a phenomenon called *hitting the wall* — at 20 miles, 6 miles short of the finish line.)

If you were stuck on an ice floe or lost in the woods for a month or so, after your body exhausts its supply of glucose, including the glucose stored in glycogen, it would start pulling energy first out of stored fat and then out of muscle. But extracting energy from body fat requires large amounts of oxygen — which is likely to be in short supply when your body has run, swum, or cycled 20 miles. So athletes have found another way to leap the wall: They load up on carbohydrates in advance.

Carbohydrate-loading is a dietary regimen designed to increase temporarily the amount of glycogen stored in your muscles in anticipation of an upcoming event. You start about a week before the event, says the University of Maine's Alfred A. Bushway, PhD, exercising to exhaustion so your body pulls as much glycogen as possible out of your muscles. Then, for three days, you eat foods high in fat and protein and low in carbohydrates to keep your glycogen level from rising again.

Three days before the big day, reverse the pattern. Now you want to build and conserve glycogen stores. What you need is a diet that's about 70 percent carbo-hydrates, providing 6 to 10 grams of carbohydrates for every kilogram (2.2 pounds) of body weight for men and women alike. And not just any carbohydrates, mind you. What you want are the complex carbohydrates in starchy foods like pasta and potatoes, rather than the simple ones more prominent in sugary foods like fruit. And of course, candy.

WARNING

This carb-loading diet isn't for everyday use, nor will it help people competing in events of short duration. It's strictly for events lasting longer than 90 minutes.

What about while you're running, swimming, or cycling? Will consuming simple sugars during the race give you extra short-term bursts of energy? Yes. Sugar is rapidly converted to glycogen and carried to the muscles. But you don't want plain table sugar (candy, honey) because it's *hydrophilic* (*hydro* = water; *philic* = loving), which means that it pulls water from body tissues into your intestinal tract. This can increase dehydration and trigger nausea. Getting the sugar you want from sweetened athletic drinks, which provide fluids along with the energy, is safer, especially since the athletic drink also contains salt (sodium chloride) to replace the salt that you lose when perspiring heavily. Turn to Chapter 13 to find out why this is important.

Dietary Fiber: The Non-Nutrient in Carbohydrate Foods

Dietary fiber is a group of complex carbohydrates that aren't a source of energy for human beings. Because human digestive enzymes can't break the bonds that hold fiber's sugar units together, fiber adds no calories to your diet and can't be converted to glucose.

Ruminants (animals, such as cows, that chew the cud) have a combination of digestive enzymes and digestive microbes that enable them to extract the nutrients from insoluble dietary fiber (cellulose and some hemicelluloses). But not even these creatures can pull nutrients out of lignin, an insoluble fiber in plant stems and leaves and the predominant fiber in wood. As a result, the U.S. Department of Agriculture specifically prohibits the use of wood or sawdust in animal feed.

But just because you can't digest dietary fiber doesn't mean it isn't a valuable part of your diet. The opposite is true. Dietary fiber is valuable *because* you can't digest it!

Defining the two kinds of dietary fiber

Nutritionists classify dietary fiber as either insoluble fiber or soluble fiber, depending on whether it dissolves in water.

>> **Insoluble dietary fiber** includes cellulose, some hemicelluloses, and lignin found in whole grains and other plants. This kind of dietary fiber is a natural laxative. It absorbs water, helps you feel full after eating, and stimulates your intestinal walls to contract and relax. These natural contractions, called *peristalsis*, move solid materials through your digestive tract.

   By moving food quickly through your intestines, insoluble fiber may help relieve or prevent digestive disorders such as constipation or diverticulitis (infection that occurs when food gets stuck in small pouches in the wall of the colon). Insoluble fiber also bulks up stool and makes it softer, reducing your risk of developing hemorrhoids and lessening the discomfort if you already have them.

>> **Soluble dietary fiber** includes pectins (found in most fruit), and beta-glucans (found in oats and barley), and gums such as guar, fenugreek and locust bean gums derived from seeds and used as thickeners in various prepared food

products. Soluble dietary fiber seems to lower the amount of cholesterol circulating in your blood (your *cholesterol level*), which is why a diet rich in fiber appears to lower cholesterol levels and thus offer some protection against heart disease.

TIP

Here's a benefit for dieters: Soluble fiber forms gels in the presence of water, which is what happens when apples and oat bran reach your digestive tract. So, like insoluble fiber, soluble fiber can make you feel full without adding calories.

TECHNICAL STUFF

Ordinary soluble dietary fiber can't be digested, so your body doesn't absorb it. But in 2002, researchers at Detroit's Barbara Ann Karamonos Cancer Institute fed laboratory mice a form of soluble dietary fiber called *modified citrus pectin*. The fiber, which is made from citrus fruit peel, can be digested. When fed to laboratory rats, it appeared to reduce the size of tumors caused by implanted human breast and colon cancer cells. The researchers believe that the fiber prevents cancer cells from linking together to form tumors. Today, modified citrus pectin is being sold as a dietary supplement, but the American Cancer Society notes on its website that this fiber's effects on human bodies (and human cancers) remain unproven.

Getting dietary fiber from food

You'll find absolutely no fiber in foods from animals: meat, fish, poultry, milk, milk products, and eggs. But you will find lots of dietary fiber in all plant foods — fruits, vegetables, and grains.

A balanced diet with plenty of foods from plants gives you both insoluble and soluble fiber. Most foods that contain fiber have both kinds, although the balance usually tilts toward one or the other. For example, the predominant fiber in an apple is pectin (a soluble fiber), but an apple peel also has some cellulose, hemi-cellulose, and lignin.

Table 8-1 shows you which foods are particularly good sources of specific kinds of fiber. A diet rich in plant foods (fruits, vegetables, and grains) gives you adequate amounts of dietary fiber.

Determining how much fiber you need

According to the U.S. Department of Agriculture, the average American woman gets about 12 grams of fiber a day from food; the average American man gets about 17 grams. Those figures are well below the Institute of Medicine (IOM) recommendations that I conveniently list here:

TABLE 8-1

Food Sources of Different Kinds of Fiber

Fiber	Where the Fiber's Found
Soluble fiber	
Pectin	Fruits (apples, strawberries, citrus fruits)
Beta-glucans	Oats, barley
Gums	Beans, cereals (oats, rice, barley), seeds, seaweed
Insoluble fiber	
Cellulose	Leaves (cabbage), roots (carrots, beets), bran, whole wheat, beans
Hemicellulose	Seed coverings (bran, whole grains)
Lignin	Plant stems, leaves, and skin

>> 25 grams a day for women age 19 to 50

>> 38 grams a day for men age 19 to 50

>> 21 grams a day for women older than 50

>> 30 grams a day for men older than 50

The amounts of dietary fiber recommended by IOM are believed to give you the benefits you want without causing fiber-related unpleasantries. Unpleasantries? Like what? And how will you know if you've got them? Trust me: If you eat more than enough fiber, your body will tell you right away. All that roughage may irritate your intestinal tract, which will issue an unmistakable protest in the form of intestinal gas or diarrhea. In extreme cases, if you don't drink enough liquids to moisten and soften the fiber you eat so it easily slides through your digestive tract, the dietary fiber may form a mass that can end up as an intestinal obstruction. (For more about water, see Chapter 12.)

TIP

If you decide to up the amount of fiber in your diet, follow this advice:

>> **Do it *very* gradually, a little bit more every day.** That way, you're less likely to experience intestinal distress. In other words, if your current diet is heavy on no-fiber foods such as meat, fish, poultry, eggs, milk, and cheese, and low-fiber foods such as white bread and white rice, don't load up on bran cereal (35 grams dietary fiber per 3.5-ounce serving) or dried figs (9.3 grams per serving) all at once. Start by adding a serving of cornflakes

(2.0 grams dietary fiber) at breakfast, maybe an apple (2.8 grams) at lunch, a pear (2.6 grams) at midafternoon, and a half cup of baked beans (7.7 grams) at dinner. Four simple additions, and already you're up to 15 grams dietary fiber.

>> **Always check the nutrition label whenever you shop.** (For more about the wonderfully informative guides, see Chapter 17.) When choosing between similar products, just take the one with the higher fiber content per serving. For example, white pita bread generally has about 1.6 grams dietary fiber per serving. Whole wheat pita bread may have as much as 7.4 grams.

Here's a carb word to the wise: Check the serving size. What may look like a serving with tons of fiber could just be a large serving.

>> **Get enough liquids.** Dietary fiber is like a sponge. It sops up liquid, so increasing your fiber intake may deprive your cells of the water they need to perform their daily work. (For more about how your body uses the water you drink, see Chapter 12.) That's why the American Academy of Family Physicians (among others) suggests checking to make sure you get plenty of fluids when you consume more fiber. How much is enough? Back to Chapter 12.

Table 8-2 shows the amounts of all types of dietary fiber — insoluble plus soluble — in a 100-gram (3.5-ounce) serving of specific foods. By the way, nutritionists like to measure things in terms of 100-gram portions because that makes comparing foods at a glance possible.

To find the amount of dietary fiber in your own serving, divide the gram total for the food shown in Table 8-2 by 3.5 to get the grams per ounce, and then multiply the result by the number of ounces in your portion. For example, if you're having 1 ounce of cereal, the customary serving of ready-to-eat breakfast cereals, divide the gram total of dietary fiber by 3.5; then multiply by 1. If your slice of bread weighs 1/2 ounce, divide the gram total by 3.5; then multiply the result by 0.5 (1/2).

FIBER FACTOID

The amount of fiber in a serving of food may depend on whether the food is raw or cooked. For example, as you can see from Table 8-2, a 3.5-ounce serving of plain dried prunes has 7.2 grams of fiber while a 3.5-ounce serving of stewed prunes has 6.6 grams of fiber.

Why? When you stew prunes, they plump up, which means they absorb water. The water adds weight but (obviously) no fiber. So a serving of prunes-plus-water has slightly less fiber per ounce than a same-weight serving of plain dried prunes.

TABLE 8-2

Dietary Fiber Content in Common Foods

Food	Grams of Fiber in a 100-Gram (3.5-Ounce) Serving
Bread	
Bagel	2.1
Bran bread	8.5
Pita bread (white)	1.6
Pita bread (whole wheat)	7.4
White bread	1.9
Cereals	
Bran cereal	35.3
Bran flakes	18.8
Cornflakes	2.0
Oatmeal	10.6
Wheat flakes	9.0
Grains	
Barley, pearled (minus its outer covering), raw	15.6
Cornmeal, whole grain	11.0
Degermed	5.2
Oat bran, raw	6.6
Rice, raw (brown)	3.5
Rice, raw (white)	1.0–2.8
Rice, raw (wild)	5.2
Wheat bran	15.0
Fruits	
Apple, with skin	2.8
Apricots, dried	7.8
Figs, dried	9.3
Kiwi fruit	3.4
Pear, raw	2.6

(continued)

TABLE 8-2 *(continued)*

Food	Grams of Fiber in a 100-Gram (3.5-Ounce) Serving
Prunes, dried	7.2
Prunes, stewed	6.6
Raisins	5.3
Vegetables	
Baked beans (vegetarian)	7.7
Chickpeas (canned)	5.4
Lima beans, cooked	7.2
Broccoli, raw	2.8
Brussels sprouts, cooked	2.6
Cabbage, white, raw	2.4
Cauliflower, raw	2.4
Corn, sweet, cooked	3.7
Peas with edible pods, raw	2.6
Potatoes, white, baked, with skin	5.5
Sweet potato, cooked	3.0
Tomatoes, raw	1.3
Nuts	
Almonds, oil-roasted	11.2
Coconut, raw	9.0
Hazelnuts, oil-roasted	6.4
Peanuts, dry-roasted	8.0
Pistachios	10.8
Other	
Corn chips, toasted	4.4
Tahini (sesame seed paste)	9.3
Tofu	1.2

Provisional Table on the Dietary Fiber Content of Selected Foods (Washington, D.C.: U.S. Department of Agriculture, 1988)

Or you can just look at the nutrition label on the side of the package because it lists the amounts of the nutrients per serving.

Finally, the amounts in Table 8-2 are averages. Different brands of processed products (breads, some cereals, cooked fruits, and vegetables) may have more (or less) fiber per serving.

FIBER AND YOUR HEART: THE CONTINUING SAGA OF OAT BRAN

Oat bran is the second chapter in the fiber fad that started with wheat bran around 1980. Wheat bran, the fiber in wheat, is rich in the insoluble fibers cellulose and lignin. Oat bran's gee-whiz factor is the soluble fiber beta-glucans. For more than 30 years, scientists have known that eating foods high in soluble fiber can lower your cholesterol, although nobody knows exactly why. Fruits and vegetables (especially dried beans) are high in soluble fiber, but ounce for ounce, oats have more. In addition, beta-glucans are a more effective cholesterol-buster than pectin and gum, which are the soluble fibers in most fruits and vegetables.

By 1990, researchers at the University of Kentucky reported that people who add ½ cup dry oat bran (*not* oatmeal) to their regular daily diets can lower their levels of low-density lipoproteins (LDLs), the particles that carry cholesterol into your arteries, by as much as 25 percent (see Chapter 7 for more on cholesterol).

Recently, scientists at the Medical School of Northwestern University, funded by Quaker Oats, enlisted 208 healthy volunteers whose normal cholesterol readings averaged about 200 milligrams per deciliter for a study involving oat bran. The volunteers' total cholesterol levels decreased an average of 9.3 percent with a low-fat, low-cholesterol diet supplemented by 2 ounces of oats or oat bran every day. About one-third of the cholesterol reduction was credited to the oats.

Oat cereal makers rounded the total loss to 10 percent, and the National Research Council said that a 10 percent drop in cholesterol could produce a 20 percent drop in the risk of a heart attack.

Do I have to tell you what happened next? Books on oat bran hit the bestseller list. Cheerios elbowed Frosted Flakes aside to become the number-one cereal in America. And people added oat bran to everything from bagels to orange juice.

(continued)

(continued)

Today scientists know that although a little oat bran can't hurt, the link between oats and cholesterol levels is no cure-all.

As a general rule, a cholesterol level higher than 240 milligrams per deciliter is considered to be *high.* A cholesterol reading between 200 and 239 milligrams per deciliter is considered *borderline high.* A cholesterol level below 200 milligrams per deciliter is considered *desirable.*

If your cholesterol level is above 240 milligrams per deciliter, lowering it by 10 percent through a diet that contains oat bran may reduce your risk of heart attack without the use of medication. If your cholesterol level is lower than that to begin with, the effects of oat bran are less dramatic. For example:

- If your cholesterol level is below 240 milligrams per deciliter, a low-fat, low-cholesterol diet alone may push it down 24 points into the moderately risky range, but doesn't take you into "safe" territory, under 200 milligrams per deciliter.

- If your cholesterol is already low, say 199 milligrams per deciliter or less, a low-fat, low-cholesterol diet plus oats may drop it to 180 milligrams per deciliter, but the oats account for only a third of your loss.

Recognizing oat bran's benefits, the Food and Drug Administration now permits health claims on oat product labels. For example, the product label may say: "Soluble fiber from foods such as oat bran, as part of a diet low in saturated fat and cholesterol, may reduce the risk of heart disease." And to prove the staying power of this story, consider this: As recently as 2015, continuing studies continue to point to the benefits of oats.

Note: The soluble pectin in apples and the soluble beta-glucans (gums) in beans and peas also lower cholesterol levels. The insoluble fiber in wheat bran does not.

Chapter **9**

Alcohol: Another Form of Grape and Grain

A lcohol beverages are among mankind's oldest home remedies and simple pleasures, so highly regarded that the ancient Greeks and Romans called wine a "gift from the gods," and when the Gaels — early inhabitants of Scotland and Ireland — first produced whiskey, they named it *uisge beatha* (whis-key-ba), a combination of the words for "water" and "life." Today, although you may share their appreciation for the product, you know that alcohol may have risks as well as benefits.

When microorganisms (yeasts) digest (ferment) the sugars in carbohydrate foods, they make two byproducts: a liquid and a gas. The gas is carbon dioxide. The liquid is *ethyl alcohol*, also known as *ethanol*, the intoxicating ingredient in alcohol beverages.

This biochemical process is not an esoteric one. In fact, it happens in your own kitchen every time you make yeast bread. Remember the faint, beerlike odor in the air while the dough is rising? That odor is from the alcohol the yeasts make as they chomp their way through the sugars in the flour. (Don't worry; the alcohol evaporates when you bake the bread.) As the yeasts digest the sugars, they also produce carbon dioxide, which makes the bread rise.

In this chapter, I explain how alcohol beverages are made, discuss what ABV means, show you what happens to your body when you drink alcohol, and discuss the health benefits and risks of imbibing.

Creating Alcohol Beverages

Alcohol beverages are produced either through fermentation or through a combination of fermentation plus distillation. Beer, wine, and spirits professionals call these products "alcohol beverages" not "alcoholic beverages." The first is accurately descriptive; the second is colorful but conjures up the image of tipsy bottles dancing on a shelf rather than respected members of the food and drink family.

Fermented alcohol products

Fermentation is a simple process in which yeasts or bacteria are added to carbohydrate "starter" foods such as corn, potatoes, rice, or wheat. The microorganisms digest the sugars in the food, leaving liquid (alcohol); the liquid is filtered to remove the solids, and water is usually added to dilute the alcohol, producing — voilà — an alcohol beverage.

TECHNICAL
STUFF

Beer is made this way. So is wine. *Kumiss,* a fermented milk product, is slightly different because it's made by adding yeasts and friendly bacteria called *lactobacilli* (*lacto* = milk) to mare's milk. The microorganisms make alcohol, but it remains in the milk, creating a fizzy, fermented beverage.

Distilled alcohol products

The second way to make an alcohol beverage is through *distillation.*

As with fermentation, yeasts are added to starter foods to make alcohol from the sugars. But yeasts can't thrive when the concentration of alcohol is higher than 20 percent, as occurs in most distilled products. To concentrate the alcohol and separate it from the rest of the ingredients in the fermented liquid, distillers pour the fermented liquid into a *still,* a large vat with a wide column-like tube on top. The still is heated so that the alcohol, which boils at a lower temperature than everything else in the vat, turns to vapor, which rises through the column on top of the still, to be collected in containers where it condenses back into a liquid.

The condensed liquid, called *neutral spirits,* is the base for the alcohol beverages called spirits or distilled spirits: gin, rum, tequila, whiskey, and vodka. Brandy is a special product, a spirit distilled from wine. Fortified wines, such as Port and Sherry, are wines with brandy added.

The foods used to make beverage alcohol

Beverage alcohol can be made from virtually any carbohydrate food, most commonly cereal grains, fruit, honey, molasses, or potatoes. Table 9-1 shows which foods are used to produce the different kinds of alcohol beverages.

TABLE 9-1

Foods Used to Make Alcohol Beverages

Original Food	Alcohol Beverage Produced
Fruit and fruit juice	
Agave plant	Tequila
Apples	Hard cider
Grapes and other fruits	Wine
Grain	
Barley	Beer, various distilled spirits, kvass
Corn	Bourbon, corn whiskey, beer
Rice	Sake (a distilled product), rice wine
Rye	Whiskey
Wheat	Distilled spirits, beer
Others	
Honey	Mead
Milk	Kumiss (koumiss), kefir
Potatoes	Vodka
Sugar cane	Rum

On its own, alcohol provides energy (7 calories per gram) but no nutrients, so distilled spirits, such as whiskey or plain unflavored vodka, serve up nothing but calories. Beer, wine, cider, and other fermented beverages contain some of the food from which they're made, so they may deliver (very) small amounts of proteins, carbohydrates, vitamins, and minerals.

Checking How Much Alcohol Is in That Bottle

No alcohol beverage is 100 percent alcohol. It's alcohol plus water, and — if it's a wine or beer — some residue of the foods from which it was made.

The label term ABV or Alc/Vol (alcohol by volume) shows the amount of alcohol as a percentage of all the liquid in the container. For example, if your bottle or can holds 10 ounces of liquid and 1 ounce of that is alcohol, the product is 10 percent ABV — the alcohol content divided by the total amount of liquid multiplied by 100. Like this:

$1 / 10 = 0.1 \times 100 = 10$ percent

Proof — an older term to describe alcohol content —is two times the ABV. For example, an alcohol beverage that is 10 percent alcohol by volume is 20 proof.

Right now, alcohol beverages, which are regulated by the Alcohol and Tobacco Trade and Tax Bureau (ATT) rather than the Food and Drug Administration (FDA), are the only food and drink products not required by law to carry a Nutrition Facts Label. However, in 2013, ATT announced that beer, wine, and spirits companies may voluntarily list serving size and nutrients per serving on their bottles.

Budweiser was quick to adopt a consumer-friendly label, followed by other domestic and some international brewers (as of 2020, Stella Artois and Michelob are two notable holdouts). Among distillers, in 2015, Diageo, the world's largest producer of alcohol beverages, announced that it would put complete Nutrition Facts Labels on every one of its products, relatively quickly followed by other major companies such as Bacardi and Jack Daniels.

Following Alcohol through Your Body

Other foods must be digested before being absorbed by your cells, but alcohol flows directly through your stomach and gastrointestinal tract into your blood-stream, which carries it to body tissues and organs. Here's a road map to show you the route traveled by the alcohol in every drink you take:

>> **Starting at the mouth:** Alcohol is an *astringent;* it coagulates proteins on the surface of the lining of your mouth to make it "pucker." Some alcohol is absorbed through the lining of the mouth and throat, but most spills into

your stomach, where an enzyme called *gastric alcohol dehydrogenase* (gADH) begins to metabolize (digest) it.

How much of this enzyme and a similar one produced by your liver (next paragraph) your body churns out is influenced by your ethnicity and your gender. For example, Asians, Native Americans, and Inuits appear to secrete less than do most Caucasians, and the average woman (regardless of her ethnicity), less than the average man. As a result, more unmetabolized alcohol flows from her stomach into her bloodstream, which is why the average woman is likely to feel the effects of alcohol more quickly than the average man does. For both men and women, a certain amount of unmetabolized alcohol flows through the stomach walls into the bloodstream and on to the small intestine.

>> **Stopping at the liver:** Most of the alcohol you drink is absorbed through the *duodenum* (the first part of the small intestine), from which it flows through a large blood vessel (the portal vein) into the liver. There, ADH, an enzyme similar to gADH, metabolizes the alcohol, which is then converted to energy by a coenzyme called *nicotinamide adenine dinucleotide* (NAD). NAD is also used to convert the glucose derived from other carbohydrates (see Chapter 8) to energy, so while NAD is being used for alcohol, glucose conversion grinds to a halt.

   The normal, healthy liver can process about ½ ounce of pure alcohol (that's 6 to 12 ounces of beer, 5 ounces of wine, or 1 ounce of spirits) in an hour. The rest flows on to your heart.

>> **Breathing in and out:** Entering the heart, alcohol reduces the force with which the heart muscle contracts. You pump out slightly less blood for a few minutes, blood vessels all over your body relax, and your blood pressure goes down temporarily. The contractions soon return to normal, but the blood vessels may remain relaxed and blood pressure lower for as long as half an hour.

   At the same time, alcohol flows in blood from the heart through the pulmonary vein to the lungs. Now you breathe out a tiny bit of alcohol every time you exhale, and your breath smells of liquor. Then the newly oxygenated, still alcohol-laden blood flows back through the pulmonary artery to your heart, and up and out through the *aorta* (the major artery that carries blood out to your body).

   As it circulates in the blood, alcohol raises the level of "good" cholesterol, the high-density lipoprotein (HDLs) that reduce your risk of heart disease, although not necessarily the specific ones that carry cholesterol out of your body. (For more about lipoproteins, see Chapter 7.) Alcohol also makes blood less likely to clot, temporarily reducing the risk of heart attack and stroke.

>> **Rising to the surface:** Alcohol makes blood vessels expand, so more warm blood flows up from the center of your body to the surface of the skin. You feel warmer for a while and, if your skin is fair, you may flush and turn pink. (Asians, who tend to make less alcohol dehydrogenase than do Caucasians, often experience a characteristic flushing when they drink even small amounts of alcohol.) At the same time, tiny amounts of alcohol ooze out through your pores, and your perspiration smells of alcohol.

>> **Hitting curves in the road:** Alcohol is a depressant. When it reaches your brain, it slows the transmission of impulses between nerve cells that control your ability to think and move.

TECHNICAL STUFF

Do you feel a sudden urge to urinate? That's because alcohol reduces your brain's production of *antidiuretic hormones,* chemicals that keep you from making too much urine. You may lose lots of liquid, plus vitamins and minerals. You also grow very thirsty, and your urine may smell faintly of alcohol.

>> **Ending the process:** This cycle continues as long as you have alcohol circulating in your blood, or in other words, until your liver can manage to produce enough ADH to metabolize all the alcohol you've consumed. How long is that? Most people need an hour to metabolize the amount of alcohol (½ ounce) in one drink within an hour, but that's an average. Some people may have alcohol circulating in their blood for up to three hours after only one drink. What's one drink? See the next section.

Understanding How Alcohol Affects Your Health

Beverage alcohol offers both benefits and risks. The benefits are strongly linked to what is commonly called *moderate drinking* — no more than one drink a day for a woman, two drinks a day for a man.

TIP

What's one drink? Easy: 5 ounces of wine, 12 ounces of beer, 1.5 ounces of hard liquor such as whiskey, vodka, tequila, or gin.

Moderate amounts of alcohol not only reduce stress but also have beneficial effects on various parts of the human body. For example, as noted by the Mayo Clinic, moderate drinking may

>> Reduce your risk of developing and/or dying from *coronary artery disease (CAD),* the form of heart disease due to narrowed or blocked blood vessels

A LOT AND A LITTLE VERSUS THE MIDDLE

When scientists talk about the relationship between alcohol and heart disease, the words *J-curve* often pop up. What's a J-curve? A statistical graph in the shape of the letter J.

In terms of heart disease, the lower peak on the left of the J shows the risk among teeto-talers, the high spike on the right shows the risk among those who drink too much, and the curve in the center shows the risk in the moderate middle. In other words, the J-curve says that people who drink moderately have a lower risk of heart disease than people who drink too much or not at all.

>> Reduce your risk of *ischemic stroke* — that is, stroke due to narrowed or blocked blood vessels in your brain

>> Reduce your risk of developing diabetes

That's the good news. Here's the bad news: Although the evidence isn't conclusive, some studies that applaud the effects of moderate drinking on heart health are less reassuring about the relationship between alcohol and cancer. For example, the Department of Health and Human Services' National Toxicology Program labels alcohol beverages a human carcinogen. The National Cancer Institute says that people who smoke and drink are at higher risk for cancers of the mouth, throat (esophagus, pharynx, larynx), and liver. And American Cancer Society (ACS) statistics suggest a 20 percent higher risk of breast cancer among women who have more than three drinks a week compared with women who do not drink at all.

The physical effects of excessive drinking

Alcohol abuse is a term generally taken to mean drinking so much that it interferes with your ability to have a normal, productive life. *Excessive drinking,* including binge drinking (see the sidebar "Binge drinking: A behavioral no-no," later in this chapter), can also make you feel terrible the next day. *The morning after* is not fic-tion. A hangover is a miserable physical fact:

>> You're thirsty because you lost excess water through copious urination.

>> Your stomach hurts and you're queasy because even small amounts of alcohol irritate your stomach lining, causing it to secrete extra acid and lots of *histamine,* the same immune system chemical that makes the skin around a mosquito bite red and itchy.

>> Your muscles ache and your head pounds because processing alcohol through your liver requires an enzyme — nicotinamide adenine dinucleotide (NAD) — normally used to convert *lactic acid,* a byproduct of muscle activity, to other chemicals that can be used for energy. The extra, unprocessed lactic acid piles up painfully in your muscles.

Alcoholism: An addiction disease

No one knows exactly why some people are able to have a drink once a day or once a month or once a year, enjoy it, and move on, while others become addicted to alcohol. In the past, alcoholism has been blamed on "bad genes," lack of will-power, or even a nasty childhood.

As science continues to unravel the mysteries of body chemistry, it's reasonable to expect that researchers will eventually come up with a rational scientific explanation for the differences between social drinkers and people who can't safely use alcohol. It just hasn't happened yet.

What is clear, however, is that *alcoholics* are people who find it difficult to control their drinking. This situation, if left untreated, may lead to life-threatening situations, such as acute alcohol poisoning that paralyzes body organs, including the heart and lungs, liver damage (cirrhosis), or malnutrition.

Alcoholics are often emaciated, with such visible symptoms of malnutrition as problem skin, broken nails, and dull hair. Less visible symptoms of vitamin and mineral deficiencies may hide underneath the surface because

>> Alcohol depresses appetite.

>> An alcoholic may substitute alcohol for food, getting calories but no nutrients.

>> Even if the alcoholic eats a balanced, nutritious diet, the alcohol in his tissues can prevent the proper absorption of vitamins (notably the B vitamins), minerals, and other nutrients.

>> Alcohol may also reduce the alcoholic's ability to synthesize proteins.

This set of problems can't be resolved simply by downing a multivitamin with the alcohol; it requires medical attention to understand and treat the primary cause — drinking too much, much too often.

BINGE DRINKING: A BEHAVIORAL NO-NO

The Federal Centers for Disease Control and Prevention (CDC) calls binge drinking, which they describe as four or more drinks in one hour (extreme binge drinking is 10 drinks per hour), as "the most common, costly, and deadly pattern of excessive alcohol use in the United States." Binge drinkers, sometimes labeled as "once-in-a-while alcoholics," don't drink every day, but when they do indulge, they go so far overboard that they sometimes fail to come back up. After downing so much beer, wine, or spirits, the amount of alcohol in their blood rises to lethal levels that, in the worst case, may lead to death by alcohol poisoning.

Binging on alcohol is most common among younger adults, age 18 to 34, often on college campuses. Efforts to stamp out binge drinking may rely on guilt or shame to change behavior, but a 2008 study at the Kellogg School of Management at Northwestern University found that binge drinkers are already uncomfortable with their behavior. Attempting to make them more so doesn't work. Instead, the researchers suggested couching anti-binge messages in simple, intelligent language focusing on how to avoid situations that lead to binge drinking rather than the nasty effects of the overindulgence.

As in other areas of modern life, money matters here, at least to grown-ups. In 2015, scientists at Boston University's School of Public Health published a report in the journal *Addiction,* showing that a simple 1 percent increase in the tax on alcohol beverages lowered the proportion of adult binge drinkers by 1.4 percent. Its other economic impact is on the country's economy. In 2010, for example, the CDC estimated that binge drinking cost the United States $249 billion.

There seemed to be one small bright spot in this picture. In 2014, the Monitoring the Future study, funded by the National Institute on Drug Abuse, found that the rate of self-reported college-age extreme binge drinking had fallen from 44 percent in 1980 to 35 percent in 2014. But barely six years later, in the summer of 2020, the CDC reported that 29 percent of American high school students were drinking alcohol beverages, with nearly two-thirds reporting binge drinking, girls more frequently than boys.

Who shouldn't drink

WARNING

No one should drink to excess. But some people shouldn't drink at all, not even in moderation. They include

>> **People who plan to drive or do work that requires both attention and skill:** Alcohol slows reaction time and makes your motor skills — operating a sewing machine or turning the wheel of a car — less precise, which make you

more likely to end up with a needle through the hand or a head through the windshield.

» **Women who are pregnant or who plan to become pregnant in the near future:** *Fetal alcohol syndrome* (FAS) is a collection of birth defects including low birth weight, heart defects, cognitive delays, and facial deformities documented only in babies born to female alcoholics.

No evidence links FAS to casual drinking — that is, one or two drinks during a pregnancy, or even one or two drinks a week. In fact, for years before FAS was identified and diagnosed, pregnant women were routinely advised to drink beer as a source of nutritious calories.

However, it's not clear yet whether there's any completely safe level of alcohol during pregnancy. In 2005, the U.S. Surgeon General urged women who are pregnant or may become pregnant to abstain from alcohol. This advice remains in effect not only in the United States but also in other countries, including Australia, Canada, France, and New Zealand.

» **People who take certain prescription drugs or over-the-counter medication:** Alcohol makes some drugs stronger, increases some drugs' side effects, and renders other drugs less effective. At the same time, some drugs make alcohol a more powerful sedative or slow down the elimination of alcohol from your body.

Table 9-2 shows some of the interactions known to occur between alcohol and some common prescription and over-the-counter drugs. This short list gives you an idea of some of the general interactions likely to occur between alcohol and drugs. But the list is far from complete. Today, by law, drugs that interact with alcohol usually carry a warning on the label, but if you're taking any kind of medication — over-the-counter or prescription — and you're not sure of the possibility of interactions, check with your doctor or pharmacist.

Alcohol and age

As you grow older, changes in the body's ability to metabolize food may lower your tolerance for alcohol, increasing the risk of problems associated with excessive drinking.

On the other hand, moderate drinking remains a pleasant experience for people healthy enough to indulge. Like everyone else, senior citizens are likely to find a moderate amount of alcohol relaxing and — believe it or not — beneficial for the aging brain. For more on that subject, check out Chapter 24.

TABLE 9-2

Drug and Alcohol Interactions

Drug	Possible Interaction with Alcohol
Acetaminophen	Increased liver toxicity
Aspirin and other nonsteroidal inflammatory drugs (NSAIDs)	Increased stomach bleeding; irritation
Anti-arthritis drugs	Increased stomach bleeding; irritation
Antidepressants	Increased drowsiness/intoxication; high blood pressure
Antihypertension drugs	Very low blood pressure
Diabetes medications	Very low blood sugar
Diet pills	Excessive nervousness
Diuretics	Low blood pressure
Isoniazid (anti-tuberculosis drug)	Decreased drug effectiveness; higher risk of hepatitis
Sleeping pills	Increased sedation
Tranquilizers	Increased sedation

Advice from the Sages: Moderation

Good advice is always current.

Who could improve on this from the Romans — actually, one Roman writer named Terence (Publius Terentius Afer): "Moderation in all things."

Or this, from the authors of Ecclesiastes (31:27): "Wine is as good as life to a man, if it be drunk moderately: what life is then to a man that is without wine? for it was made to make men glad."

Intelligent. Sensible. Enjoy.

Chapter **10**

Validating Vitamins

Vitamins are *organic chemicals*, substances that contain carbon, hydrogen, and oxygen — elements essential for life. As a result, organic chemicals, including some vitamins, occur naturally in all living things: flowers, trees, birds, bees, chickens, fish, cows, and you. The virtue of vitamins is that they regulate a variety of bodily functions, such as the extraction of nutrients from food, and help build tissues and organs, such as bones and teeth, skin and nerves, and blood. Finally, they prevent certain deficiency diseases and generally promote good health.

This chapter explains how vitamins work, where you find them, and exactly how much you need each day.

Understanding What Vitamins Your Body Needs

For optimum health, your body requires at least 11 vitamins: vitamin A, vitamin D, vitamin E, vitamin K, vitamin C, and the members of the B vitamin family — thiamin (vitamin B1), riboflavin (B2), niacin, vitamin B6, folate, and vitamin B12. Two more B vitamins (biotin and pantothenic acid) and two unusual compounds, choline (a compound similar to the B vitamins) and carnitine (a name for three compounds that help convert fatty acids to energy), are also valuable.

Although your body needs these 11 vitamins, it's amazing how little of each vitamin you need. In some cases, the Recommended Dietary Allowances (RDAs) may be as small as several micrograms — 1/1,000,000, or one-one-millionth of a gram.

Modern nutrition classifies vitamins as either *fat soluble* or *water soluble*, meaning that they dissolve either in fat or in water. If you consume larger amounts of fat-soluble vitamins than your body needs, the excess is stored in body fat. With water-soluble vitamins, your body simply shrugs its shoulders, so to speak, and urinates away most of the excess.

THE FATHER OF ALL VITAMINS: CASIMIR FUNK

Vitamins are so much a part of modern life that you may have a hard time believing they were first conclusively identified and defined less than a century ago. Of course, people have long known that certain foods contain *something* special. For example, nearly 4,000 years ago, the Egyptian King Amenophis IV consumed liver to help him see clearly when the light was poor; 2,000 years later, the Greek physician Hippocrates prescribed raw liver soaked in honey for *nyctalopia* ("night blindness").

By the end of the 18th century (1795), British Navy ships carried a mandatory supply of limes or lime juice to prevent scurvy among the men on long journeys, thus earning the Brits once and forever the nickname "limeys." The Japanese, whose sailors had similar problems with beriberi (from *biribiri*, the word for *weak* in Sinhala, a language spoken in Sri Lanka), protected their men by adding whole grain barley to the normal ship's rations.

Everyone knew these remedies worked, but no one knew why until the turn of the 20th century when Casimir Funk, a Polish biochemist working first in England and then in the United States, identified "somethings" in food that he called *vitamines* (*vita* = life; *amines* = nitrogen compounds).

The following year, Funk and a fellow biochemist, Briton Frederick Hopkins, suggested that some medical conditions, such as scurvy and beriberi, were simply deficiency diseases caused by the absence of a specific nutrient in the body. Adding a food with the missing nutrient to one's diet would prevent or cure the deficiency disease. What else is there to say except *Eureka!* (which, because Funk was Polish but working in England, is probably exactly what he said).

Each entry on the following list of vitamins names a food serving that provides at least one-quarter of the adult RDA for the particular vitamin. For a complete list of RDAs, check out Chapter 3.

Fat-soluble vitamins

Vitamins A, D, E, and K have two characteristics in common: All dissolve in fat, and all are stored in your fatty tissues. But like members of any family, they also have distinct personalities. One keeps your skin moist. Another protects your bones. A third keeps reproductive organs purring happily. And the fourth enables you to make special proteins. And, yes, as noted late in this chapter, each vitamin may have more than one benefit to offer.

TIP

Medical students often use mnemonic (pronounced neh-*mah*-nic) devices — memory joggers — to remember complicated lists of body parts and symptoms of diseases. Here's one to help you remember which vitamins are fat soluble: "All Dogs Eat Kidneys," which stands for vitamins A, D, E, and K, of course.

Vitamin A

Vitamin A is the moisturizing nutrient that keeps your skin and *mucous membranes* (the slick tissue lining of the nose, mouth, throat, vagina, urethra, and rectum) smooth and supple. Vitamin A is also the vision vitamin, a constituent of 11-*cis-retinol*, a protein in the *rods* (cells in the back of your eye that enable you to see even when the lights are low) that prevents or slows the development of age-related *macular degeneration*, or progressive damage to the retina of the eye, which can cause the loss of central vision (the ability to see clearly enough to read or do fine work). Finally, vitamin A promotes the growth of healthy bones and teeth, keeps your reproductive system humming, and encourages your immune system to churn out the cells you need to fight off infection.

Your body gets its vitamin A from two classes of chemicals:

» *Retinoids* are compounds whose names all start with *ret*: retinol, retinaldehyde, retinoic acid, and so on. These fat-soluble substances are found in several foods of animal origin: liver (again!) and whole milk, eggs, and butter. Retinoids give you *preformed* vitamin A, the kind of nutrient your body can use right away.

» *Carotenoids* are *vitamin A precursors,* chemicals such as beta carotene — a deep yellow carotenoid (pigment) found in dark green, bright yellow, and orange fruits and vegetables. Your body transforms a vitamin A precursor into a retinol-like substance. So far, scientists have identified at least 500 different carotenoids. Only 1 in 10 — about 50 altogether — are considered to be sources of vitamin A.

OVERDOSE BY ACCIDENT

As the great lexicographer and essayist Samuel Johnson, or English naturalist John Ray, Saint Bernard of Clairvaux, or Publius Vergilius Maro, better known as the Roman poet Virgil, or maybe even the author of Ecclesiastes 21:10 (King Solomon?) once wrote: "The road to hell is paved with good intentions."

Although no one's really sure who said it first, clearly everyone knows they were talking about life choices. But they may as well have been talking about vitamin A.

More than enough vitamin A can be much too much. This fat-soluble vitamin dissolves in body fat, and overdoses linger in your liver, possibly triggering vision problems, bone pain, skin problems. And if the overdose is large enough and lasts long enough, you risk liver damage and increased pressure on your brain.

This is why the RDAs for vitamin A were dramatically lowered several years ago.

Fortification is still the rule in the United States, but both the German Federal Institute for Risk Assessment and the Dutch National Institute for Public Health have proposed there be no vitamin A fortification of foods at all. This remains an open question, but the mantra "more than enough is too much" is a pretty good guide.

One-half cup dried apricots or ¼ cup cooked carrots provides 25 percent of the adult RDA for vitamin A.

Vitamin D

Calcium is essential for hardening teeth and bones, but no matter how much calcium you consume, without vitamin D, your body can't absorb and use the mineral. Researchers at the Bone Metabolism Laboratory at the Jean Mayer USDA Human Nutrition Research Center on Aging at Tufts University in Boston say vitamin D may also reduce the risk of tooth loss. The mechanism? Preventing the inflammatory response that leads to periodontal disease, a condition that destroys the thin tissue (ligaments) that connects the teeth to the surrounding jawbone, a claim supported in 2018 by researchers at the Department of Dental and Oral Pathology of the Lithuanian University of Health Sciences Medical Academy. Early studies suggested that vitamin D may also offer protection against some forms of cancer, but as of 2020 these suggestions remain to be proven.

Vitamin D occurs in three forms:

» *Calciferol* is found naturally in fish oils and egg yolks. In the United States, it's added to margarines and milk.

» *Cholecalciferol* is created when sunlight hits your skin and ultraviolet rays react with steroid chemicals in body fat just underneath triggering two, yes two, conversions of the compound in order to make it available for your use. And there's this catch: To make this form of vitamin D, you need to be exposed to direct sunlight. Sitting warm and comfy in front of a glass window with sunlight streaming through won't do the trick.

» *Ergocalciferol* is synthesized in plants exposed to sunlight. Cholecalciferol and ergocalciferol justify vitamin D's nickname: the Sunshine Vitamin.

The RDA for vitamin D is measured either in International Units (IUs) or micrograms (mcg) of cholecalciferol: 10 mcg cholecalciferol = 400 IU vitamin D.

One 8-ounce cup of fortified whole milk provides 100 IU, 25 percent of the RDA; one cup of skim milk with added non-fat milk solids has 120 IU.

Vitamin E

Vitamin E, which maintains your healthy reproductive system, nerves, and muscles, is found in *tocopherols* and *tocotrienols,* two families of naturally occurring organic chemicals in vegetable oils, nuts, whole grains, and green leafy vegetables. Out of the eight naturally occurring chemical forms of vitamin E, Alpha-tocopherol is the only form that is recognized to meet human requirements.

Tocopherols, the more important source, are anticoagulants and antioxidants that reduce the blood's ability to clot. As a result, for a while, many people believed that vitamin E was the nutrient specifically designed to ward off blood clot–related heart attacks. But in 2005, data from the Heart Outcomes Prevention Evaluation (HOPE), a study with more than 9,000 at-risk subjects, showed no such vitamin E benefits. And to add insult to injury, patients taking 400 International Units (IU) of vitamin E per day were *more* likely to develop heart failure.

On the other hand, in 2013, researchers at the Minneapolis VA Health Care System reported that over a period of two to three years, Alzheimer's patients who got vitamin E experienced a slower loss of the ability to perform simple tasks, such as shopping for food and cooking dinner, than did patients taking memantime (Nemanta), a drug known to preserve nerve function for people with Alzheimer's, or a placebo. As of 2019, the claim of cause and effect is considered scientifically unreliable. (See Chapter 24 for more information on food and your brain.)

One cup of cooked greens, such as mustard greens or kale, provides about 25 percent of the adult RDA for vitamin E.

Vitamin K

Vitamin K is a group of chemicals that your body uses to make specialized proteins found in blood *plasma* (the clear fluid in blood). One such protein is prothrombin, the protein chiefly responsible for blood clotting. Like vitamin D, vitamin K is essential for healthy bones, activating at least three different proteins that take part in forming new bone cells. In 2003, a report from the long-running Framingham (Massachusetts) Heart Study showed adults consuming the least vitamin K each day are likely to have the highest incidence of broken bones, although there is no evidence that this vitamin promotes or maintains bone density.

Vitamin K is found in dark green leafy vegetables (broccoli, cabbage, kale, lettuce, spinach, and turnip greens), cheese, liver, cereals, and fruits.

There is no RDA established for vitamin K because most of what you need is produced by naturally resident colonies of friendly bacteria in your intestines (the *microbiome* described in Chapter 2).

Water-soluble vitamins

The good news about water-soluble vitamins is that it's virtually impossible to overdose on them without taking enormous amounts of supplements. The bad news is that you have to take enough of these vitamins on a more or less regular schedule to protect yourself against deficiencies. But the more good news is that you don't have to take them every day; you can take less one day and more the next, and it evens out over time.

Vitamin C

Vitamin C, also known by its chemical name *ascorbic acid*, is essential for the development and maintenance of connective tissue (the fat, muscle, and bone framework of the human body). Vitamin C speeds the production of new cells in wound healing, protects your immune system, helps you fight off infection, reduces the severity of allergic reactions, and plays a role in the syntheses of hormones and other body chemicals.

One medium-size orange or sweet potato provides at least 25 percent of the adult RDA for vitamin C.

LEMONS, LIMES, ORANGES — AND BACON?

Check the meat label. Right there it is, plain as day — vitamin C in the form of *sodium ascorbate* and/or *isoascorbate.*

Processed meats, such as bacon and sausages, are preserved with sodium nitrite, which protects the meat from *Clostridium botulinum,* microorganisms that cause the potentially fatal food poisoning known as botulism.

On its own, sodium nitrite reacts at high temperatures with compounds in meat to form carcinogens called nitrosamines. Antioxidant vitamin C prevents the chemical reaction. It also helps prevent free radicals (incomplete pieces of molecules) from hooking up with each other to form damaging compounds — in this case, *carcinogens,* substances that cause cancer.

And that is why the U.S. Food and Drug Administration (FDA) and Department of Agriculture/Food Safety and Inspection Service (USDA FISIS) require vitamin C in your bacon.

Thiamin (vitamin B1)

This sulfur *(thia)* and nitrogen *(amin)* compound, the first of the B vitamins to be isolated and identified, helps ensure a healthy appetite. It acts as a *coenzyme* (a substance that works along with other enzymes) essential to at least four different processes by which your body extracts energy from carbohydrates. It's found in every body tissue, with the highest concentrations in your vital organs — heart, liver, and kidneys.

The richest dietary sources of thiamin are unrefined cereals and grains, lean pork, beans, nuts, and seeds. Refined ("white") flours, stripped of the brown parts that contain thiamin, are popular in the United States. To make up what's lost in processing, all breads and cereals are enriched with additional B1.

Three ounces of pork, ham, or beef or pork liver provide at least 25 percent of the adult RDA for thiamine.

Riboflavin (vitamin B2)

Riboflavin, the second B vitamin to be identified, is named for its chemical structure, a carbon-hydrogen-oxygen skeleton that includes *ribitol* (a sugar) attached to a *flavonoid* (a substance from plants containing one of the orange-to-red pigments called flavones).

Like thiamin, riboflavin is a coenzyme that enables you to digest and use proteins and carbohydrates. Like vitamin A, it protects the health of mucous membranes. And like the other B vitamins, your best source for riboflavin are foods of animal origin (meat, fish, poultry, eggs, and milk), plus brewer's yeast, and whole or enriched grain products.

Three ounces of beef or pork liver or one ounce of liverwurst provide 25 percent of the adult RDA for riboflavin. Three ounces of fortified ready-to-eat puffed rice cereal, 163 percent of the RDA for a woman, 138 percent for a man.

Niacin (vitamin B3)

Niacin is found either as a preformed nutrient or acquired via your body's conversion of the amino acid tryptophan. Preformed niacin comes from meat; tryptophan comes from milk and dairy foods. There is some niacin in grains, but your body can't absorb it efficiently unless the grain has been treated with lime (the mineral, not the fruit), a practice common in Central and South American countries where lime is added to cornmeal in making tortillas. In the United States, breads and cereals are routinely fortified with niacin.

Three-fourths ounce of turkey or 1.4 ounces of fish provide 25 percent of the adult RDA for niacin.

Pantothenic acid (vitamin B5)

Pantothenic acid is employed in enzyme reactions that enable you to use carbohydrates and create steroid biochemicals such as hormones. This vitamin also helps stabilize blood sugar levels, defends against infection, and protects *hemoglobin* (the protein in red blood cells that carries oxygen through the body) as well as nerve, brain, and muscle tissue.

You get pantothenic acid from meat, fish, poultry, beans, whole grain cereals, and fortified grain products.

There is no RDA for pantothenic acid. About 1.25 ounces of shitake mushrooms or oily fish provide 25 percent of the adult Adequate Intake (AI).

Vitamin B6 (pyridoxine)

Vitamin B6 is a compound comprising three related chemicals: pyridoxine, pyridoxal, and pyridoxamine, which is a component of enzymes that take part in more than 100 actions that metabolize proteins and fats. Vitamin B6 is essential for extracting energy and nutrients from food. It also helps lower blood levels of homocysteine, an amino acid produced when you digest proteins.

The best food sources of vitamin B6 are liver, chicken, fish, pork, lamb, milk, eggs, unmilled rice (rice with the bran intact), whole grains, soybeans, potatoes, beans, nuts, seeds, dark green vegetables (such as turnip greens), and enriched grain products.

One-third cup of instant (fortified) oatmeal, 3.5 ounces skinless chicken breast or 3 ounces of beef liver provide 25 percent of the RDA for vitamin B6.

Biotin (vitamin B7)

Biotin is a component of enzymes that ferry carbon and oxygen atoms between cells. It helps you metabolize fats and carbohydrates and is essential for synthesizing fatty acids and amino acids needed for healthy growth.

The best food sources of biotin are liver, egg yolk, yeast, nuts, and beans, but if your diet doesn't give you all the biotin you need, bacteria in your gut will synthesize enough to make up the difference.

There is no RDA for biotin. Two ounces of salmon provide 25 percent of the adult Adequate Intake (AI).

Folic acid (vitamin B9)

Folic acid, also known as folate or folacin, plays a role in the synthesis of DNA, the metabolism of proteins, and the subsequent synthesis of amino acids used to produce new body cells and tissues and is directly involved in both normal growth and wound healing. This vitamin is most important for women of child-bearing age. Not only does it assist in creating new maternal and fetal tissue, an adequate supply before and during pregnancy dramatically reduces the risk of neural tube (spinal cord) birth defects such as *spina bifida* (the failure of the bones of the spine to close properly around the spinal cord).

Beans, dark green leafy vegetables, liver, yeast, and various fruits are the best natural sources of folate, but as a protective measure, all multivitamin supplements and all grain products sold in the United States must now include 400 micrograms of folate per dose/serving.

A 3.5-ounce serving of Romaine lettuce provides 136 micrograms.

Vitamin B12 (cyanocobalamin)

Vitamin B12 is unique. It's the only vitamin that contains a mineral — in this case, cobalt, the *cobal* in its name. The combination is vital for healthy red blood cells and protects *myelin*, the fatty material that covers your nerves and enables you to transmit electrical impulses (messages) between nerve cells that make it possible for you to see, hear, think, move, and do all the things a healthy body does each day.

The best natural sources of B12 are from animals: beef, pork, poultry, and fish. Fruits and veggies don't manufacture vitamin B12, but, like vitamin K, this nutrient is produced by beneficial bacteria (the *microbiome*) in the small intestine.

Three ounces of beef, pork, poultry, or fish provide 25 percent of the adult RDA for vitamin B12.

Choline

In 1998, 138 years after choline was first identified, the Institute of Medicine (IOM) finally declared it essential for human beings. The IOM had good reasons for doing so. Although choline is neither vitamin, mineral, protein, carbohydrate, nor fat, it does help keep body cells healthy.

HAND IN HAND: HOW VITAMINS HELP EACH OTHER

All vitamins have specific jobs in your body. Some have partners. Here are some examples of nutrient cooperation:

- Vitamin E keeps vitamin A from being destroyed in your intestines.
- Vitamin D enables your body to absorb calcium and phosphorus.
- Vitamin C helps folate build proteins.
- Vitamin B1 works in digestive enzyme systems with niacin, pantothenic acid, and magnesium.

Taking vitamins with other vitamins may also improve body levels of nutrients. For example, in 1993, scientists at the National Cancer Institute and the U. S. Department of Agriculture (USDA) Agricultural Research Service gave one group of volunteers a vitamin E capsule plus a multivitamin pill; a second group, vitamin E alone; and a third group, no vitamins at all. The people getting vitamin E plus the multivitamin had the highest amount of vitamin E in their blood — more than twice as high as those who took plain vitamin E capsules.

Sometimes, one vitamin may even alleviate a deficiency caused by the lack of another vitamin. People who do not get enough folate are at risk of a form of anemia in which their red blood cells fail to mature. As soon as they get folate, either by injection or by mouth, they begin making new healthy cells. That's to be expected. What's surprising is the fact that anemia caused by *pellagra,* the niacin deficiency disease, may also respond to folate treatment.

Choline is used to make *acetylcholine,* a chemical that enables brain cells to exchange messages. It protects the heart and lowers the risk of liver cancer. And new research at the University of North Carolina (Chapel Hill) shows that choline plays a role in developing and maintaining the ability to think and remember, at least among rat pups and other beasties born to lab animals that were given choline supplements while pregnant. Follow-up studies showed that prenatal choline supplements helped the animals grow bigger brain cells. As yet, no one knows whether this would also be true for human babies.

There is no RDA for choline; ¾ ounce of caviar provides the adult Adequate Intake (AI). Rarely indulge in caviar? Not to worry: One egg gives you 25 percent of the AI.

Discovering Where to Get Your Vitamins

One reasonable set of guidelines for good nutrition is the list of Recommended Dietary Allowances (RDAs) and amounts of Adequate Intakes (AI) established by the National Research Council's Food and Nutrition Board. The RDAs present safe and effective doses for healthy people.

You can find the complete chart of RDAs for adults (ages 19 and up) in Chapter 3. Photocopy this chart. Pin it on your fridge. Tape it to your organizer or appointment book. Stick it in your wallet. Think of it as the truly simple way to see how easy it is to eat healthy.

For a totally, absolutely, mind-bendingly complete list of the nutrients in thousands of foods, check out the USDA's multiple info centers at `https://fdc.nal.usda.gov`. If you can even think of a food the U.S. Department of Agriculture experts missed, let them know and they will probably add it, making this list even more totally, absolutely, mind-bendingly complete.

Too Much or Too Little: Avoiding Two Ways to Go Wrong with Vitamins

Recommended Dietary Allowances (RDAs) and Adequate Intakes (AIs) are broad enough to prevent vitamin deficiencies and avoid the side effects associated with very large doses of some vitamins. The trick is to get exactly what you need — no more, no less.

Vitamin deficiencies

Vitamin deficiencies are rare among people who have access to a wide variety of foods and know how to put together a balanced diet. For example, the only people likely to experience a vitamin E deficiency are premature and/or low-birth-weight infants or people with a metabolic disorder that keeps them from absorbing fat. A healthy adult may go as long as ten years on a vitamin E-deficient diet without developing any signs of a problem.

Aha, you say, but what about a subclinical deficiency that might sneak up on you? Nutritionists use the term *subclinical deficiency* to describe a deficit not yet far enough advanced to produce obvious symptoms. In lay terms, however, the phrase has become a handy explanation for common but hard-to-pin-down symptoms, such as fatigue, irritability, nervousness, emotional depression, allergies, and insomnia. And it's a dandy way to increase the sale of nutritional supplements.

Simply put, the RDAs protect you against deficiency. If your symptoms linger even after you take reasonable amounts of vitamin supplements, something other than a lack of any one vitamin may be to blame. Don't wait until your patience or your bank account has been exhausted to find out. Check with your doctor. While you're waiting for an appointment, check out Table 10-1 for a list of the symptoms of various vitamin deficiencies.

TABLE 10-1   ## What Happens When You Don't Get the Vitamins You Need

A Diet Low in This Vitamin...	... May Produce These Signs of Deficiency
Vitamin A	Poor night vision; dry, rough, or cracked skin; dry mucous membranes including the inside of the eye; slow wound healing; nerve damage; reduced ability to taste, hear, and smell; inability to perspire; reduced resistance to respiratory infections
Vitamin D	In children: rickets (weak muscles, delayed tooth development, and soft bones, all caused by the inability to absorb minerals without vitamin D); in adults: osteomalacia (soft, porous bones that fracture easily); fatigue
	Recent reports suggest that a vitamin D deficiency may reduce a woman's chances of conceiving while undergoing In Vitro Fertilization (IVF) and increase the risk of asthma attacks in adults.
Vitamin E	Inability to absorb fat
Vitamin K	Blood fails to clot
Vitamin C	Scurvy (bleeding gums; tooth loss; nosebleeds; bruising; painful or swollen joints; shortness of breath; increased susceptibility to infection; slow wound healing; muscle pains; skin rashes)

A Diet Low in This Vitamin...	...May Produce These Signs of Deficiency
Thiamin (vitamin B1)	Poor appetite; unintended weight loss; upset stomach; gastric upset (nausea, vomiting); mental depression; an inability to concentrate; fatigue, and the thiamine deficiency disease beriberi
Riboflavin (vitamin B2)	Inflamed mucous membranes, including cracked lips, sore tongue and mouth, burning eyes; skin rashes; anemia; fatigue
Niacin (vitamin B3)	Pellagra (diarrhea; inflamed skin and mucous membranes; mental confusion and/or dementia); fatigue
Vitamin B6 (pyridoxine)	Anemia; convulsions similar to epileptic seizures; skin rashes; upset stomach; nerve damage (in infants); fatigue
Folic acid (vitamin B9)	Anemia (immature red blood cells); fatigue
Vitamin B12	Pernicious anemia (destruction of red blood cells, nerve damage, increased risk of stomach cancer attributed to damaged stomach tissue, neurological/psychiatric symptoms attributed to nerve cell damage); fatigue
Biotin (vitamin B7)	Loss of appetite; upset stomach; pale, dry, scaly skin; hair loss; emotional depression; skin rashes (in infants younger than 6 months)

Vitamin megadoses

WARNING

Can you get too much of a good thing? Yes. In fact, some vitamins are toxic when taken in the very large amounts popularly known as *megadoses*. How much is a megadose? Nobody knows for sure. The general consensus is that a megadose is several times the RDA, but the term is so vague that it stops my spellcheck cold and isn't even in the 28th edition of Stedman's Medical Dictionary (2006), a tome that's pretty much the gold standard in medical word books.

Nonetheless, it's clear that

>> Megadoses of vitamin A (as retinol) may cause symptoms that make you think you have a brain tumor. Taken by a pregnant woman, megadoses of vitamin A may damage the fetus.

>> Megadoses of vitamin D may cause kidney stones and hard lumps of calcium in soft tissue (muscles and organs) as well as nausea and other gastro discomfort.

>> Megadoses of niacin (sometimes used to lower cholesterol levels) can damage liver tissue.

>> Megadoses of vitamin B6 can cause (temporary) damage to nerves in arms, legs, fingers, and toes.

The important fact is that, with one exception, the likeliest way to get a megadose of vitamins is to take supplements (see Chapter 13 for more on supplements) because it's pretty much impossible for you to cram down enough food to overdose on vitamins D, E, K, C, and all the Bs.

The exception is vitamin A. Liver and fish liver oils are concentrated sources of preformed vitamin A (retinol), the potentially toxic form of vitamin A. Liver contains so much retinol that early 20th century explorers to the South Pole made themselves sick on seal and whale liver. On the other hand, even very large doses of vitamin E, vitamin K, thiamin (vitamin B1), riboflavin (vitamin B2), folate, vitamin B12, biotin, and pantothenic acid appear safe for human beings. Table 10-2 lists the effects of vitamin overdoses.

TABLE 10-2   **Amounts and Effects of Vitamin Overdoses/Megadoses for Healthy People**

Vitamin	Overdose/Megadose and Possible Effect
Vitamin A	15,000 to 25,000 IU retinol a day for adults (2,000 IU or more for children) may lead to liver damage, headache, vomiting, abnormal vision, constipation, hair loss, loss of appetite, low-grade fever, bone pain, sleep disorders, and dry skin and mucous membranes. A pregnant woman who takes more than 10,000 IU a day doubles her risk of giving birth to a child with birth defects.
Vitamin D	2,000 IU a day can cause irreversible damage to kidneys and heart. Smaller doses may cause muscle weakness, headache, nausea, vomiting, high blood pressure, retarded physical growth, mental retardation in children, and fetal abnormalities.
Vitamin E	Large amounts (more than 400 to 800 IU a day) may cause upset stomach or dizziness. Similarly, in 2005 a meta-analysis (a study comparing the results of several studies) in the *Annals of Internal Medicine* showed that use of "high dose" (400 IU or more) vitamin E supplements might "increase all causes of mortality [death] and should be avoided."
Vitamin C	1,000 mg or higher may cause upset stomach, diarrhea, or constipation.
Niacin	Doses higher than the RDA raise the production of liver enzymes and blood levels of sugar and uric acid, leading to liver damage and an increased risk of diabetes and gout.
Vitamin B6	Continued use of 50 mg or more a day may damage nerves in arms, legs, hands, and feet. Some experts say the damage is likely to be temporary; others say that it may be permanent.
Choline	Very high doses (14 to 37 times the adequate amount) have been linked to vomiting, salivation, sweating, low blood pressure, and — ugh! — fishy body odor.

Acceptable Exceptions: Taking Extra Vitamins as Needed

Some people do need extra vitamins. Who? Maybe you. The RDAs are designed to protect healthy people from deficiencies, but sometimes the circumstances of your life (or your lifestyle) mean that you need something extra. For example, are you taking medication? Do you smoke? Are you on a restricted diet? Are you pregnant? Are you a nursing mother? Are you approaching menopause? Answer yes to any of these questions, and you may be a person who needs larger amounts of vitamins than the RDAs provide.

I'm taking medication

Many valuable medical drugs interact with vitamins. Some drugs increase or decrease the effectiveness of vitamins; some vitamins increase or decrease the effectiveness of drugs. For example, a woman who's using birth control pills may absorb less than the customary amount of the B vitamins. For more about vitamin and drug interactions, see Chapter 25.

I'm a smoker

Really? Still? Then you should know that you probably have abnormally low blood levels of vitamin C. More trouble: Chemicals from tobacco smoke create more free radicals in your body. Even the National Research Council, which is tough on vitamin overdosing, says that regular smokers need to take about 66 percent more vitamin C — up to 100 milligrams a day — than nonsmokers.

I never eat animals

Vegans also benefit from extra vitamin C because it increases their ability to absorb iron from plant food. Vitamin B12 enriched grains or supplements are a must to supply the nutrient found only in fish, poultry, milk, cheese, and eggs.

I'm pregnant

Keep in mind that "eating for two" means that you're the sole source of nutrients for the growing fetus, not that you need to double the amount of food you eat. If you don't get the vitamins you need, neither will your baby.

The RDAs for many nutrients are the same as those for women who aren't pregnant. But when you're pregnant, you need extra

>> **Vitamin D:** Every smidgen of vitamin D in a newborn's body comes from his or her mom. If the mother doesn't have enough vitamin D, neither will the baby. Are vitamin pills the answer? Yes. And no. The qualifier is how many pills, because although too little vitamin D can weaken a developing fetus, too much can cause birth defects. That's why until/unless new recommendations for vitamin D are issued, the second important *d*-word is *doctor* — as in, check with yours to see what's right for you.

>> **Vitamin E:** To create all that new tissue (the woman's as well as the baby's), a pregnant woman needs an extra 2 milligram alpha-tocopherol equivalents (mg alpha-TE) each day, the approximate amount in one egg.

>> **Vitamin C:** The level of vitamin C in your blood falls as your vitamin C flows across the placenta to your baby, who may — at some point in the pregnancy — have vitamin C levels as much as 50 percent higher than yours. So you need an extra 10 milligrams of vitamin C each day (½ cup cooked zucchini or two stalks of asparagus).

>> **Riboflavin (vitamin B2):** To protect the baby against structural defects, such as cleft palate or a deformed heart, a pregnant woman needs an extra 0.3 milligrams of riboflavin each day (slightly less than 1 ounce of ready-to-eat cereal).

>> **Folate:** As many as 2 of every 1,000 babies born each year in the United States have a neural tube defect such as spina bifida because their mothers didn't get enough folate to meet the RDA standard. Taking 400 micrograms of folate (also known as folic acid) daily before becoming pregnant and through the first two months of pregnancy significantly lowers the risk of giving birth to a child with cleft palate. Taking 400 micrograms of folate each day through an entire pregnancy reduces the risk of neural tube defects.

>> **Vitamin B12:** To meet the demands of the growing fetus, a pregnant woman needs an extra 0.2 micrograms of vitamin B12 each day (just 3 ounces of roasted chicken).

I'm breast-feeding

You need extra vitamin A, vitamin E, thiamin, riboflavin, and folate to produce sufficient quantities of nutritious breast milk, about 25 ounces or 750 milliliters each day. You need extra vitamin D, vitamin C, and niacin as insurance to replace the vitamins you lose — that is, the ones you transfer to your child in your milk.

I'm approaching menopause

There are RDAs and AIs for people 50 and older, but in a country where the population over 80 is growing by leaps and bounds, information about the specific vitamin requirements of older women is as hard to find as, well, information about the specific vitamin requirements of older men. Right now, just about all anybody can say for sure about the nutritional needs of older women is that they require extra calcium to stem the natural loss of bone that occurs when women reach menopause and their production of the female hormone estrogen declines. They may also need extra vitamin D to enable their bodies to absorb and use the calcium.

Gender bias alert! No similar studies are available for older men. But adding vitamin D supplements to calcium supplements increases bone density in older men as well.

I have very light skin or very dark skin

Sunlight transforms fats just under the surface of your skin to vitamin D. So getting what you need should be a cinch, right? Not necessarily. Getting enough vitamin D from sunlight is hard to do when you avoid the sun for fear of skin cancer. Safe solution? A diet with sufficient amounts of the vitamin. But you knew that.

Chapter **11**

Making Mineral Magic

M inerals are *elements*, substances composed of only one kind of atom. They're inorganic, which means they don't contain the carbon, hydrogen, and oxygen atoms found in all organic compounds, including vitamins. Minerals occur naturally in nonliving things, such as rocks and metal ores. Yes, you can find minerals in plants and animals, but they're imported. Plants absorb minerals from the soil; animals obtain minerals by eating plants.

Most minerals have names that describe where they're found or what they look like. For example, calcium comes from *calx*, the Greek word for "lime" (chalk), a source of calcium. Chlorine comes from *chloros*, the Greek word for "greenish-yellow," which just happens to be the color of the mineral. Other minerals, such as americium, curium, berkelium, californium, fermium, and nobelium, are named for where they were first identified or to honor an important scientist.

This chapter tells you which minerals your body requires, which foods provide what minerals, and how much of each mineral a healthy person needs.

Getting the Minerals You Need

Think of your body as a house. Vitamins (see Chapter 10) are like tiny little maids and butlers, scurrying about to turn on the lights and make sure the windows are closed to keep the heat from escaping. Minerals are more sturdy stuff, the mortar and bricks that strengthen the frame of the house and the current that keeps the lights running.

Nutritionists classify the minerals essential for human life, including the electrolytes described in Chapter 12, as either *major minerals* (also known as *macrominerals*) or *trace elements*.

Major Minerals	Trace Elements
Calcium	Iron
Phosphorus	Zinc
Magnesium	Iodine
Sulfur	Selenium
Sodium	Copper
Potassium	Manganese
Chloride	Fluoride
	Chromium
	Molybdenum

Both major minerals and trace elements are vital for human health. Nutritionally speaking, though, the difference between the two is the amount of the mineral you store in your body and how much you need to take in to maintain a steady supply.

For example, your body stores more than 5 grams (about 1/6 of an ounce) of each of the major minerals and principal electrolytes (sodium, potassium, and chloride). To maintain a healthful level of these nutrients, you need to consume more than 100 milligrams (3.5 ounces) a day of each. You need much less of the trace elements whose Recommended Dietary Allowances (RDAs) are commonly measured not in milligrams (1/100 of a gram) but in micrograms (1/1,000,000 of a gram).

AN ELEMENTARY GUIDE TO MINERALS

The early Greeks thought that all material on Earth was constructed of a combination of four basic elements: earth, water, air, and fire. Centuries later, alchemists looking for the formula for precious metals, such as gold, decided that the essential elements were sulfur, salt, and mercury. Wrong again.

In 1669, a group of German chemists isolated phosphorus, the first mineral element to be accurately identified. After that, things moved a bit more swiftly. By the end of the 19th century, scientists knew the names and chemical properties of several elements. Today, there are 118 elements on the periodic table, and the American Mineralogical Association has officially recognized more than 5,000 minerals.

The classic guide to chemical elements is the periodic table, a chart devised in 1869 by Russian chemist Dimitri Mendeleev, for whom *mendelevium* is named. The table was revised by British physicist Henry Moseley, who came up with the concept of *atomic numbers,* numbers based on the number of *protons* (positively charged particles) in an elemental atom.

The periodic table is a clean, crisp way of characterizing the elements, and if you are now or ever were a chemistry, physics, or premed student, you can testify firsthand to the joy (maybe that's not the best word) of memorizing the information it provides. Personally, I'd rather be forced to watch reruns of *Real Housewives*.

The major minerals

This section covers three major minerals — calcium, phosphorus, and magnesium — which build bones and regulate many system functions such as keeping your blood pressure on an even keel.

As you read this section, you may notice a few important minerals missing. Sodium, potassium, and chloride, also known as the principal electrolytes, aren't included here because they are the principal electrolytes covered in Chapter 12. And although sulfur, a major mineral, is an essential nutrient for human beings, you'll rarely find it in nutrition books and/or charts because it's an integral part of all proteins. Any diet that provides adequate protein also provides adequate sulfur. (For more on proteins, check out Chapter 6.)

Here are the rest, each with an example of a food serving that provides one-quarter of the Recommended Dietary Allowance (RDA) or the alternative Adequate Intake (AI) for healthy adults described in Chapter 3.

Calcium

When you step on the scale in the morning, you can assume that about 3 pounds of your body weight is calcium, most of it packed into your bones and teeth. Calcium is also present in extracellular fluid (the liquid around body cells), where it

>> Regulates fluid balance by controlling the flow of water in and out of cells

>> Enables cells to send messages back and forth from one to another

>> Keeps muscles moving smoothly and cramp free

>> Helps release hormones and enzymes that keep our body in working order.

Calcium also helps control blood pressure, and sometimes not just for the person who takes the calcium directly. Some studies suggest that if a pregnant woman gets a sufficient amount of calcium, her baby's blood pressure stays lower than average for at least the first seven years of life, meaning a lower risk of developing high blood pressure later on. This suggestion, although tantalizing, remains to be confirmed.

CALCIUM: THE BONE TEAM PLAYER

Like all body tissues, bones are constantly being replenished. Old bone cells break down, and new ones are born. Specialized cells called *osteoclasts* start the process by boring tiny holes into solid bone so that other specialized cells, called *osteoblasts,* can refill the open spaces with fresh bone. At that point, crystals of calcium, the best-known dietary bone builder, hook onto the network of new bone cells to harden and strengthen the bone.

Calcium begins its work on your bones while you're still in your mother's womb. But it's not the only mineral at play. Think iron and zinc. Based on a survey of 242 pregnant women in Peru, where zinc deficiency is common, Johns Hopkins researchers found the babies born to women who got prenatal supplements with iron, folic acid, and zinc had longer, stronger leg bones than did babies born to women who got the same supplement minus the zinc.

After you're born, calcium continues to build your bones but only with the help of vitamin D, which produces a calcium-binding protein that enables you to absorb the calcium in milk. To make sure you get your vitamin D, virtually all milk sold in the United States is fortified with the vitamin. And because you may outgrow your taste for milk but never outgrow your need for calcium, calcium supplements for adults frequently include vitamin D. Milk also contains *lactoferrin* (*lacto* = milk; *ferri* = iron), an iron compound that stimulates the production of the cells that promote bone growth.

Your best food sources of calcium are milk and dairy products as well as fish, such as canned sardines and salmon *with the bones* that have been softened and made edible by processing. (*Caution:* Bones in fresh fish are definitely *not* edible.) You can also get calcium from dark green leafy vegetables, but this form of the mineral is bound tightly into compounds that make it hard for your body to absorb.

Eight ounces of 2-percent milk provides 300 milligrams of calcium, about one-third of the RDA, and 1 cup cooked broccoli provides 200 milligrams, about one-fifth the RDA.

Phosphorus

Like calcium, phosphorus is essential for strong bones and teeth. Phosphorus also enables a cell to transmit the *genetic code* (genes and chromosomes that carry information about your special characteristics) to the new cells created when a cell divides and reproduces. In addition, phosphorus

>> Helps maintain the pH balance of blood — that is, keeps blood from being too acidic or too alkaline

>> Is used to metabolize carbohydrates, synthesizing proteins and ferrying fats and fatty acids among tissues and organs

>> Is part of *myelin,* the fatty sheath that surrounds and protects each nerve cell

Almost every item on a normal menu contains phosphorus, but the best sources are high-protein foods, such as meat, fish, poultry, eggs, and milk. For vegetarians, grains, nuts, seeds, and dry beans also provide respectable amounts.

Eight ounces of milk provide one-quarter of the adult RDA for phosphorus.

Magnesium

Your body uses magnesium to make body tissues, especially bone. The adult human body contains about an ounce of magnesium; three-quarters of that is in the bones. Magnesium also is part of more than 300 different enzymes that trigger chemical reactions throughout your body and helps to

>> Move nutrients in and out of body cells

>> Send messages between cells

>> Transmit the genetic code (genes and chromosomes) when cells divide and reproduce

Chlorophyll contains magnesium, so plant foods such as dark green fruits and vegetables are excellent food sources; whole seeds and grains as well as nuts and beans are also magnesium-rich.

Four slices of whole wheat bread or one cup (uncooked) dry beans, which puff up to 3 cups when cooked, provide one-quarter of the RDA for magnesium.

The trace elements

As noted, trace elements are essential but in much smaller amounts than major minerals. Here's a list of the trace minerals with an example of a food serving that provides one-quarter of the RDA or AI.

Iron

Iron is an essential constituent of *hemoglobin* and *myoglobin*, two proteins that store and transport oxygen. Hemoglobin (*hemo* = blood) is what makes red blood cells red; *myoglobin* (*myo* = muscle) does the same for muscle tissue. You also find in iron dozens of enzymes required for such processes as digesting food.

The best food sources of iron are organ meats (liver, heart, kidneys), red meat, egg yolks, wheat germ, and oysters, all of which provide *heme* (*heme* = blood) iron, iron attached to a specific protein. This is the form of iron your body absorbs most easily.

Whole grains, wheat germ, raisins, nuts, seed, prunes and prune juice, and potato skins contain *non-heme* iron, iron without the protein attachment. Because plants contain substances called *phytates,* which bind this iron into compounds, your body has a hard time getting at the iron. Eating plant foods with meat or with foods such as tomatoes that are rich in vitamin C increases your body's ability to split away the phytates and extract the iron from plant foods.

One ounce of cold cereal or 1 cup of dried apricots each provides one-quarter of the RDA for iron.

Zinc

Zinc protects nerve and brain tissue, bolsters the immune system, and is essential for healthy growth. Like other minerals, it is also part of the enzymes (and hormones such as insulin) that metabolize food.

I'M LOOKING FOR AN IRON SUPPLEMENT. WHAT'S THIS "FERROUS" STUFF?

The iron in iron supplements comes in several different forms, each one composed of elemental iron (the kind of iron your body actually uses) coupled with an organic acid that makes the iron easy to absorb.

The iron compounds commonly found in iron supplements are

- Ferrous citrate (iron plus citric acid)
- Ferrous fumarate (iron plus fumaric acid)
- Ferrous gluconate (iron plus a sugar derivative)
- Ferrous lactate (iron plus lactic acid, an acid formed in the fermentation of milk)
- Ferrous succinate (iron plus succinic acid)
- Ferrous sulfate (iron plus a sulfuric acid derivative)

In your stomach, these compounds dissolve at different rates, yielding different amounts of elemental iron. So supplement labels list the compound and the amount of elemental iron it provides, like this:

Ferrous gluconate 300 milligrams, Elemental iron 34 milligrams

This tells you that the supplement has 300 milligrams of the iron compound ferrous gluconate, which gives you 34 milligrams of usable elemental iron. If the label just says "iron," that's shorthand for elemental iron. The elemental iron number is what you look for in judging the iron content of a vitamin/mineral supplement.

You can fairly call zinc the macho male mineral because the largest quantities of zinc in the human body are in the testes, where it's used in making a continuous supply of *testosterone,* the hormone a man needs to produce plentiful amounts of healthy, viable sperm and maintain muscle mass. Without enough zinc, male fertility falters. And, yes, several studies have confirmed that sucking on lozenges containing one form of zinc (zinc gluconate) shortens a cold — by a day or two. Other studies show no effect. Your choice.

In addition to oysters, meat, liver, and eggs are all good sources of zinc. So are nuts, beans, miso, pumpkin and sunflower seeds, whole grain products, and wheat germ. However, as with iron, the zinc in plant foods occurs in compounds that your body absorbs less efficiently than the zinc in foods from animals.

The zinc RDA for women is 8 milligrams; for men, 11. Three ounces of beef serves up 7 milligrams; 3 ounces dark meat chicken, 2.5 milligrams.

Iodine

Iodine is a component of the thyroid hormones thyroxine and triiodothyronine, which help regulate cell activities. These hormones are also essential for protein synthesis, tissue growth (including the formation of healthy nerves and bones), and reproduction.

The best natural sources of iodine are seafood and plants grown near or in the ocean, but modern Americans are most likely to get the iodine they need from iodized salt (plain table salt with iodine added). And here's an odd nutritional note: You may get some iodine from commercial breads because iodine compounds are used as dough conditioners, the additives that make dough more pliable.

Seafood is our best source of iodine, but one slice of enriched white(!) bread provides 185 micrograms, 35 more than the 150 micrograms RDA.

Selenium

Selenium was identified as an essential human nutrient in 1979 when Chinese nutrition researchers discovered that people with low body stores of selenium were at increased risk of *Keshan disease,* a disorder of the heart muscle with symptoms that include rapid heartbeat, enlarged heart, and (in severe cases) heart failure.

Although fruits and vegetables grown in selenium-rich soils are rich in this mineral, the best sources of selenium are seafood, meat and organ meats (liver, kidney), eggs, and dairy products.

One ounce of Brazil nuts provides ten times the RDA; 1/2 ounce of oysters provides one-quarter of the RDA for selenium.

Copper

Copper is an antioxidant found in enzymes that deactivate free radicals (pieces of molecules that can link up to form compounds that damage body tissues) and make it possible for your body to absorb and use iron. In addition, copper

>> Promotes the growth of strong bones
>> Protects the health of nerve tissue

>> Prevents your hair from turning gray prematurely. But, no, no, a thousand times, no: Large amounts of copper absolutely will not turn gray hair back to its original color. Worse yet, megadoses of copper are potentially toxic.

You can get the copper you need from organ meats such as liver and heart, seafood, nuts, and dried beans, including chocolate, which is made, of course, from cacao beans.

One cup of dried prunes or one cup of cooked lentils each provides one-quarter of the RDA for copper.

Manganese

Most of the manganese in your body is in your glands (pituitary, mammary, pancreas), organs (liver, kidneys, intestines), and bones. The mineral is also found in enzymes that metabolize carbohydrates and synthesize fats. Manganese promotes a healthy reproductive system, and during pregnancy, manganese enhances proper growth of fetal tissue.

Your best dietary sources of manganese are whole grains, cereal products, fruits, and vegetables. Oolong tea is also rich in manganese with slightly more than twice as much as green tea and nearly three times as much as black tea.

One ounce of almonds or peanuts provides at least one-quarter of the AI for manganese.

Fluoride

Fluoride is the form of the element fluorine found in drinking water. Your body stores fluoride in bones and teeth. Although some question whether fluoride is an essential nutrient, there is no doubt that it hardens dental enamel, reducing your risk of getting cavities; many researchers suspect (but can't prove) that some forms of fluoride strengthen bones.

All soil, ground water, plants, and animal tissue contain small amounts of fluoride, but the most reliable source of fluoride is fluoridated drinking water, which provides the AI for this mineral.

Chromium

Very small amounts of *trivalent chromium,* a digestible form of the very same metallic element that decorates your car and household appliances, are essential for several enzymes that you need to metabolize fat.

Chromium also partners with glucose tolerance factor (GTF), a group of chemicals that enables the pancreatic enzyme insulin to regulate your use of glucose, the end product of metabolism and the basic fuel for every body cell (see Chapter 3).

Chromium occurs naturally in meat and potatoes, cheese, whole grain cereals and baked goods, brewer's yeast, some vegetables such as broccoli, and hard water — that is, water with natural minerals.

One egg yolk, 1 cup yogurt or cottage cheese, or 1 ounce of broccoli each provides one-quarter of the AI for chromium.

Molybdenum

Molybdenum (pronounced mo-*lib*-de-num) is a constituent of several enzymes that metabolize proteins. You get molybdenum from beans and grains and, because cows eat grains, from milk and cheeses as well. Molybdenum also leeches into drinking water from surrounding soil, so the molybdenum content of plants and drinking water depends entirely on how much molybdenum is in the soil.

One cup of yogurt or cottage cheese provides one-quarter of the RDA for molybdenum.

Knowing What's Too Much and What's Too Little

The Recommended Dietary Allowances (RDAs) and Adequate Intakes (AIs) for minerals and trace elements are generous allowances, large enough to prevent deficiency but not so large that they trigger toxic side effects. In the following sections, you find out exactly how much of what works best for every body.

Avoiding mineral deficiency

Some minerals, such as phosphorus, magnesium, and sulfur, are so widely available in food that deficiencies are rare to nonexistent. Most drinking water contains adequate fluoride, and Americans get so much copper (can it be from chocolate bars?) that deficiency is practically unheard of in the United States. Finally, no nutrition scientist has yet been able to identify a naturally occurring deficiency of manganese, chromium, or molybdenum in human beings with access to a normal varied diet.

But other minerals are more problematic and include the following:

>> **Calcium:** Without enough calcium, a child's bones and teeth don't grow strong and straight and an adult's bones lose minerals and weaken. Adequate vitamin D assures that you're absorbing the calcium you get from food or supplements, which is why milk sold in American is fortified with vitamin D.

>> **Iron:** If you don't get enough iron, your body can't manufacture the hemoglobin required to carry energy-sustaining oxygen to every organ and tissue, a condition called — not surprisingly — *iron deficiency anemia,* most commonly characterized by unrelieved fatigue. Mild iron deficiency may also inhibit intellectual performance. In one Johns Hopkins study, high school girls scored higher verbal, memory, and learning test scores when they took supplements providing RDA amounts of this mineral.

>> **Zinc:** An adequate supply of zinc is vital for making testosterone and healthy sperm; men who don't get enough zinc may be temporarily infertile. Zinc deficiency may also lead to loss of appetite and the ability to taste food and weaken the immune system, increasing your risk of infections and slowing the healing of wounds, including the tissue damage caused by working out. In plain language: If you don't get the zinc you need, your charley horse may linger longer.

>> **Iodine:** Even a moderate iodine deficiency may lead to *goiter* (a swollen thyroid gland) and reduced production of thyroid hormones. A more severe deficiency early in life may cause a form of mental and physical retardation called *cretinism.*

>> **Selenium:** Not enough selenium in your diet? Watch out for muscle pain or weakness. To protect against selenium problems, make sure you get the vitamin E you need. Some animal studies show that a selenium deficiency responds to vitamin E supplements. And vice versa.

Understanding the risks of overdoses

Like all health products, some vitamins and minerals are potentially toxic in large doses known commonly as *megadoses.* How much is a mineral megadose? As Chapter 10 says about vitamins, there is no standard measure. (In fact, the word *megadose* is still so new that many spellcheck programs don't recognize it. Go ahead. Try it for yourself.) The consensus is that a megadose is several times larger than a normal RDA or AI and that as U.S. Supreme Court Justice Potter Stewart once famously said of pornography, you will know it when you see it.

For example:

- >> **Calcium:** No one has shown any problems with getting lots of calcium from food, but the story changes when you get your calcium from supplements. For example:

  - Constipation, bloating, nausea, and intestinal gas are common side effects among healthy people taking supplements equal to 1,500 to 4,000 milligrams of calcium a day.

  - Doses higher than 4,000 milligrams a day may be linked to kidney damage.

  - Megadoses of calcium can bind with iron and zinc, making it harder for your body to absorb these two essential trace elements.

- >> **Phosphorus:** Too much phosphorus may lower your body stores of calcium.

- >> **Magnesium:** Megadoses of magnesium appear safe for healthy people, but if you have kidney disease, the magnesium overload can cause weak muscles, breathing difficulty, irregular heartbeat, and/or cardiac arrest (your heart stops beating).

- >> **Iron:** Thinking of adding iron supplements? Stop! Before you plunk down a penny for the pills, check with your doctor, who can run the simple blood test to determine your actual iron state. About 1 in every 200 Americans has hemochromatosis, a common but often-undiagnosed genetic condition that may lead to an increased absorption of iron resulting in an increased risk of arthritis, heart disease, and diabetes, plus infectious diseases and maybe even cancer (both microorganisms and cancer cells thrive in an iron-rich environment).

WARNING

  Even if you don't have hemochromatosis, taking too much iron can lead to iron overload with some of the results listed above. Worse yet, overdosing on iron supplements can be deadly for young children for whom the lethal dose may be as low as 3 grams (3,000 milligrams) elemental iron at one time. This is the amount in 60 tablets with 50 milligrams elemental iron each. To foil small fingers and prevent accidental overdose, FDA requires individual blister packaging for supplements containing more than 30 milligrams of iron.

- >> **Zinc:** Moderately high doses of zinc (up to 25 milligrams a day) may slow your body's absorption of copper. Doses 27 to 37 times the RDA (11 milligrams for males; 8 milligrams for females) may interfere with your immune function and make you more susceptible to infection, the very thing that normal doses of zinc protect against. Gram doses (2,000 milligrams/2 grams) of zinc cause zinc poisoning: vomiting, gastric upset, and irritation of the stomach lining.

- >> **Iodine:** Overdoses of iodine may trigger exactly the same problems as iodine-deficiency: goiter. How can that be? When you consume very large amounts of iodine, the mineral stimulates your thyroid gland, which swells in a furious attempt to step up its production of thyroid hormones. This reaction is rare, most likely to occur among people who eat lots of dried seaweed for long periods of time.

>> **Selenium:** Doses as high as 5 milligrams of selenium a day (90 times the RDA) have been linked to thickened but fragile nails, hair loss, and perspiration with a garlicky odor.

>> **Fluoride:** Despite decades of argument, no scientific proof exists that the fluorides in drinking water increase the risk of cancer in human beings. But there's no question that large doses of fluoride — for example, from heavily fluoridated well or groundwater in the western United States — leads to *fluorosis* (brown patches on your teeth), brittle bones, fatigue, and muscle weakness. Over long periods of time, high doses of fluoride may also cause *outcroppings* (little bumps) of bone on the spine.

>> **Molybdenum:** Doses of molybdenum two to seven times the AI (45 micrograms) may increase the amount of copper you excrete in urine.

Figuring Out When You May Need More than the RDA

If your diet provides enough minerals to meet the RDAs, you're in pretty good shape most of the time. But a restrictive diet, the circumstances of your reproductive life, and just plain getting older can increase your need for minerals. Here are some possible scenarios.

You're a strict vegetarian

Vegetarians who pass up fish, meat, and poultry must get their iron either from fortified grain products, such as breakfast cereals and commercial breads, or naturally from foods, such as seeds, nuts, blackstrap molasses, raisins, prune juice, potato skins, green leafy vegetables, tofu, miso, and brewer's yeast. Because iron in plant foods is bound into compounds that are difficult for the human body to absorb, iron supplements are considered pretty much standard fare.

Vegans (vegetarians who avoid all foods from animals, including dairy products) have a similar problem getting enough calcium. While many green veggies, such as kale, collard and turnip greens, and seaweed, do have calcium, like iron, this calcium is bound into hard-to-absorb compounds. Luckily, there are good non-animal foods with calcium, such as soybean milk fortified with calcium, orange juice with added calcium, and tofu processed with calcium sulfate.

You live inland, away from the ocean

Seafood and plants grown near or in the ocean absorb iodine from the seawater. Freshwater fish, plants grown far from the sea, and the animals that feed on these fish and plants do not, so people who live inland and get all their food from local gardens and farms probably can't get the iodine they need from food.

American nutrition savvy and technology solved this problem in 1924 with the introduction of iodized salt. Then came refrigerated railroad cars and trucks to carry food from both coasts to every inland city and state. Together, enriched salt and efficient shipment have virtually eliminated the iodine-deficiency disease goiter in the United States.

You're a man

Just as women lose iron during menstrual bleeding, men lose zinc at ejaculation. Men who are extremely active sexually may need extra zinc. The problem is that no one has ever written down standards for what constitutes "extremely active." Check this one out with your doctor, not your locker-room buddies.

You're a woman

Women lose blood and iron with each menstrual period; the heavier the flow, the greater the loss. Add to that the fact that many American women follow diets that provide fewer than 2,000 calories a day, a level at which it may be virtually impossible to get the iron needed for good health, and you can see how easy it would be to develop a mild iron deficiency.

Women who use an intrauterine device (IUD) may have a similar problem because IUDs irritate the lining of the uterus and cause a small but significant loss of blood and iron.

You're pregnant or nursing

Pregnant women need extra nutrients, not simply to build fetal tissues but also the new tissues and blood vessels in their own bodies. Nursing mothers need extra calcium, phosphorus, magnesium, iron, zinc, and selenium to protect their own bodies while producing nutritious breast milk. Happily, the same supplements that provide extra nutrients for pregnant women will meet a nursing mother's needs.

THE CALCIUM CONUNDRUM

Nutritionists once believed that your body's ability to absorb calcium ended in your middle 20s, thus making it impossible to reduce the age-related loss of bone density due to a decline in the natural production of the sex hormones estrogen and testosterone.

Now they know better. An increased consumption of calcium and vitamin D supplements appears to help, although who should take these supplements and in what quantities remains a question.

As its website explains, the U.S. Preventive Services Task Force (USPSTF; www. uspreventiveservicestaskforce.org) is an independent panel of experts in prevention and evidence-based medicine created in 1984 "to offer recommendations about preventive services for healthy people — that is, those with no signs or symptoms of the specific disease or condition under consideration."

In February 2015, USPSTF announced that healthy older women shouldn't take calcium and vitamin D supplements to prevent bone fractures. Low doses, it explained, appeared ineffective as preventives but increased the risk of kidney stone formation. The effectiveness of higher doses, it said, was "up in the air" based on a plethora of conflicting studies.

This recommendation contradicted that of the Institute of Medicine (IOM), the nongovernmental organization founded in 1970, under the congressional charter of the National Academy of Sciences. IOM recommends that most adults, healthy or not, should get 1,000 milligrams of calcium a day, and that women older than 50 and men older than 70 should get 1,200 milligrams.

Remember: These are proposals for healthy adults — that is, those with no sign of clinical bone loss. Is that you? Do you need supplements? Only your doctor knows for sure — so ask her.

Chapter **12**

The Wonder of Water

The human body is mostly water. The usual figure is 50 to 70 percent, but exactly how much water your own body contains depends on how much muscle and fat you have. Muscle tissue has more water than fat tissue, so, because the average male body has proportionately more muscle than the average female body, it also has more water. For the same reason (more muscle), a young body has more water than an older one.

You definitely won't enjoy the experience, but if you have to, you can live without food for weeks at a time, obtaining subsistence levels of nutrients by digesting your own muscle and fat. But water's different. Without it, you'll die in a matter of days — more quickly in a place warm enough to make you perspire and lose water more quickly.

This chapter explains why water is so important and offers some pointers on how to keep your body's water level *level*.

Investigating the Many Ways Your Body Uses Water

Water is a solvent. It dissolves other substances and carries nutrients and other material (such as blood cells) around the body, making it possible for every organ to do its job. You need water to

>> Digest food, dissolving nutrients so they can pass through the intestinal cell walls into your bloodstream, and move food along through your intestinal tract

>> Carry waste products out of your body

>> Provide a medium in which biochemical reactions, such as metabolism (digesting food, producing energy, and building tissue), occur

>> Send electrical messages between cells so your muscles can move, your eyes can see, your brain can think, and so on

>> Regulate body temperature — cooling your body with moisture (perspiration) that evaporates on your skin

>> Lubricate your moving parts

>> Protect your spinal cord and other sensitive tissues

Maintaining the Right Amount of Water in Your Body

As much as three-quarters of the water in your body is in *intracellular fluid*, the liquid inside body cells. The rest is in *extracellular fluid*, which is all the other body liquids, such as

>> Interstitial fluid (the fluid between cells)

>> Blood plasma (the clear liquid in blood)

>> Lymph (a clear, slightly yellow fluid collected from body tissues that flows through your lymph nodes and eventually into your blood vessels)

>> Bodily secretions such as sweat, seminal fluid, and vaginal fluids

>> Urine

FLUORIDATED WATER: THE REAL TOOTH FAIRY

Except for the common cold, dental cavities are the most common human medical problem.

You get cavities from *mutans streptococci,* bacteria that live in dental plaque. The bacteria digest and ferment carbohydrate residue on your teeth (plain table sugar is the worst offender), leaving acid that eats away at the mineral surface of the tooth. This eating away is called *decay.* When the decay gets past the enamel to the softer pulp inside of the tooth, your tooth hurts. And you head for the dentist even though you hate it so much you'd almost rather put up with the pain. But almost doesn't count, so off you go.

Brushing and flossing help prevent cavities by cleaning your teeth so that bacteria have less to feast on. Another way to reduce your susceptibility to cavities is to drink *fluoridated water* — water containing the mineral fluorine.

Fluoride — the form of fluorine found in food and water — combines with other minerals in teeth and makes the minerals less soluble (harder to dissolve). You get the most benefit by drinking water containing 1 part fluoride to every 1 million parts water (1 ppm) from the day you're born until the day you get your last permanent tooth, usually around age 11 to 13.

Some drinking water, notably in the American Southwest, is fluoridated naturally when it flows through rocks containing fluorine. In fact, sometimes this water contains so much fluoride that it causes a brownish spotting (or mottling) while teeth are developing and accumulating minerals. This doesn't happen with artificially fluoridated drinking water, which has only the approved 1 part fluoride to every 1 million parts of water.

By 2018, 73 percent of Americans with community water systems had access to adequately fluoridated public water supplies. Because fluorides are absorbed into bone, early on, some had feared that this might lead to an increased risk of cancer from fluoridated water. That has proved to be completely untrue. Today, the result of drinking fluoridated water has been an entirely healthful, lifelong 50 percent to 70 percent reduction in cavities. Another good reason why both American and Canadian healthful eating rules say, "Ditch the alternatives, and make water your beverage of choice."

A healthy body must have just the right amount of fluid inside and outside each cell, a situation described as *fluid balance.* Maintaining your fluid balance is essential to life. If there is too little water inside a cell, the cell shrivels and dies. If there's too much water, the cell bursts.

The body maintains its fluid balance through the action of substances called *electrolytes*, mineral compounds that, when dissolved in water, become electrically charged particles called *ions*.

Many minerals, including calcium, phosphorus, and magnesium, form compounds that dissolve into charged particles. But nutritionists generally use the term *electrolyte* to describe sodium, potassium, and chlorine. The most familiar electrolyte is the one found on every dinner table: sodium chloride — plain old table salt whose molecules dissolve in water into two ions: one sodium ion and one chloride ion. (For the non-chemists, an *ion* is an electrically charged atom.)

The electrolytes' primary job

Under normal circumstances, the fluid inside your cells has more potassium than sodium and chloride. The fluid outside is just the opposite: more sodium and chloride than potassium. The cell wall is a *semipermeable membrane*; some things pass through, but others don't. Water molecules and small mineral molecules flow through freely, unlike larger molecules such as proteins.

HOW DOES WATER KNOW WHERE TO GO?

Osmosis is the process governing how water flows through a semipermeable membrane, such as the one surrounding a body cell. It allows water to flow through the membrane from the side where the liquid solution is least dense to the side where it is more dense, thus equalizing the density on both sides of the cellular wall.

You may ask, "How does the water know which side is more dense?" That one's easy: Wherever the sodium content is higher, the fluid is more dense. When more sodium is present inside the cell, more water flows in to dilute it. When more sodium is in the fluid outside the cell, water flows out of the cell to dilute the liquid on the outside.

So when the Ancient Mariner complained, "Water, water everywhere, and not a drop to drink," he wasn't kidding. He was talking about the osmotic process that occurs if you drink seawater, causing liquid to flow out of your cells to dilute the denser salty liquid in your intestinal tract. The more seawater you drink, the more water you lose from your cells as you literally drink yourself into dehydration.

The process by which sodium flows out and potassium flows in to keep things on an even keel is called the *sodium pump.* If this process were to cease, sodium ions would build up inside your cells. Because sodium attracts water, if there is more than a normal amount of sodium inside the cell, extra water will flow in, eventually, bursting and killing the cell. Happily, the sodium pump, regular as a clock, prevents this, allowing you to move along, blissfully unaware of those efficient, electric ions that tell the water in your body where to go. (See the nearby sidebar "How does water know where to go?")

Of course, the same thing happens — though certainly to a lesser degree — when you eat salted pretzels or nuts. The salt in your mouth makes your saliva saltier, drawing liquid out of the cells in your cheeks and tongue, which feel uncomfortably dry. Solution: A glass of water.

Other tasks electrolytes perform

In addition to maintaining fluid balance, sodium, potassium, and chloride (the form of chlorine found in food) ions create electrical impulses that enable cells to send messages back and forth between themselves so you can think, see, move, and perform all the bioelectrical functions that you take for granted.

Sodium, potassium, and chloride are also major minerals (see Chapter 11) and essential nutrients. Like other nutrients, they're useful in these bodily processes:

>> Sodium helps your body digest proteins and carbohydrates and keeps your blood from becoming too acidic or too alkaline.

>> Potassium is used in digestion to synthesize proteins and starch; it's also a major constituent of muscle tissue.

>> Chloride is a constituent of the hydrochloric acid (stomach acid) that breaks down food in your stomach. It's also used by white blood cells to make *hypochlorite,* a natural antiseptic.

Getting the Water You Need

Because the body doesn't store water, you need to take in a new supply every day, enough to replace what you lose when you breathe, perspire, urinate, and defecate. On average, this adds up to 1,500 to 3,000 milliliters (50 to 100 ounces, or 6 to 12.5 cups) a day. Here's how:

>> 850 to 1,200 milliliters (28 to 40 ounces) is lost in breath and perspiration.

>> 600 to 1,600 milliliters (20 to 53 ounces) is lost in urine.

>> 50 to 200 milliliters (1.6 to 6.6 ounces) is lost in feces.

Toss in some extra ounces for a safe margin, and you come up with the anecdotal eight 8- or 10-ounce glasses of water a day. But, in fact, not all the water your body requires has to come from plain water.

For starters, about 15 percent of the water that you need is created when you digest and metabolize food, producing carbon dioxide (a waste product that you breathe out of your body) and water composed of hydrogen from food and oxygen from the air that you breathe. The rest of your daily water comes directly from what you eat and drink.

Next, as nutritionists know, some of the water you require is right there in your food. Fruits and vegetables are full of water. Lettuce, for example, is 90 percent water. Even foods that you'd never think of as water sources provide water, including hamburger (more than 50 percent), cheese (the softer the cheese, the higher the water content — Swiss cheese is 38 percent water; skim milk ricotta, 74 percent), a plain, hard bagel (29 percent water), milk powder (2 percent), and butter and margarine (10 percent). In fact, the only foods with no water are pure oils.

In 2008, the National Institutes of Health bypassed the eight-glass rule, saying that women get enough water from about 91 ounces (2.7 liters) of water a day from all sources; men, about 125 ounces (3.7 liters) a day. And the usual qualifier holds: Everybody is individual, so these are only guidelines. Two years later, three dermatologists at the Kaplan Medical Center of the Hebrew University-Hadassah Medical School in Jerusalem added that while beauty books and "experts" claim that you need six to eight glasses of water to keep your skin smooth, bright, and wrinkle free, they "have found no scientific proof for this recommendation; nor is there proof, we must admit, that drinking less water does absolutely no harm. The only certainty about this issue is that, at the end of the day, we still await scientific evidence to validate what we know instinctively to be true — namely, that is all a myth."

WARNING

Not all liquids are equally liquefying. The caffeine in coffee and tea and the alcohol in beer, wine, and spirits are *diuretics*, chemicals that make you urinate more copiously. Although caffeinated and alcohol beverages provide water, they also increase its elimination from your body — which is why you feel thirsty the morning after you've had a glass or two of wine.

BAD NEWS BOTTLES

Most people in the United States get their drinking water straight from the tap, but a steadily growing number of Americans get theirs in plastic bottles.

Exactly how many people buy exactly how many bottles of water may vary a bit from source to source, but according to the International Bottled Water Association, by 2019, Americans were downing 14.411 billion gallons of bottled water a year, up from about 4.7 billion in 2000. That number translates to nearly 43.7 gallons of bottled water per year for every man, woman, and child in the country.

Those gallons don't come cheap. The National Resource Defense Council estimates that bottled water costs anywhere from 240 to 10,000 (!) times as much as safe tap water. They're also expensive for the environment. Every year, Americans tossed away 38 billion plastic water bottles to live forever in landfills or make their way out to sea. Worldwide, the United Nations estimates that every single square mile of ocean on the planet contains 48,000 pieces of floating plastic. And the World Economic Forum suggests that by the year 2050, there will be more plastic bottles in the sea than there are fish.

Container recycling laws, local bans on bottled water, and newly reusable bottles offer hope of some relief from the tons of plastic garbage. So does new technology suggesting that ultraviolet light and heat may render plastic bottles degradable.

Finally, not all bottled water is fluoridated. So, the better bet is to buy a lightweight thermos and carry tap water. Your wallet, your planet, and your teeth will thank you.

In other words, a healthy adult in a temperate climate who isn't perspiring heavily can get enough water simply by drinking only when he or she is thirsty.

Evaluating Electrolytes

The electrolytes sodium, potassium, and chlorine are chemicals that dissolve in water, separating into atoms called ions that conduct electricity. In your body, electrolytes enable the transfer of messages back and forth between cells so keeping them balanced is essential to maintaining the normal function of your organs, tissues, and cells.

Sodium

The Centers for Disease Control (CDC) estimated that most American adults consume an average 3,400 milligrams (about 1.5 teaspoons) of sodium a day. These are levels of consumption many experts such as the American Heart Association consider protective against hypertension (high blood pressure) and other forms of heart disease.

Certainly, people who are sensitive to sodium or have certain medical conditions, such as diabetes, may indeed end up with high blood pressure that can be lowered if they reduce their sodium intake. For more about high blood pressure, check out *High Blood Pressure For Dummies,* by Alan L. Rubin, MD (Wiley).

The question is whether extra sodium is hazardous to *everyone.* The answer is, maybe not. Like several vitamins, electrolytes dissolve in water, so they're excreted in urine. The amount of electrolytes you put out in your urine is a measure of how much sodium, potassium, and chloride you consumed in food and beverages. The more you take in, the more you put out.

This simple formula proved useful in August 2014, when a team of scientists published a report in the *New England Journal of Medicine* based on data from a Prospective Urban Rural Epidemiology (PURE) survey of more than 100,000 people. Their analysis showed that people at both ends of the excretion spectrum — very low levels and very high levels — had a higher risk of death and cardiovascular disease than those in the middle. Naturally, this has led to many interesting discussions among nutritionists and other experts; the end result is not yet in sight.

Potassium and chloride

Potassium and chloride are found in so many foods that here, too, a dietary deficiency is a rarity. In fact, the only recorded case of chloride deficiency was among infants given a formula liquid from which the chloride was inadvertently omitted. The AI for potassium and chloride are 3,400 milligrams for men age 19 to 70 and 2,600 milligrams for women of the same age.

When you need more

Most Americans get plenty of water and the electrolytes as a matter of course, but sometimes you actually need extra, such as in the following instances.

When you're sick to your stomach

Repeated vomiting or diarrhea drains your body of water and electrolytes. Similarly, you also need extra water to replace the liquid lost in perspiration when you have a high fever.

When you lose enough water to be dangerously dehydrated, you also lose the electrolytes you need to maintain fluid balance, regulate body temperature, and trigger dozens of biochemical reactions. Plain water doesn't replace those electrolytes. Check with your doctor for a drink that will hydrate your body without upsetting your tummy.

When you're exercising or working hard in a hot environment

When you're warm, your body perspires. The moisture evaporates and cools your skin so that blood circulating up from the center of your body to the surface is cooled. The cooled blood returns to the center of your body, lowering the temperature (your *core temperature*) there, too.

WHEN PLAIN WATER IS TOO PLAIN

Serious dehydration calls for serious medicine, such as the World Health Organization's electrolyte replacement formula:

- 6 level teaspoons sugar
- 0.5 teaspoon salt
- 1 quart fluid (approx. 1 liter)

The best fluid is plain, clean water. In an emergency — or in a place where the water is less than perfectly safe — the formula allows substitutes, such as freshly poured coconut water or clear consommé or unsweetened weak tea or fruit juice. If only questionable water is available, boil it.

Warning: If you're reading this while lying in bed exhausted by some variety of *turista* — the traveler's diarrhea acquired from impure drinking water — don't make the formula without absolutely clean glasses, washed in bottled water. Better yet, get paper cups.

If you don't cool your body down, you continue losing water. If you don't replace the lost water, things can get dicey because not only are you losing water, but you're also losing electrolytes. The most common cause of temporary sodium, potassium, and chloride depletion is heavy, uncontrolled perspiration.

WARNING

Deprived of water and electrolytes, your muscles cramp, you're dizzy and weak, and perspiration, now uncontrolled, no longer cools you. Your core body temperature begins rising, and without relief — air conditioning or a cool shower, plus water, ginger ale, or fruit juice — you may progress from heat cramps to heat exhaustion to heat stroke. The latter is potentially fatal.

When you're on a high-protein diet

You need extra water to eliminate the nitrogen compounds in protein. This is true of infants on high-protein formulas and adults on high-protein weight-reducing diets. See Chapter 6 to find out why too much protein may be so harmful.

When you're taking certain medications

Because some medications interact with water and electrolytes, always ask whether you need extra water and electrolytes whenever your doctor prescribes the following:

>> **Diuretics:** These drugs increase the loss of sodium, potassium, and chloride.

>> **Neomycin (an antibiotic):** This medicine binds sodium into insoluble compounds, making it less available to your body.

>> **Colchicine (an antigout drug):** This medicine lowers your body's absorption of sodium.

Dehydration: When the Body Doesn't Get Enough Water

Every day, you lose an amount of water equal to about 4 percent of your total weight. If you don't take in enough water to replace it, warning signals go off loud and clear.

First signs

Early on, when you've lost just a little water, equal to about 1 percent of your body weight, you feel thirsty. If you ignore thirst, it grows more intense.

When water loss rises to about 2 percent of your weight, your appetite fades. Your circulation slows as water seeps out of blood cells and blood plasma. And you experience a sense of emotional discomfort, a perception that things are, well, not right.

Worsening problems

By the time your water loss equals 4 percent of your body weight (5 pounds for a 130-pound woman; 7 pounds for a 170-pound man), you're slightly nauseated, your skin is flushed, and you're very, very tired. With less water circulating through your tissues, your hands and feet tingle, your head aches, your temperature rises, you breathe more quickly, and your pulse quickens.

Really bad trouble

After this, things go downhill more quickly. When your water loss reaches 10 percent of your body weight, your tongue swells, your kidneys start to fail, and you're so dizzy that you can't stand on one foot with your eyes closed. In fact, you probably can't even try: Your muscles are in spasm.

When you lose enough water to equal 15 percent of your body weight, you're deaf and pretty much unable to see out of eyes that are sunken and covered with stiffened lids. Your skin has shrunk, and your tongue has shriveled.

The crash

When you've lost water equal to 20 percent of your body weight, your body is at the limit of its endurance. Deprived of life-giving liquid, your skin cracks, and your organs grind to a halt. And so do you.

Ave atque vale, or as the Romans say when in the United States, Canada, Great Britain, Australia, or any place where English is the mother tongue: "Hail and Farewell."

WATER WORDS

Chemically speaking, H$_2$O (one molecule hydrogen, two molecules oxygen) is a queer duck, the only substance on earth that exists as a liquid (water) and a solid (ice) — but never as a bendable plastic material. No, as chemistry teachers explain each year to first-year chemistry students, snow is not plastic water. It's a collection of solids (ice crystals). Semantically speaking, water is also challenging. For starters, water may be hard or soft, but these terms have nothing to do with how the water feels on your hand. They describe the liquid's mineral content:

- *Hard water* has lots of minerals, particularly calcium and magnesium. This water rises to the Earth's surface from underground springs, picking up calcium carbonate as it moves up through the ground.

- *Soft water* has fewer minerals. In nature, soft water is surface water, the runoff from rain-swollen streams or rainwater that falls directly into reservoirs. *Water softeners* are products that attract and remove the minerals in water.

What you get at the supermarket is another list of water words:

- *Distilled water* is tap water that has been *distilled,* or boiled until it turns to steam, which is then collected and condensed back into a liquid free of impurities, chemicals, and minerals. The term *distilled* is also used to describe a liquid produced by *ultrafiltration,* a process that removes everything from the water except water molecules. Distilled water makes clean, clear ice cubes and serves as a flavor-free mixer or base for tea and coffee. It won't clog a steam iron, and it's valuable for chemical and pharmaceutical processing.

- *Spring water* is water from springs relatively near the Earth's surface. This water has fewer mineral particles and what some people describe as a "cleaner taste" than mineral water.

- *Mineral water* is water from deeper down; it picks up minerals on its journey upwards. Mineral spring water is naturally alkaline, which makes it a natural antacid and a mild diuretic.

- *Still water* is spring water that flows up to the surface on its own. *Sparkling water* is pushed to the top by naturally occurring gases in the underground spring. So, you ask, what's the big difference? Sparkling water has bubbles; still water doesn't.

- *Springlike* or *spring fresh* are terms designed to make the water in the bottle seem more prestigious. Products labeled with these terms aren't spring water; they're most likely to be filtered tap water, the liquid that flows out when you turn on the faucet (see *distilled water,* earlier in this list).

Chapter **13**

Added Attractions: Supplements

Dietary supplements are a *big* business. In 2017 alone, Americans spent more than $8 billion on everything from herbal supplements to concentrated caffeine powder and cannabis oil, the latest entrant onto the scene. By 2024, the figure for *nutraceuticals* (foods that act like medicines) is expected to cross the $100 billion line.

You can stir up a good food fight in any group of nutrition experts simply by asking whether all these products are (a) necessary, (b) economical, or (c) safe. But when the argument's over, you still may not have a satisfactory *official* answer, so this brief chapter aims to provide the information you need to make your own sensible choices.

Introducing Dietary Supplements

Your daily vitamin pill is a dietary supplement. So are the calcium antacids many American women consider standard nutrition and the vanilla, chocolate, or strawberry liquid your granny chug-a-lugs each afternoon before setting out on her power walk. In fact, according to the Food and Drug Administration, any tablet, capsule, powder, or liquid you take by mouth that contains a dietary ingredient is a dietary supplement. That includes

>> Vitamins

>> Minerals

>> Herbs and spices, such as echinacea, which presumes to ward off colds, and ginger, which is said to relieve seasickness

>> Amino acids (the "building blocks of protein" described in Chapter 6)

>> Enzymes, such as lactase, the one that turns lactose (milk sugar) into lactic acid (see Chapter 2 for how enzymes empower your digestive tract)

>> Organ tissue, such as dried liver

>> Some hormones, such as melatonin, the purported sleep aid

>> Metabolites (substances produced when nutrients are digested)

>> Extracts

Dietary supplements may be single-ingredient products, such as vitamin E capsules, or they may be combination products, such as multivitamin and mineral pills, or the ubiquitous and controversial "energy drinks" whose "energy" is mostly caffeine-fueled. In a country where food is plentiful and affordable, you have to wonder why so many people opt to rely on these products instead of just plain food.

MORE THAN FOOD, LESS THAN MEDS

As mentioned earlier in the chapter, nutraceuticals are foods with medical properties. Two simple examples are fish oil, which is reputed to improve heart health, and probiotics, whose claim to fame is their ability to help regulate the gastrointestinal system. (More about probiotics in Chapter 2.) Some nutraceuticals have been tested and show promise in benefiting human health. Others are considered safe but not proven effective. Both may be safe for some but potentially harmful to others. For example, some protein powders contain casein, a protein found in milk which can trigger allergic reactions in people sensitive to dairy products. Like food and dietary supplements, nutraceuticals are the province of the Food and Drug Administration (FDA) in the United States. (In Canada, these products are regulated by the Natural and Non-prescription Health Products Directorate [NNHPD].)

Examining Two Reasons to Use Dietary Supplements

Many people consider supplements a quick and easy way to get nutrients without much shopping and kitchen time and without all the pesky fats and sugars in food. Others take supplements as nutritional insurance. (For more on Recommended Dietary Allowances of vitamins and minerals, see Chapters 10 and 11.) And some use supplements as substitutes for medical drugs.

TIP

In general, nutrition experts, including the American Dietetic Association, the National Academy of Sciences, and the National Research Council, prefer that you invest your time and money whipping up meals and snacks that supply the nutrients you need in a balanced diet of real food.

Nonetheless, every expert admits that supplements may be valuable for people with specific nutritional needs and as an insurance policy in certain circumstances.

When food isn't enough

Some metabolic disorders and diseases of the digestive organs (liver, gallbladder, pancreas, and intestines) and some medicines interfere with the normal digestion of food and the absorption of nutrients, meaning you may need supplements to make up the difference. People who suffer from certain chronic diseases or who have experienced a major injury (such as a serious burn), or who have just been through surgery may also need more nutrients than they can get from food.

WARNING

To be safe, check with your doctor before opting for a supplement you hope will have medical effects (make you stronger, smooth your skin, ease your anxiety, and so forth). Your doctor, the person most familiar with your health, knows what medications you're taking and can caution you about potential side effects.

Supplementing aging appetites

As you grow older, your appetite may decline and your sense of taste and smell may falter. If food no longer tastes as good as it once did, if you have to eat alone all the time and don't enjoy cooking for one, or if dentures make chewing difficult, you may not be taking in all the foods that you need to get the nutrients you need, and dietary supplements may be the answer.

Meeting a woman's special needs

At various stages of her reproductive life, a woman may benefit from supplements. For example:

» **Before menopause:** Women, who lose iron each month through menstrual bleeding, rarely get sufficient amounts of iron from a typical American diet providing fewer than 2,000 calories a day. For them, and for women who are on a weight-loss diet, iron supplements may be the only practical answer. Deciding which iron pill to choose? Check out Chapter 11.

» **During pregnancy and lactation:** Before and during pregnancy, supplements of the B vitamin folate are known to decrease a woman's risk of giving birth to a child with a neural tube defect (a defect of the spinal cord and column). While pregnant, women often need supplements to provide the nutrients they need to build new maternal and fetal tissue; once the baby is born, supplements provide the nutrients needed to produce healthful breast milk.

WARNING

Don't self-prescribe while pregnant. Even simple nutrients may be hazardous for your baby. For example, megadoses of vitamin A while pregnant may increase the risk of birth defects.

» **Through adulthood:** True, women older than 19 can get the calcium they require (1,000 milligrams per day) from four 8-ounce glasses of nonfat skim milk, three 8-ounce or four 6-ounce containers of yogurt made with nonfat milk, 22 ounces of canned salmon (with the soft edible bones; definitely not the hard bones in fresh salmon!), or any proportional combination of the above. However, expecting women to do this nutritional balancing act every single day may be unrealistic. The simple alternative is calcium supplements.

Boosting a special diet

Vitamin B12 is found only in food from animals, such as meat, milk, and eggs. (Some seaweed does have B12, but the suspicion is that the vitamin comes from microorganisms living in the plant.) Once upon a time, *vegans* (people who eat only plant foods — no dairy foods or eggs allowed) would almost certainly have had to get their B12 from supplements. Today, fortified grains may do the trick, but some vegans still add B12 to be sure.

Using supplements as insurance

Some healthy people who eat a nutritious diet still choose supplements to make sure they're getting adequate nutrition.

At first glance, it seemed they might be right. In 2002, the American Medical Association (AMA), which for decades had turned thumbs down on vitamin supplements, changed its collective mind after a review of 26 years' worth of scientific studies relating vitamin levels to the risk of chronic illness. Robert H. Fletcher and Kathleen M. Fairfield, the Harvard-based authors of the study, which was published in the *Journal of the American Medical Association (JAMA),* noted that while true vitamin-deficiency diseases such as scurvy and beriberi are rare in Western countries, *suboptimal vitamin levels* — sciencespeak for slightly less than you need — are a real problem. If "slightly less than you need" sounds slightly less than important, consider this:

>> Suboptimal intake of folate and two other B vitamins (B6 and B12) may raise your risk of heart disease, colon cancer, breast cancer, and birth defects.

>> Suboptimal vitamin D intake means a higher risk of rickets and osteoporosis.

However, there is no evidence that swallowing large amounts of some vitamins will reduce your risk of cancer. In fact, in 2009, a report in *The Archives of Internal Medicine* summarizing data from an analysis of more than 150,000 women showed that taking multivitamins every day had no effect on the risk for breast cancer, colorectal cancer, endometrial cancer, lung cancer, ovarian cancer, heart attack, stroke, blood clots, or mortality. The study's author, Marian L. Neuhouser, a nutritional epidemiologist with the Fred Hutchinson Cancer Research Center in Seattle, was quoted as concluding that "buying more fruits and vegetables might be a better choice." Tastes better, too.

Who takes dietary supplements? Seventy-seven percent of all U.S. adults take dietary supplements of some kind. Here's a further breakdown:

>> 79 percent of female adults

>> 74 percent of male adults

>> 70 percent of adults 18–34

>> 81 percent of adults 35–54

>> 79 percent of adults 55+

>> 76 percent of retired adults

>> 81 percent of adults who are married

>> 73 percent of adults who live in the Northeast

>> 74 percent of adults who live in the Midwest

>> 80 percent of adults who live in the South

Exploring Supplement Safety: An Iffy Proposition

As its name implies, the Food and Drug Administration (FDA) regulates drugs *and* food. Before the agency allows a new food or a new drug on the market, the manufacturer must submit proof that the product is safe. Drug manufacturers must also meet a second test, showing that their new medicine is *efficacious,* meaning that it works and that the drug and the dosage in which it's sold will cure or relieve the condition for which it's prescribed.

Nobody says the drug-regulation system is perfect. Reality dictates that manufacturers test a drug only on a limited number of people for a limited period of time. So you can bet that some new drugs will trigger unexpected, serious, maybe even life-threatening side effects when used by thousands of people or taken for longer than the testing period. For proof, look no further than the multiple recalls FDA has issued over the last decades. But at least the FDA can require that premarket safety and/or effectiveness info be displayed on foods and drugs. Unfortunately, the agency has no such power when it comes to dietary supplements. In 1994, Congress passed and President Clinton signed into law the Dietary Supplement Health and Education Act, which limits the FDA's control over dietary supplements. Under this law, the FDA can't

» Require premarket tests to prove that supplements are safe and effective.

» Limit the dosage in any dietary supplement.

» Halt or restrict sales of a dietary supplement unless evidence shows that the product has caused illness or injury *when used according to the directions on the package;* in other words, if you experience a problem after taking slightly more or less of a supplement than directed on the label, the FDA can't help you.

As a result, the FDA has found it virtually impossible to take products off drugstore shelves even after reports of illness and injury. The classic example is that of supplements containing the herb *ephedra,* once sold for their reputed ability to enhance weight loss and sports performance. More than 600 reports of illness and at least 100 deaths were linked to the use of ephedra supplements. The herb was banned by professional football and college athletics in the United States and by the Olympics. However, the FDA didn't act until February 2003, following the death of Baltimore Orioles pitcher Steve Bechler, who reportedly had been using ephedra products to control his weight. Bechler's untimely death rang warning bells across the country, including in Washington, D.C., where the FDA ruled that henceforth every bottle of ephedra must carry strong warnings that the popular herb can cause potentially lethal heart attacks or strokes. In the sports world, ephedra was immediately forbidden in minor-league but not major-league baseball. The FDA then banned all ephedra products, and despite a challenge from an ephedra manufacturer, the ban was upheld by the U.S. Court of Appeals for the Tenth Circuit in 2006.

More recently, in April 2019, the FDA issued warning letters to companies selling supplements containing DMHA (also known as dimethylhexylamine and octodrine), a central nervous system simulant often marketed for sports performance and weight loss. A second set of warning letters was issued for products containing phenibut, sometimes marketed for uses such as a sleep aid, although it does not meet the definition of a dietary supplement.

WARNING

Of course, these are not the only problematic herbal supplements. For a list of some well-known offenders, see Table 13-1.

TABLE 13-1 ## Some Potentially Hazardous Herbal Products

Herbal Product	Possible Side Effects and Interactions
Acacia rigidula (also known as acacia blackbrush, Chaparro Prieto, Vachellia rigidula)	Rapid heartbeat, palpitations, cardiac arrest, hypertension.
Concentrated caffeine powders and liquids	One teaspoon of pure caffeine powder may be equal to 28 cups of regular coffee, a toxic amount that may cause rapid or erratic heartbeat, seizures, gastric upset (vomiting, diarrhea) disorientation, and (in extreme cases) death.
Cayenne	Increased risk of bleeding for people taking blood thinners such as warfarin (Coumadin) and clopidogrel (Plavix)
Cesium (cesium salts)	Irregular heartbeat, lowered potassium, seizures, fainting, and (rarely) death.
Dong quai	Increased risk of bleeding for people taking blood thinners such as warfarin (Coumadin) and clopidogrel (Plavix)
Echinacea	Decreased effectiveness of immunosuppressant drugs, leading to transplant rejection
	Can be toxic and can cause copper deficiency when taken with zinc

(continued)

TABLE 13-1 *(continued)*

Herbal Product	Possible Side Effects and Interactions
Garlic	Increased risk of bleeding for people taking blood thinners such as warfarin (Coumadin) and clopidogrel (Plavix)
	Increased effect of hypoglycemic drugs used to control blood sugar levels
	Decreased effectiveness of immunosuppressant drugs, leading to transplant rejection
	Decreased effectiveness of oral contraceptives
Ginkgo	Increased risk of bleeding for people taking blood thinners such as warfarin (Coumadin) and clopidogrel (Plavix)
Ginseng	Increased risk of bleeding for people taking blood thinners such as warfarin (Coumadin) and clopidogrel (Plavix)
Glucosamine	Increased insulin resistance in people using hypoglycemic drugs used to control blood sugar levels
Licorice	Decreased effectiveness of the blood thinner warfarin (Coumadin)
St John's Wort	Added rise in serotonin levels, leading to possible fever, muscle rigidity, and altered mental responses for people using antidepressants such as fluoxetine (Prozac and paroxetine (Paxil)
Valerian	Increased sedative effects in people using alcohol, and other sedatives

Sources: The Mayo Clinic, the University of Miami School of Medicine, Food and Drug Administration

Choosing the Most Effective Supplements

Okay, you've read about the virtues and drawbacks of supplements. You've decided which supplements you think may do you some good. Now what you really want to know is how to choose the safest, most effective products. The following guidelines can help:

>> **Pick a well-known brand.** Even though the FDA can't require manufacturers to submit safety and effectiveness data, a respected name on the label offers some assurance of a quality product. It also promises a fresh product; well-known brands generally sell out more quickly. The initials *USP* (U.S. Pharmacopoeia, a reputable testing organization) are another quality statement, and so are the words "release assured" or "proven release," which mean the supplement is easily absorbed by your body.

>> **Look for the expiration date.** Over time, all dietary supplements become less potent. Always choose the product with the longest useful shelf life. Pass

on the ones that will expire before you can use all the pills, such as the 100-pill bottle with an expiration date 30 days from now.

>> **Read the storage requirements.** Even when you buy a product with the correct expiration date, it may be less effective if you don't keep it in the right place. Some supplements must be refrigerated; the rest you need to store, like any food product, in a cool, dry place. Avoid putting dietary supplements in a cabinet above the stove or refrigerator — true, the fridge is cold inside, but the motor pulsing away outside emits heat.

>> **Stick with a safe dose.** Unless your doctor prescribes a dietary supplement as medicine, you don't need products marked "therapeutic," "extra-strength," or any variation thereof. Pick one that gives you no more than the RDA for any ingredient.

>> **Avoid hype.** When the label promises something that's too good to be true, you know it's too good to be true. The FDA doesn't permit supplement marketers to claim that their products cure or prevent disease (that would make them medicines and require premarket testing). But the agency does allow claims that affect function, such as "maintains your cholesterol" (the medical claim would be "lowers your cholesterol").

Another potential hype zone is the one labeled "natural," as in "natural vitamins are better." If you took Chem 101 in college, you know that the ascorbic acid (vitamin C) in oranges has exactly the same chemical composition as the ascorbic acid some nutritional chemist cooks up in her lab. To be fair, the ascorbic acid in a "natural" vitamin pill may come without additives, such as coloring agents or fillers used in "regular" vitamin pills. In other words, if you aren't sensitive to the coloring agents or fillers in plain old pills, don't spend the extra dollars for "natural." If you are sensitive, do. What could be simpler? (For more on "natural" versus "synthetic" food ingredients, see Chapter 22.)

>> **Check the ingredient list.** In the early 1990s, the FDA introduced the consumer-friendly nutrition food label with its mini-nutrition guide to nutrient content, complete ingredient listings, and dependable information about how eating certain foods may affect your risk of chronic illnesses, such as heart disease and cancer. Read it.

TIP

Like foods, supplement labels must list all ingredients. The label for vitamin and mineral products must give you the quantity per nutrient per serving plus the *%DV* (percentage daily value), the percentage of the RDA (Recommended Dietary Allowance). The listings for other dietary supplements, such as botanicals (herbs), must show the quantity per serving plus the part of the plant from which the ingredient is drawn (root, leaves, and so on). A manufacturer's own proprietary blend of two or more botanicals must list the weight of the total blend.

THE BOOST IN A BOTTLE

It all started with Gatorade. In the summer of 1965, a football coach at the University of Florida asked a team of university physicians to explain why so many players wilted in the heat. The answer: loss of fluid and electrolytes (see Chapter 12) when sweating. The result: a thirst-quenching hydrating fluid replacement beverage that soon had the Florida Gators walking over their opponents to end up with a winning season and a win at the Orange Bowl in 1966. (In 2010, Gatorade introduced a new generation of sugar-free products and re-labeled the original as Gatorade G.)

Nothing succeeds like success, of course. Fairly soon, other universities began ordering up some Gatorade for their teams, pro teams bought in, and, by 1983, Gatorade was the official sports drink of the NFL; today it is the official thirst quencher for an entire alphabet including the AFGL, NFL, MLB, NBA, WNBA, USA Basketball, NHL, Association of Volleyball Professionals, and NASCAR.

Eventually, the hydrating liquid for serious athletes morphed into an "energy drink" for amateur athletes with nutrient-packed beverages promising to increase performance and, sometimes, just keep a person awake and alert. To no one's surprise, the most common ingredient in these beverages is the original awake-and-alert substance, caffeine, as in coffee or guarana, a caffeinated berry native to Brazil and Venezuela. Again to no one's surprise, nutrition experts questioned the virtue of adding large amounts of caffeine to one's daily diet to produce a nervous, irritable insomniac with a rapid heartbeat and maybe even high blood pressure. And this is not a minor matter: According to a 2003 report from the *Journal of the American Pharmaceutical Association,* at least four case reports resulted in caffeine-associated deaths and four documented cases of seizures were associated with energy drinks. By 2010, the FDA total was up to 53 illnesses, two permanent disabilities, and five deaths linked directly to two band-name products. Nine years later, in 2019, the Consortium for Health and Military Performance weighed in, recommending that service members from all branches of the Armed Services limit their caffeine intake to no more than 200 milligrams every four hours and no more than 800 milligrams a day.

But in between, to everyone's surprise, a group of consumers sued one of the energy drinks complaining that it didn't have *enough* caffeine. In 2013, the makers of Red Bull agreed to pay out $14.8 million to settle a class action lawsuit claiming that Red Bull's advertising — "Red Bull gives you wings" — was false not because it didn't grow wings on your back, but because one can of the drink contained less caffeine than a cup of Starbucks coffee.

Anyone here want a glass of water? Plain, delicious, and nutritious, as described in Chapter 12.

Figure 13-1 shows an example of the supplement labels.

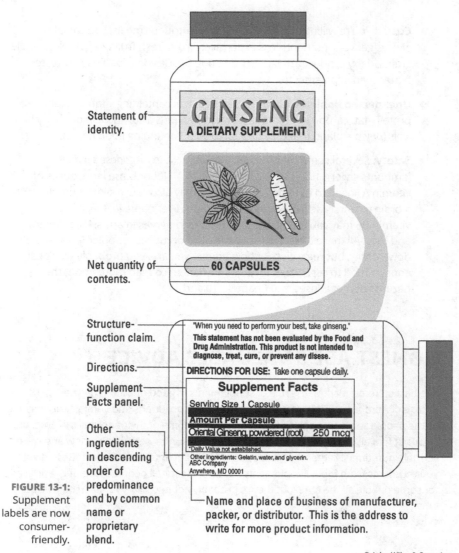

Nutrition Labeling for Dietary Supplements

(Effective March 1999)

Statement of identity.

GINSENG
A DIETARY SUPPLEMENT

Net quantity of contents.

60 CAPSULES

Structure-function claim.

"When you need to perform your best, take ginseng."

This statement has not been evaluated by the Food and Drug Administration. This product is not intended to diagnose, treat, cure, or prevent any disese.

Directions.

DIRECTIONS FOR USE: Take one capsule daily.

Supplement Facts panel.

Supplement Facts

Serving Size 1 Capsule

Amount Per Capsule

Oriental Ginseng, powdered (root)   250 mcg*

*Daily Value not established.

Other ingredients: Gelatin, water, and glycerin.
ABC Company
Anywhere, MD 00001

Other ingredients in descending order of predominance and by common name or proprietary blend.

Name and place of business of manufacturer, packer, or distributor. This is the address to write for more product information.

© John Wiley & Sons, Inc.

FIGURE 13-1: Supplement labels are now consumer-friendly.

Getting Nutrients from Food Rather Than Supplements

Finally, having presented facts in favor of supplements and how to choose the most effective ones, here is why people with no underlying chronic or temporary (think pregnancy) medical conditions or need may be better off getting all or most of their nutrients from food:

» **Cost:** If you're willing to plan and prepare nutritious meals, you can almost always get your nutrients less expensively from fresh fruits, vegetables, whole grains, dairy products, meat, fish, and poultry. Besides, food usually tastes better than supplements.

» **Unexpected bonuses:** Food is a package deal containing vitamins, minerals, protein, fat, carbohydrates, and dietary fiber, plus a cornucopia of phytochemicals (*phyto* = plant) that may be vital to your continuing good health.

» **Safety:** Several common nutrients may be toxic in *megadose servings* (amounts several times larger than the RDAs). Not only are large doses of vitamin A linked to birth defects, but they may also cause symptoms similar to a brain tumor. Niacin megadoses may cause liver damage. Megadoses of vitamin B6 may cause (temporary) damage to nerves in arms, legs, fingers, and toes. All these effects are more likely to occur with supplements. Pills slip down easily, but regardless of how hungry you are, you probably won't eat enough food to reach toxic levels of nutrients. (To read more about the hazards of megadoses, see Chapters 10 and 11.)

HONEST ABE'S VALUABLE ADVICE

The best statement about the role of supplements in good nutrition may be a paraphrase of Abraham Lincoln's famous remark about politicians and voters: "You may fool all the people some of the time; you can even fool some of the people all the time; but you can't fool all of the people all the time." If Honest Abe were with us now and were a sensible nutritionist rather than a president, he might amend his words: "Best to get your nutrients from food. Supplements are valuable for all people some of the time and for some people all the time, but they're probably not necessary for all people all the time."

3

Hunger, Health, and Habits

Chapter **14**

Why You Eat When You Eat

B ecause you need food to live, your body has multiple ways of letting you know that it's ready for breakfast, lunch, dinner, and maybe a few snacks in between. This chapter explains the signals that send you to the kitchen, your favorite fast-food joint, or that pernicious vending machine down the hall.

Underlining the Difference between Hunger and Appetite

People eat for two basic reasons. The first is hunger; the second is appetite. Hunger and appetite are *not* synonyms. In fact, hunger and appetite are entirely different processes.

PAVLOV'S PERFORMING PUPPIES

Ivan Petrovich Pavlov (1849–1936) was a Russian scientist who won the Nobel Prize in physiology/medicine in 1904 for his research on the digestive glands. Pavlov's Big Bang, though, was his identification of respondent conditioning — a fancy way of saying that you can train people to respond physically (or emotionally) to an object or stimulus that simply reminds them of something they love or hate.

Pavlov tested respondent conditioning on dogs. He began by ringing a bell each time he offered food to his laboratory dogs so that the dogs learned to associate the sound of the bell with the sight and smell of food.

Then he rang the bell without offering the food, and the dogs responded as though food were on tap — salivating madly, even though the dish was empty.

Respondent conditioning applies to many things other than food, such as the emotional response someone may experience to the sight of his national flag. Nutrition-wise, the insidious truth is that food companies are great at using respondent conditioning to encourage you to buy their products. One tasty example: When you see a picture of a deep, dark, rich chocolate bar, doesn't your mouth start to water, and — hey, come back! Where are you going?

Hunger is the *need* for food. It is

>> A physical reaction that includes chemical changes in your body related to a naturally low level of glucose in your blood several hours after eating

>> An instinctive, protective mechanism that makes sure your body gets the fuel it requires to function

Appetite is the *desire* for food. It is

>> A sensory or psychological reaction (looks good! smells good!) that stimulates an involuntary physiological response (salivation, stomach contractions)

>> A conditioned response to food (see the nearby sidebar on Pavlov's dogs)

The practical difference between hunger and appetite is this: When you're hungry, you eat one hot dog. After that, your appetite may lead you to eat two more hot dogs just because they look appealing or taste good.

In other words, appetite is the basis for the familiar saying: "Your eyes are bigger than your stomach." Not to mention the well-known advertising slogan: "Bet you can't eat just one." Hey, like Pavlov (see that sidebar again), these guys know their customers.

Refueling: The Cycle of Hunger and Satiety

Your body does its best to create cycles of activity that parallel a 24-hour day. Like sleep, hunger occurs at pretty regular intervals, although your lifestyle may make it difficult to follow this natural pattern.

Recognizing hunger

The clearest signals that your body wants food, right now, are physical reactions from your stomach. An empty one has absolutely no manners. If you don't fill it right away, it will issue an audible, sometimes embarrassing, call for food, the rumble called a *hunger pang.*

Hunger pangs are muscle contractions. When your stomach is full, these contractions and their continual waves down the entire length of the intestine — known as *peristalsis* — move food through your digestive tract (see Chapter 2 for more about digestion). When your stomach is empty, the contractions just squeeze air, and that makes noise.

TECHNICAL STUFF

This phenomenon was first observed in 1912 by an American physiologist named Walter B. Cannon. (Cannon? Rumble? Could you make this up?) Cannon convinced a fellow researcher to swallow a small balloon attached to a thin tube connected to a pressure-sensitive machine. Then Cannon inflated and deflated the balloon to simulate the sensation of a full or empty stomach. Measuring the pressure and frequency of his volunteer's stomach contractions, Cannon discovered that the contractions were strongest and occurred most frequently when the balloon was deflated and the stomach empty. Cannon drew the obvious conclusion: When your stomach is empty, you feel hungry.

Identifying the hormones that say, "I'm hungry" and "I'm full"

Like so many other body functions, hunger is influenced by hormones — in this case, *ghrelin, insulin, PYY* (peptide tyrosine-tyrosine), and *leptin.* These natural chemicals act on the satiety center in your brain (see Figure 14-1) to make sure you get enough to eat — and (perhaps) know when to stop.

>> **Ghrelin:** Ghrelin (pronounced *grel*-in) is a hormone secreted primarily by cells in the lining of the stomach; smaller amounts are secreted by the hypothalamus. Ghrelin is an appetite stimulant that elicits messages from your brain that say, "I'm hungry." If you're fasting or simply cutting back on food to lose weight, your body responds by producing more than normal amounts of ghrelin, triggering a higher than normal desire to eat. This is one way to explain why dieters find it difficult to stick to a reduced-calorie regimen.

>> **Insulin:** Every time you eat, your pancreas secretes *insulin*, a hormone that enables you to transform the food you eat into *glucose*, the simple sugar on which the body runs, and then to move the glucose into body cells. The higher level of insulin temporarily suppresses appetite, but when the amount of glucose circulating in your blood declines again, you may feel empty, which prompts you to eat. Most people experience the natural rise and fall of glucose — and the consequent secretion of insulin — as a relatively smooth pattern that lasts about four hours. ***Note:*** People with Type 1 (insulin dependent) diabetes don't produce the insulin needed to process glucose, so the glucose continues to circulate around the body and is eventually excreted in sugary urine.

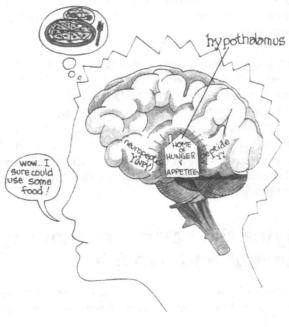

FIGURE 14-1:
Your hypothalamus is in charge of your appetite!

© *John Wiley & Sons, Inc.*

>> **PYY (peptide tyrosine-tyrosine):** After you've eaten, this hormone, secreted by your small intestine and in lesser amounts by cells in other parts of your digestive tract, acts as an appetite suppressant that cancels out ghrelin's appetite-stimulating effects. Some overweight or obese people seem to have an inability to receive PYY's message, which is, "You're full; stop eating."

>> **Leptin:** Leptin, identified in 1995 at Rockefeller University in New York, is produced in the body's fat cells, a source of stored energy. Leptin is an appetite suppressant; if your body loses a lot of fat, you also lose leptin. The result? An increase in the desire for food to increase your store of body fat.

Beating the four-hour hungries

Throughout the world, the cycle of hunger (glucose and insulin rising and falling as described in the preceding section) prompts a feeding schedule that generally provides four meals during the day: breakfast, lunch, a mid-afternoon snack, and supper.

In the United States, a three-meal-a-day culture forces people to fight this natural eating pattern by going without food from lunch at around noon to supper at 6 p.m. or later. The unpleasant result is that when glucose levels go south around 4 p.m. (and people in other countries are enjoying afternoon tea), many Americans get really testy, growl at their coworkers, make mistakes they'll have to correct the next day, or try to satisfy their natural hunger by grabbing the nearest food, usually a high-fat, high-calorie snack. (For a list of calorie-acceptable mid-afternoon snacks, see Chapter 18.)

The better way: Five or six small meals

In 1989, David Jenkins, MD, PhD, and Tom Wolever, MD, PhD, of the University of Toronto, set up a "nibbling study" designed to test the idea that if you even out digestion — by eating several small meals rather than three big ones — you can spread out insulin secretion and keep the amount of glucose in your blood on an even keel all day long.

The theory turned out to be right. People who ate five or six small meals rather than three big ones felt better and experienced an extra bonus: lower cholesterol levels. After two weeks of nibbling, the people in the Jenkins-Wolever study showed that people on the multi-meal regimen had lower levels of cholesterol and lost more weight than people who ate exactly the same amount of food divided into three big meals. (For more on lipoproteins and cholesterol levels, check out Chapter 7. For more on weight control, see Chapter 4.) As a result, some diets designed to help you lose weight now emphasize a daily regimen of several small meals rather than the basic big three. To be fair about it, though, several studies show no beneficial effect, so this is an if-it-works-for-you-do-it issue.

In 2015, scientists at the Salk Institute for Biological Studies in San Diego, California, added another wrinkle: Nibble or gorge, eating within an 8-hour or 12-hour window makes for better bodies. At least in mice. When the researchers allowed their animals to eat anything they wanted but only in a specific 8- or 12-hour window, the mice stayed slimmer and sleeker than their brothers and sisters on the same number of calories that were allowed to eat throughout the 24-hour day.

In 2017, researchers at the university of Alabama, Birmingham, published the results of a small (11-person) study of what they called "early time restricted feeding." What they meant was that their study subjects, all of whom were over-weight, consumed a full day's calories between the hours of 8 a.m. and 2 p.m., a regimen known as *intermittent fasting*. The results were striking: Insulin levels fell, some subjects lost weight, but to everyone's surprise, not a single person felt hungry. Three years later, in the summer of 2020, Miriam Merad, Director of the Precision Immunology Institute at New York's Mt. Dina Hospital's Icahn School of Medicine, reported that in addition to waylaying hunger, helping to control blood pressure, increasing insulin sensitivity, and — yay! — peeling off some pounds, intermittent fasting also seemed to reduce chronic inflammation, such as what people with arthritis experience. Working with both human and mouse cells, Merad discovered that passing up food for a defined, limited period of time appeared to reduce the release of *monocytes*, cells which both fight off invaders such as bad bugs and trigger inflammation. Given the long list of inflammatory conditions, the study results led to the obvious conclusion: "There is enormous potential in investigating the anti-inflammatory effects of controlled fasting."

TIP

Now, most people know they should be sleeping 7 to 8 hours a night. That leaves 16 to 17 hours of wake-time for eating. Want to try intermittent fasting on your own? Set a time limit, say breakfast at 8 a.m. and last snack at 8 p.m., or an hour later in the morning and an hour earlier at night on the 8-hour regimen. And no cheating.

Maintaining a healthy appetite

TIP

The best way to deal with hunger and appetite is to recognize and follow your body's natural cues.

If you're hungry, eat — in reasonable amounts that support a realistic weight. And remember: Nobody's perfect. Make one day's indulgence guilt-free by reducing your calorie intake proportionately over the next few days.

A little give here, a little take there, and you'll stay on target overall.

Responding to Your Environment on a Gut Level

Your physical and psychological environments definitely affect appetite and hunger, sometimes leading you to eat more than normal, sometimes less.

Baby, it's cold outside

Think of the foods that tempt you in winter — stews, roasts, thick soups — versus those you find pleasing on a simmering summer day — salads, chilled fruit, simple sandwiches.

This difference is no accident. Food gives you calories. Calories keep you warm. Yes, you will need more energy if you're running a marathon in the summer than if you're sitting quietly all day in front of the TV while the snow piles up outside.

But as a general rule, to get the energy it needs to keep you warm, your body will say, "I'm hungry," more frequently when it's cold outside. In addition, you process food faster in a cold environment. Your stomach empties more quickly as food speeds along through the digestive tract, which means those old hunger pangs show up sooner than expected so you eat more and stay warmer.

Exercising more than your mouth

Everybody knows that working out gives you a big appetite, right? Well, everybody's wrong. People who exercise regularly are definitely likely to have a healthy (*read:* normal) appetite, but they're rarely hungry immediately after exercising because

>> Exercise pulls stored energy — glucose and fat — out of body tissues, so your glucose levels stay steady and you don't feel hungry.

>> Exercise slows the passage of food through the digestive tract. Your stomach empties more slowly, and you feel fuller longer.

   Caution: If you eat a heavy meal right before heading for the gym or the stationary bike in your bedroom, the food sitting in your stomach may make you feel stuffed. Sometimes, you may develop cramps or — as Ken DeVault, MD, and I explain in *Heartburn & Reflux For Dummies* (Wiley) — heartburn.

>> Exercise (including mental exertion) reduces anxiety. For some people, that means less desire to reach for a snack.

Taking medicine that changes your appetite

Some drugs affect your appetite, leading you to eat more (or less) than usual. This side effect is rarely mentioned when doctors hand out prescriptions, perhaps because it isn't life-threatening and usually disappears when you stop taking the drug or simply because your doctor doesn't know about it. Some examples of appetite uppers are certain antidepressants, antihistamines (allergy pills), diuretics (drugs that make you urinate more frequently), steroids (drugs that fight inflammation), and tranquilizers (calming drugs). Medicines that may reduce your appetite include some antibiotics, anticancer drugs, antiseizure drugs, blood pressure medications, and cholesterol-lowering drugs.

WARNING

Not every drug in a particular class of drugs has the same effect on appetite. For example, the antidepressant drug amitriptyline (Elavil) increases your appetite while fluoxetine (Prozac) may either increase or decrease your desire for food.

Revealing Unhealthy Relationships with Food

This chapter, as the title says, is about why you eat when you eat. Up until this point, the reasons have been physiological: Your hormones say you're hungry or full, or perhaps the weather says you need more food (or less) for energy. But sometimes, the decision to eat or not eat is triggered by an *eating disorder,* a psychological illness that leads you to eat either too much or too little or to regard food as your enemy or your savior.

Indulging in a hot fudge sundae or two once in a while isn't an eating disorder. Neither is dieting for three weeks so you can fit into last year's dress this New Year's Eve. Nor is the determination to eat a healthful diet. The difference between these behaviors and an eating disorder is that these are medically acceptable while eating disorders are potentially life-threatening illnesses that require immediate medical attention.

For some people, food is not simply a meal. It is the object of love or loathing, a way to relieve anxiety or an anxiety provoker. As a result, human beings may experience various eating disorders — *obesity, anorexia nervosa, bulimia,* and *binge eating* — which I describe in the following sections.

WARNING

Eating disorders are serious, potentially life-threatening conditions. If you (or someone you know) experience any of the signs and symptoms described in the following sections, the safest course is to seek immediate medical advice and treatment. For more info about eating conditions, contact the National Eating Disorders Association, 165 West 46th Street, Suite 402, New York, NY 10036; national helpline 1-800-931-2237; website www.nationaleatingdisorders.org.

Obesity

Although everyone knows that there's a worldwide increase in obesity (spelled out in Chapter 4), not everyone who is larger or heavier than the current ideal body has an eating disorder. Human bodies come in many different sizes, and some healthy people are just naturally larger or heavier than others. But an eating disorder may be present when

» A person continually confuses the desire for food (appetite) with the need for food (hunger)

» A person who has access to a normal diet experiences psychological distress when denied food

>> A person uses food to relieve anxiety provoked by what he or she considers a scary situation — a new job, a party, ordinary criticism, or a deadline

Traditionally, doctors find it difficult to treat obesity, but in recent years, some studies have suggested that some people overeat in response to irregularities in the production of chemicals that regulate satiety (the feeling of fullness). This research may open the path to new kinds of drugs that can control extreme appetite, thus reducing the incidence of obesity-related disorders, such as arthritis, diabetes, high blood pressure, and heart disease.

Anorexia nervosa

Anorexia is voluntary starvation, a condition often considered an affliction of affluence, most likely to strike the young and well-to-do, men as well as women, although more commonly women.

TIP

The signs of anorexia are weight less than 85 percent of the normal weight, a fear of gaining weight, an obsession with one's appearance, and the belief that one is fat regardless of the true weight. For young women, anorexia can lead to the absence of menstrual cycles.

Up to 40 percent of people with anorexia develop *bulimia nervosa*; up to 30 percent develop *binge eating disorder*, the next two problems in this section. Left untreated, anorexia nervosa may be fatal.

Until recently, anorexia was considered simply a psychiatric disorder, but in 2019 a new possibility emerged. Comparing DNA from nearly 17,000 anorectics and more than 55,000 healthy "controls," researchers at King's College, London, and the University of North Carolina at Chapel Hill discovered eight common genes linking anorexia to genes involved in the body's ability to burn fat, be physically active, and sustain a resistance to Type 2 diabetes. In short, said King's College geneticist Gerome Breen: "We can no longer treat anorexia, and perhaps other eating disorders, as purely psychiatric or psychological."

Bulimia nervosa

Unlike people with anorexia, individuals with bulimia don't refuse to eat, but they don't want to hold on to the food they've consumed. They may use laxatives to increase defecation, or they may simply retire to the bathroom after eating to take *emetics* (drugs that induce vomiting) or stick their fingers into their throats to make themselves throw up. Like anorexics, bulimics may develop *binge eating disorder*.

Either way, danger looms. Repeated regurgitation can severely irritate or even tear through the lining of the esophagus (throat). Acidic stomach contents also damage teeth, which is why dentists are often the first medical personnel to identify a bulimic. Finally, the continued use of emetics may result in a life-threatening loss of potassium that triggers irregular heartbeat or heart failure.

Binge eating disorder

The criterion for a diagnosis of binge eating disorder is consuming enormous amounts of food — a whole chicken, several pints of ice cream, an entire loaf of bread — in one sitting twice a week for up to six months. Some binge eaters become overweight; others stay slim by regurgitating. Either way, binge eating, like other eating disorders, is hazardous behavior.

Binge eaters who regurgitate experience adverse effects similar to those associated with bulimia. Binge eaters who don't regurgitate risk not only obesity but also, paradoxically, malnutrition. Why? Because the foods they choose may be high in calories but low in vital nutrients. (Think hot fudge sundae again, and again, and again.) More dramatically, the enormous quantities of food they consume may dilate or even rupture the stomach or esophagus, a potentially fatal medical emergency.

FROM FINGERS TO FORKS

For most people, the words "food processing" means cooking, smoking, freezing, canning or vacuum packing food. But the most important step in processing food is processing it from your plate to your mouth, Our earliest ancestors used their hands, but as man (and woman) advanced, so did their table tools. First came the stone knife to spear and slice. Next, the clay, bone, or wooden spoon. Sticks came somewhere in between, with rounded ends in China and pointed ones in Japan, both perfectly suited to capturing and lifting the small pieces in Asian cuisine. Finally, we invented our most complicated serving piece, the fork, first used, like spoons and sticks to stir the pot. But with time, forks multiplied into multiple shapes to match different foods. True, there's the simple dinner fork used for, well, dinner, and the similar but smaller luncheon fork. There are also oyster forks, pickle forks, spaghetti forks designed to twist pasta strands into a liftable unit, and finally, the Spork, a spoon with tines trademarked in the 1960s. Sure beats trying to scoop up ice cream with your fingers.

Chapter **15**

Why You Like the Foods You Like

N utritionally speaking, *taste* is the ability to perceive flavors in food and beverages. *Preference* is the appreciation of one food and distaste of another. Decisions about taste are physical reactions that are dependent on specialized body organs called taste buds. Although your culture has a decided influence on what you think is good to eat, decisions about food preferences may also depend on your genes, your medical history, and your personal reactions to specific foods.

Tackling Taste: How Your Brain and Tongue Work Together

Your *taste buds* are sensory organs that enable you to perceive different flavors in food — in other words, to taste the food you eat.

Taste buds (also referred to as *taste papillae*) are tiny bumps on the surface of your tongue (see Figure 15-1). Each one contains groups of receptor cells that anchor an antenna-like structure called a *microvillus,* which projects up through a gap (or pore) in the center of the taste bud, sort of like a thread sticking through the hole in Life Savers candy. (For more about the microvilli and how they behave in your digestive tract, see Chapter 2.)

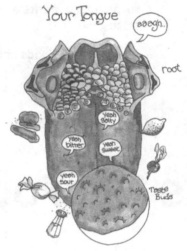

FIGURE 15-1:
Your tongue up close.

The microvilli in your taste buds transmit messages from flavor chemicals in the food along nerve fibers to your brain, which translates the messages into perceptions: "That's good," or "That's awful."

The five basic flavors

Your taste buds recognize five basic flavors: *sweet, sour, bitter, salty,* and *umami* — the last a Japanese word describing richness or a savory flavor associated with glutamate (or glutamic acid), the amino acid responsible for the distinctive flavor of soy products, such as soybeans, tofu, and tempeh.

TECHNICAL STUFF

At first, scientists believed that people had specific taste buds for specific flavors: sweet taste buds for sweets, sour taste buds for sour, and so on. Modern science proposes that groups of taste buds work together so that flavor chemicals in food link up with chemical bonds in taste buds to create patterns that you recognize as sweet, sour, bitter, salty, and, yes, umami. The technical term for this process is *across–fiber pattern theory of gustatory coding.* Receptor patterns for the sweet, sour, bitter, and salty have been tentatively identified, but the pattern for umami remains elusive.

Having named the five basic flavors, nutrition researchers now suggest that there are also taste bud patterns to recognize six more:

>> *Calcium,* which many describe as "bitter and chalky" on its own, a flavor camouflaged by the fat in dairy products.

>> *Carbon dioxide (CO2),* the gas that gives soft drinks and champagne their fizz. In 2009, researchers discovered an enzyme on mouse sour tasting cells specific to tasting C02. Whether this is true in humans as well remains a question.

>> *Coolness,* the fresh minty flavor of peppermint transmitted to your brain, which translates as something cool.

>> *Fat,* which is either a flavor or a creamy sensation. People who are sensitive to the flavor (or creaminess) of fat are less likely to be overweight, probably because a little high-calorie fatty food is just enough.

>> *Kokumi,* the Japanese word meaning "hearty," for an ingredient that interacts with calcium to enhance other flavors.

>> *Piquancy,* a "hot" flavor detected when receptors in the tongue called *molecular thermometers* come in contact with a spicy ingredient, such as the capsaicin in hot pepper.

The way we experience these six flavors remains to be conclusively identified so stay tuned: You never know what other wonders your sensory system may eventually reveal.

Your health and your taste buds

Some illnesses, including the common cold and the notorious COVID-19, alter your ability to taste foods. The result may be partial or total *ageusia* (the medical term for loss of taste). Or you may experience *flavor confusion* — meaning that you mix up flavors, translating sour as bitter, or sweet as salty, or vice versa.

Table 15-1 lists some medical conditions that affect your sense of taste.

TABLE 15-1 **Things That Make It Difficult to Taste Your Food**

This Condition	May Do This
A bacterial or viral infection of the tongue	Produce secretions that block your taste buds
Injury to your mouth, nose, or throat	Damage nerves that transmit flavor signals
Radiation therapy to mouth and throat	Damage nerves that transmit flavor signals

Some meds also affect your sense of taste. For example, some stimulants, such as Adderall and methylphenidate (Ritalin), make bitter flavors more intense. The antibiotics penicillin, amoxicillin, Augmentin, Ancef, and Keflex may affect your body's absorption of zinc creating a deficiency that leaves a metallic taste in your mouth. Some other antibiotics, such as Biaxin, Flagyl, and tetracycline plus Lithium (a drug used to treat bipolar disorder) also leave you tasting metal, but no one actually knows why. If you are taking Accutane to treat severe acne, best pass up the lemon drops — this med interrupts the sensory channels that let you taste sour. Finally, there are the meds which totally temporarily wipe out your sense of taste. The list includes the anti-seizure drugs Tegretol, Carbatrol, and Equetro; Bentyl and Levsin, which are prescribed to alleviate irritable bowel syndrome (IBS); Diltiazem and hydrochlorothiazide (HCTZ) to lower blood pressure; the diuretic Aldactone; and last but not least, Lamisil, which treats fingernail and toenail fungus.

THE NOSE KNOWS — AND THE EYES HAVE IT

As Chapter 2 explains, your nose is important to your sense of taste. Just like the taste of food, the aroma of food also stimulates sensory messages. Think about how you sniff your brandy before drinking and how the wonderful aroma of baking bread warms the heart and stirs the soul — not to mention the salivary glands. When you can't smell, you can't really taste. As anyone who's ever had a cold knows, when your nose is stuffed and your sense of smell is deadened, almost everything tastes like plain old cotton. Don't have a cold? You can test this theory by closing your eyes, pinching your nostrils shut, and having someone put a tiny piece of either a raw onion or a fresh apple into your mouth. Bet you can't tell which is which without looking — or sniffing!

Food color is also an important clue to what you'll enjoy eating. Repeated studies show that when testers change the expected color of foods, people find them (the foods, not the testers) less appealing. For example, blue mashed potatoes or green beef lose to plain old white mashed potatoes and red meat every time.

One famous food taste experiment is performed with gelatin whose flavor doesn't match its color. Without even thinking twice, more than half the volunteers in the test will say the gelatin tastes like the flavor associated with its color — for example, green gelatin tastes like lime and orange like oranges — even when the flavors are actually the opposite.

Tricking your taste buds

Combining foods can short-circuit your taste buds' ability to identify flavors correctly. For example, when you sip wine (even an apparently smooth and silky one), your taste buds taste something sharp. Take a bite of cheese first, though, and the wine tastes smoother (less acidic) because the cheese's fat and protein molecules coat your receptor cells so that acidic wine molecules can't connect.

A similar phenomenon occurs during serial wine tastings (sampling many wines, one after another). Try two equally dry, acidic wines, and the second seems mellower because acid molecules from the first one fill up space on the chemical bonds that perceive acidity. Drink a sweet wine after a dry one, and the sweetness often is more pronounced.

Here's another way to fool your taste buds: Eat an artichoke. The meaty part at the base of the artichoke leaves contains *cynarin*, a sweet-tasting chemical that makes any food you taste after the artichoke taste sweeter.

Determining Deliciousness

When it comes to deciding what tastes good, all human beings and most animals have four things in common: They like sweets, crave salt, go for the fat, and avoid the bitter (at least at first).

These choices are rooted deep in biology and evolution. In fact, you can say that whenever you reach for something that you consider good to eat, the entire human race — especially your own individual ancestors — reaches with you.

Listening to your body

Here's something to chew on: The foods that taste good — sweet foods, salty foods, fatty foods — are essential for a healthy body.

>> Sweet foods are a source of quick energy because their sugars can be converted quickly to glucose, the molecule that your body burns for energy. (Check out Chapter 8 for an explanation of how your body uses sugars.)

Better yet, sweet foods make you feel good. Eating them tells your brain to release natural painkillers called *endorphins*. Sweet foods may also stimulate an increase in blood levels of *adrenaline*, a hormone secreted by the adrenal glands. Adrenaline sometimes is labeled the *fight-or-flight hormone* because it's secreted more heavily when you feel threatened and must decide whether to stand your ground — *fight* — or hurry away — *flight.*

>> Salt is vital to life. As Chapter 12 explains, salt enables your body to maintain its fluid balance and to regulate chemicals called electrolytes that give your nerve cells the power needed to fire electrical charges that energize your muscles, power up your organs, and transmit messages from your brain.

>> Fatty foods are even richer in calories (energy) than sugars. So the fact that you want them most when you're very hungry comes as no surprise. (Chapters 5 and 7 explain how you use fats for energy.)

>> Which fatty food you want may depend on your gender. Numerous studies suggest that women like their fats with sugar (think chocolate). Men, on the other hand, seem to prefer their fat with salt (think fries).

One explanation for the increase in obesity among Americans (see Chapter 4) may be the food industry's manipulating our natural desire for rich foods by creating layered products: sugar on top of fat on top of salt. Or vice versa. Need proof? Look no further than the diabolically delicious pretzel M&Ms introduced in 2010: sugar coating on top of fatty chocolate on top of salty pretzel dishing up 150 calories, 4.5 grams fat, 24 grams carbohydrates (17 of them sugars) per ounce. Yum? Or yipes?

Loving the food you're with: Geography and taste

Marvin Harris was an anthropologist with a special interest in the history of food. In his perfectly delightful classic book, *Good to Eat: Riddles of Food and Culture* (Simon & Schuster, 1998), Harris posed this interesting situation.

Suppose that you live in a forest where someone has pinned $20 and $1 bills to the upper branches of the trees. Which will you reach for? The $20 bills, of course. But wait. Suppose that only a couple of $20 bills are pinned to branches among millions and millions of $1 bills.

Now, substitute chickens for $20 bills and large insects for $1 bills, and you can see why people who live in places where insects far outnumber the chickens spend their time and energy picking off the plentiful high-protein bugs rather than chasing after the occasional chicken — although they wouldn't turn it down if one fell into the pot.

CREEPY CRAWLY NUTRIENTS

Who's to say grilled grasshopper is less appetizing than a lobster? After all, both have long skinny bodies and plenty of legs. The surprising difference is in the nutrients: The bug beats the lobster hands (legs?) down.

Food 3.5 oz	Protein (g)	Fat (g)	Carbohydrates (g)	Iron (mg)
Water beetle	19.8	8.3	2.1	13.6
Red ant	13.9	3.5	2.9	5.7
Cricket	12.9	5.5	5.1	9.5
Small grasshopper	14.3	3.3	2.2	3.0
Large grasshopper	20.6	6.1	3.9	5.0
Lobster	22	<1	<1	0.4
Blue crab	20	<1	0	0.8

USDA and Iowa State University (www.ent.iastate.edu/misc/insectnutrition.html).

Therefore, the first rule of food choice is that people tend to eat and enjoy what is easily available, which explains the differences in cuisines in different parts of the world.

Here's a second rule: For a food to be appealing (good to eat), it must be both nutritious *and* relatively easy or economical to produce.

A food that meets one test but not the other is likely to be off the list. For example:

>> The human stomach cannot extract nutrients from the indigestible dietary fiber cellulose in grass. So even though grass grows here, there, and everywhere, under ordinary circumstances, it never ends up in your salad.

>> Cows are harder to raise than plants, especially under the hot South Asian sun; pigs eat what people do, so they compete for your food supply. In other words, although they're highly nutritious, sometimes neither the cow nor the pig is economical to produce, a reasonable — though not the only — explanation for why some cultures and some religious beliefs take exception to the use of pigs and cows as food.

Taking offense to food and flavors

You may truly dislike the flavor of a particular food because (a) your genes tell you to, or (b) your past experience with the food was unpleasant. Being allergic to a certain food isn't really a taste disqualifier, but in some cases, your stomach may make the decision for you.

You blame it on your genes

Virtually everyone instinctively dislikes bitter foods, at least at first tasting. This dislike is a protective mechanism. Bitter foods are often poisonous, so disliking stuff that tastes bitter is a primitive but effective way to eliminate potentially toxic food.

According to Linda Bartoshuk, of the University of Florida Institute of Food and Agricultural Sciences and Human Nutrition (Gainesville), about two-thirds of all human beings carry a gene that makes them especially sensitive to bitter flavors. This gene may have given their ancestors a leg up in surviving their evolutionary food trials.

TECHNICAL STUFF

People with this gene can taste very small concentrations of a chemical called phenylthiocarbamide (PTC). You can test for the trait by having people taste a piece of paper impregnated with 6-n-propylthiouracil, a thyroid medication whose flavor and chemical structure are similar to PTC. People who say the paper tastes bitter are called *PTC tasters*. People who taste only paper are called *PTC nontasters*.

If you're a PTC taster, you're likely to find the taste of saccharin, caffeine, the salt substitute potassium chloride, and the food preservatives sodium benzoate and potassium benzoate really nasty. The same is true for the flavor chemicals common to cruciferous vegetables — members of the mustard family, including broccoli, Brussels sprouts, cabbage, cauliflower, and radishes.

Another group of people who don't like what they taste includes those for whom the green herb cilantro tastes like soap. Yes, soap. Here's the connection: The chemicals that create the flavor of cilantro include fragments of fat molecules called *aldehydes*. Making soap requires breaking up fat molecules, a process that produces, yes, aldehydes.

Although nobody has yet pinned down the genetic trait that makes some people loathe the smell and taste of aldehydes, the scientists at the Monell Chemical Senses Center in Philadelphia believe that further research will eventually identify it. In the meantime, if you're in the anti-cilantro camp, the solution is simple: Substitute parsley.

You once ate this food and it made you sick

People who've gotten truly sick — I'm talking nausea and vomiting here — after eating a specific food, definitely remember the experience. Sometimes, says psychologist Alexandra W. Logue, author of *The Psychology of Eating and Drinking* (Routledge, 2014), a person's revulsion may be so strong that they'll never try the food again — even when they know that what actually made them ill was something else entirely, like riding a roller coaster just before eating, or having the flu, or taking a drug whose side effects include an upset stomach.

You're allergic, but you love the food

If you're allergic to a food or have a metabolic problem that makes digesting it hard for you, you may eat the food less frequently, but you'll enjoy it as much as everyone else does. For example, people who can't digest *lactose*, the sugar in milk, may end up gassy every time they eat ice cream, but they still like the way the ice cream tastes.

Your digestive system says no

Does digestion depend on whether you like your food? To some extent, yes. The simple act of putting food into your mouth needs to stimulate the flow of saliva and the secretion of enzymes that you need to digest the food. Some studies suggest that if you really like your food, your pancreas may release as much as 30 times its normal amount of digestive enzymes. However, if you truly loathe what you're eating, your body may refuse to take it in. No saliva flows, and your mouth becomes so dry that you may not even be able to swallow the food. If you do manage to choke it down, your stomach muscles and your digestive tract may convulse in an effort to be rid of the awful stuff.

Changing the Menu: Adapting to Exotic Foods

New foods are an adventure. Some people dive right in to the dish. They like new foods and flavors the first time they try them. Others may not like them the first time around, but in time what once seemed strange can become just another entry on the dinner menu.

Learning to like unusual foods

Exposure to different people and cultures expands your taste horizons. Some taboos — horsemeat, snake, dog — may simply be too emotion-laden to be overcome. Others with no emotional baggage tend to fall to experience. On first taste, people often dislike very salty, very bitter, very acidic, or very slippery foods, such as caviar, coffee, and oysters, but many later learn to enjoy them.

Coming to terms with these foods can be both physically and psychologically rewarding:

» Several bitter foods, such as coffee and unsweetened chocolate, are relatively mild stimulants that temporarily improve mood and physical performance.

» Strongly flavored foods, such as salty caviar, offer a challenge to the taste buds.

» Foods such as oysters, which may seem totally disgusting the first time you see or taste them, are symbols of wealth or worldliness. Trying them implies a certain sophistication in the way you face life.

Happily, an educated, adventurous sense of taste can be a pleasure that lasts as long as you live. Professional tea tasters, wine tasters, and others who develop the ability to discern even the smallest differences among flavors continue to enjoy their gift well into old age as long as they continue to provide stimuli in the form of tasty, well-seasoned food.

In other words, as they say about adult life's other major sensory delight, "Use it or lose it."

Stirring the stew: The culinary benefits of immigration

If you're lucky enough to live in a place that attracts many immigrants, your dining experience is flavored by the favorite foods of other people (meaning the foods of other cultures). In the United States, for example, the *melting pot* isn't an idle phrase. American cooking literally bubbles with contributions from every group that's ever stepped ashore here.

Table 15-2 lists some of the foods and food combinations characteristic of specific ethnic/regional cuisines. Imagine how few you might sample living in a place where everybody shares exactly the same ethnic, racial, or religious background. Just thinking about it is enough to make you stand up and shout, "Hooray for diversity at the dinner table!" (Check out Figure 15-2 for the visuals!)

TABLE 15-2   ## Geography and Food Preference

If Your Ancestors Came From	You're Likely Familiar with This Flavor Combination
Central and Eastern Europe	Sour cream and dill or paprika
China	Soy sauce plus wine and ginger
Germany	Meat roasted in vinegar and sugar
Greece	Olive oil and lemon
India	Cumin and curry
Italy	Tomatoes, cheese, and olive oil
Japan	Soy sauce plus rice wine and sugar
Korea	Soy sauce plus brown sugar, sesame, and chili
Mexico	Tomatoes and chili peppers
Middle Europe	Milk and vegetables
Puerto Rico	Rice and fish
West Africa	Peanuts and chili peppers

A. W. Logue, *The Psychology of Eating and Drinking, 2nd Edition* (New York: W. H. Freeman and Company, 1991)

Of course, enjoying other people's foods doesn't mean Americans don't have their own cuisine. Table 15-3 is a list of made-in-America taste sensations, many created by immigrant chefs whose talents flowered in America's kitchens.

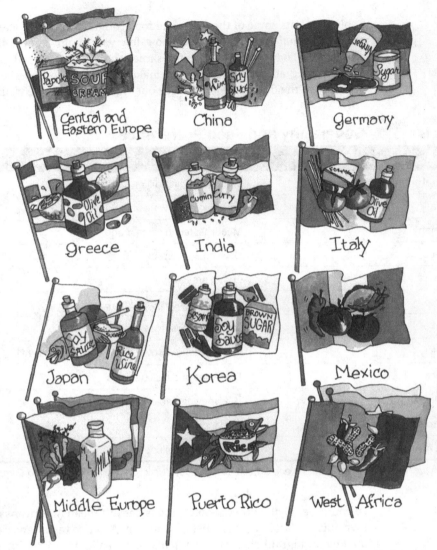

FIGURE 15-2: Ethnic and regional cuisines abound.

Central and Eastern Europe

China

Germany

Greece

India

Italy

Japan

Korea

Mexico

Middle Europe

Puerto Rico

West Africa

© John Wiley & Sons, Inc.

TABLE 15-3   **Foods Born in the United States**

This Food Item	Was Born Here
Baked beans	Boston (Pilgrim adaptation of Native American dish)
Buffalo wings	Buffalo, New York, 1960s
Chocolate chip cookies	Created by Massachusetts baker Ruth Wakefield in the 1930s and named for her family's inn
Clam chowder	Boston (the word *chowder* comes from the French *la chaudière,* the large copper soup pot used by fishermen to make a communal soup)
Corn bread	Native American dish
Hamburger	Everywhere (originally called a Hamburg steak by everyone except the citizens of Hamburg, Germany)
Jambalaya	Louisiana (combination of French Canadian [Cajun] with native coastal cookery)
Peanut butter	Created by George Washington Carver and introduced in 1904 at the World's Fair in St. Louis
Potato chips	Saratoga Springs, New York (credited to George Crum, a Native American/African American chef at the Moon Lake Lodge resort in Saratoga Springs, New York, in 1853)
Ranch dressing	Created by Steve Henson of California's Hidden Valley Ranch in the 1950s
Spoon bread	Southern United States (adapted from Native American corn pudding)
Vichyssoise	New York (commonly attributed to Louis Diat, chef at the Ritz Carlton Hotel in New York in 1917, who is said to have named the cold potato-and-cream soup in honor of the city of his birth, Vichy, France)

James Trager, The Foodbook (New York: Grossman Publishers, 1970); About.com, http://cookingfortwo. about.com/od/soupssaladssandwiches/r/Vichyssoise.htm

IN THIS CHAPTER

» Introducing the 2020–2025 *Dietary Guidelines for Americans*

» Adding information from the 2019 Canadian version

» Adopting smart food choices

» Using the *Guidelines* in real life

Chapter **16**

Building Your New and Improved Healthful Diet

There is no end to the list of really good people who want to help you find a diet that will make it possible for you to live healthy and practically forever. The American Heart Association says to edit your consumption of fats. The American Cancer Society says to eat more fruits and veggies. The American Diabetes Association says to eat regular meals so your blood sugar stays even. The Food Police pretty much say if it tastes good, forget it!

Happily, one group puts it all together. The U.S. Departments of Agriculture and Health and Human Services' 2020–2025 *Dietary Guidelines for Americans* makes it possible to make and enjoy food choices that both taste good and benefit your body.

Discovering the Dietary Guidelines for Americans

The *Dietary Guidelines for Americans* is a collection of sensible nutrition suggestions first published by the U.S. Departments of Agriculture and Health and Human Services (USDA/HHS) as a skinny, 20-page booklet in 1980.

Since then, USDA and HHS have published eight revised editions (1985, 1990, 1995, 2000, 2005, 2010, 2015, and now 2020). The one in 2010 weighed in at a hefty 110 pages, with so many words, sentences, and paragraphs — some repeated several times — that it was not released until January 31, 2011, one month into the timetable for the next edition.

The 2020–2025 edition of the *Guidelines* held to the schedule, arriving the second week in December 2020, making it onto the Internet nearly a month ahead of the previous one.

Surprisingly, the most user-friendly of the *Guidelines* remains the 2000 version, which seemed to have been written by real people who actually like real food. You could see this philosophy right upfront in the first sentence in the first paragraph: "Eating is one of life's greatest pleasures."

Contrast that with the first sentence of the *Dietary Guidelines for Americans 2005*: "The *Dietary Guidelines for Americans,* first published in 1980, provides science-based advice to promote health and reduce risk for chronic disease through diet and physical activity." Alas, what you saw was what you got: a frankly cranky, bare-bones, chilly presentation of the facts.

The 2010 edition was a verbose but directed pull-up-your-bootstraps-and-get-with-the-program document with a single-minded focus on the fact that too many Americans weigh too much (see Chapter 4). The take-away message could not be more clear: *Control what you eat to control your weight to control your health.*

The 2015–2020 edition, with three multi-section chapters, 14 appendices, and 19 tables and 24 figures, some of which compare Americans' performance to the recommendations to show exactly how bad people are at following dietary directions, delivers pretty much a similar common-sense dietary message but with a few important changes tossed in for flavor.

The 2020–2025 edition has lots of new stuff (which I lay out for you in this chapter). The language is science-speak in some places and human-speak in others, a mix much like our multi-culti American diet.

Note: Throughout this chapter, when you read "see Chapter X," it means the chapter in this book, not in the *Guidelines*.

Finding What's New in the 2020–2025 Edition

In general, the changes in the *Guidelines* over the years can be tracked in subtle shifts in emphasis. For example, from 1980 to 1995, the *Guidelines* offered the simple admonition to "Eat a variety of foods." Then, in 2000, that advice was expanded to suggest using the Food Guide Pyramid (see Chapter 17) to make nutritious choices including a variety of grains, fruits, and vegetables. In 2010, the My Plate diagram arrived to push the Pyramid off the table, a move some consumers still regret.

The 2020–2025 edition serves up a sort of blended dish: Dietary Patterns, the new way to manage food choices detailed in Chapter 17. For the moment, let's concentrate on what's new in 2020–2025. Following are the ten takeaways from the *Guidelines* experts to help you "make every bite count":

1. **The *Dietary Guidelines* is developed to help all Americans.**

   The science-based recommendations are for everyone, healthy people as well as those of us who are either living with a food-related problem such as celiac disease (check out Chapter 1) or at risk for one such as obesity, anorexia, or bulimia (see Chapter 14).

2. **There are four overarching guidelines in the 2020–2025 edition:**

   - An aim to make it easy for you to eat healthy at every stage of life

   - A framework you can customize to your own special needs and food favorites

   - Information on how to get the nutrients you need within the calorie limits that keep you fit and trim

   - Warnings to stay away from foods and beverages high in added sugars, saturated fat, and sodium and to limit alcohol beverages

3. **There are key recommendations supporting the four guidelines, including quantitative recommendations on limits that are based on the body of science reviewed.**

   The 2020-2025 *Guidelines* recommend limiting intakes of added sugars, saturated fats, sodium, and alcohol beverages in line with the 2015–2020 edition. That means keeping consumption of added sugars to less than 10 percent of your daily calories; limiting saturated fat to less than 10 percent (for further fats facts, check out Chapter 7); limiting sodium intake to less than 2,300 milligrams per day (as noted in Chapter 12); and, if you drink alcohol beverages, no more than two drinks a day for a man and one for a woman (for more on the two sides of alcohol beverages turn to Chapter 9).

4. **This is the first time the *Dietary Guidelines* has provided guidance by stage of life, from birth to older adulthood, including pregnancy and lactation.**

When they say "everyone," they really mean it. This edition of the *Guidelines* offers guidance organized by chapters for each life stage, thus emphasizing the fact that it is never too early or too late to follow a healthful diet.

5. **This edition has a call to action: "Make Every Bite Count with the *Dietary Guidelines*."**

Like all good cheerleaders, the experts who wrote the newest *Guidelines* have a catchy new slogan. Yay, team!

6. **Making choices rich in nutrients should be the first choice.**

Need to know how much nutrition — read "nutrients" — you need? Chapter 3 has the answers.

7. **It's about the pattern of eating, not just healthy choices here and there.**

Forget the original pyramid. Toss the 2015–2020 plate. Time to set your table by following a pattern based on overall healthful choices as outlined in Chapter 17.

8. **Most Americans still do not follow the *Dietary Guidelines*.**

The average American diet scores a 59 out of 100 on the Healthy Eating Index (HEI), which measures how closely a diet aligns with the *Dietary Guidelines*. (See the nearby sidebar for more on the HEI.) Three-fourths of us don't eat enough fruit, veggies and airy foods. About two-thirds of us gorge on added sugars; 77 percent exceed the suggested limits for saturated fat, and a whopping 90 percent of us overdo salty foods.

9. **There are three key dietary principles:**

- Get your nutrients from food and drink, not supplements.

- Choose a variety of foods in every group such as fruits and veggies and grains.

- Be careful when you fill your plate: Portion size counts.

10. **The *Dietary Guidelines* is meant to be adaptable to personal preferences, cultural foodways, and budgetary considerations.**

As you read at the top of these ten points, the *Guidelines* are for everyone, so use the suggestions they offer to tailor a healthful diet to your own needs and especially your own personal and cultural preferences. In other words, set your table with food patterns that satisfy. (Read more about that in Chapter 17.)

THE HEALTHY EATING INDEX

The Healthy Eating Index (HEI) lists 13 components of a healthful diet: individual foods such as whole fruit, food groups such as protein foods, and individual nutrients such as saturated fats. You can calculate the nutritional value of your own diet by adding up the points each of these contributes. A higher score on the foods labeled "adequate" means a healthier diet; a higher score on the components labeled "moderate" means a lower score. And the closer your entire menu aligns with the *Dietary Guidelines for Americans*, the higher the HEI score will be.

HEI-2015[1] Components and Scoring Standards

Component	Maximum points	Standard for maximum score	Standard for minimum score of zero
Adequacy:			
Total Fruits[2]	5	≥0.8 cup equivalent per 1,000 kcal	No Fruit
Whole Fruits[3]	5	≥0.4 cup equivalent per 1,000 kcal	No Whole Fruit
Total Vegetables[4]	5	≥1.1 cup equivalent per 1,000 kcal	No Vegetables
Greens and Beans[4]	5	≥0.2 cup equivalent per 1,000 kcal	No Dark-Green Vegetables or Legumes
Whole Grains	10	≥1.5 ounce equivalent per 1,000 kcal	No Whole Grains
Dairy[5]	10	≥1.3 cup equivalent per 1,000 kcal	No Dairy
Total Protein Foods[4]	5	≥2.5 ounce equivalent per 1,000 kcal	No Protein Foods
Seafood and Plant Proteins[4,6]	5	≥0.8 ounce equivalent per 1,000 kcal	No Seafood or Plant Proteins
Fatty Acids[7]	10	(PUFAs + MUFAs) / SFAs ≥2.5	(PUFAs + MUFAs)/SFAs ≤1.2
Moderation:			
Refined Grains	10	≤1.8 ounce equivalent per 1,000 kcal	≥4.3 ounce equivalent per 1,000 kcal
Sodium	10	≤1.1 grams per 1,000 kcal	≥2.0 grams per 1,000 kcal
Added Sugars	10	≤6.5% of energy	≥26% of energy
Saturated Fats	10	≤8% of energy	≥16% of energy

[1] Intakes between the minimum and maximum standards are scored proportionately.
[2] Includes 100% fruit juice.
[3] Includes all forms except juice.
[4] Includes legumes (beans and peas).
[5] Includes all milk products, such as fluid milk, yogurt, and cheese, and fortified soy beverages.
[6] Includes seafood; nuts, seeds, soy products (other than beverages), and legumes (beans and peas).
[7] Ratio of poly- and mono-unsaturated fatty acids (PUFAs and MUFAs) to saturated fatty acids (SFAs).

Source: Food and Nutrition Service, U.S. Department of Agriculture

TECHNICAL STUFF

If you feel like reading all the actual words they wrote, check out www.dietaryguidelines.gov/resources/2020-2025-dietary-guidelines-online-materials/top-10-things-you-need-know-about-dietary.

Factor in the fats

The 2020–2025 *Guidelines* simply say to be smart but not obsessive: Just avoid the saturated fats and keep cholesterol consumption low.

As in the previous edition of the *Guidelines*, this simple statement is driven by the fact that when told to cut back on fats, most people just cut back on fats — good, bad, and in between. But some fats, such as those found in certain plant foods like avocados and nuts (check out Chapter 29 for more on these superstar foods), are good for you.

Word to the fat-wise #1: You can reduce your intake of solid fats in food, and thus your intake of saturated fats, simply by wielding a sharp knife to cut away as much visible fat as possible from meat and poultry as well as stripping off the fat-laden poultry skin.

Word to the fat-wise #2: Liquid fats, otherwise known as oils, are mixtures of saturated fats and unsaturated fats. See Chapter 7 to find out which oils are high in saturated fatty acids and which are not.

IS IT FAT OR IS IT WATER WEIGHT?

Got a bathroom scale at home? Here's an interesting three-day experiment that shows how a high-salt/sodium diet may affect your weight.

On Day One, weigh yourself as soon as you awake. For the rest of the day, go ahead, eat your little heart out — sorry, American Heart Association — binge away on high-salt/sodium potato chips and sausages.

On Day Two, you Surprise! probably weigh one, two, or even three pounds more than you did on Day One. Why? Sodium is *hydrophilic* (*hydro* = water; *philic* = loving). It doesn't increase the amount of fat in your body, but it does hold water in your tissues, which increases your weight.

Happily, the gain is temporary. Go back to your normal diet, cut out the extra salt/sodium, and on Day Three, your weight should be back to what it was on Day One.

Subtract the added sugar

Once again, the *Guidelines* recommend avoiding foods with added sweeteners. Notice the word *added* because this means editing your diet to reduce foods to which sugar is added, such as cakes and cookies — or coffee with three spoons of sugar — *not* to avoid foods with naturally occurring sugars such as fruits. (For the skinny on substitute sweeteners, your guide is Chapter 19.)

"NO CALORIES" MAY NOT MEAN "DIET-SAFE"

Diet sodas don't make the *Guidelines'* list of recommended sugar-free beverages. Why? Because some studies suggest that rather than helping you lose weight, these drinks actually lead to weight gain, perhaps by leading you to eat things you wouldn't otherwise have chosen ("I had a diet soda, so I can have a brownie").

In 2005, a team of researchers at the University of Texas Health Science Center, San Antonio, released data from an 8-year, 1,550-person study showing that among people drinking sodas sweetened with sugar, the risk of becoming overweight or even obese was

- 26 percent for those drinking up to ½ can daily
- 30.4 percent at ½ to 1 can daily
- 32.8 percent at 1 to 2 cans daily
- 47.2 percent at more than 2 cans daily

No surprise there. But look at the risk for people drinking diet soft drinks:

- 36.5 percent for those drinking up to ½ can daily
- 37.5 percent at ½ to 1 can daily
- 54.5 percent at 1 to 2 cans daily
- 57.1 percent at more than 2 cans daily

In others words — unpleasant ones — statistically speaking, your risk of packing on the pounds rises with each can of diet soda you drink each day. Makes water look better and better, doesn't it?

Get adequate essential nutrients

For various reasons, even an adequate diet may be deficient in specific nutrients. One example is the fact that as we age, our bodies may be less able to absorb vitamin B12 from food, meaning that supplements are sensible.

As always, this edition of the *Guidelines* stresses the need to obtain adequate amounts of important nutrients.

For the recommended amounts of each nutrient, as well as a more detailed explanation of their benefits, check out Chapter 8 (dietary fiber), Chapter 10 (vitamins), and Chapter 11 (minerals).

Go fish for good food

Finding a balance in what fish to eat and how much can be challenging. On the one hand, fish provides undeniably beneficial omega-3 fatty acids EPA and DHA, whose benefits are listed in Chapter 7. On the other hand, some fish is contaminated with methylmercury, a toxic metal that can wreak neurological and cardiovascular havoc, particularly in the fetus and in children.

Taking this into account, the *Guidelines* recommend that most healthy people consume about 8 ounces of fish and seafood a week to get the 250 milligrams per day of EPA and DHA associated with a lower risk of death from heart disease among otherwise healthy people and an improved outcome for newborns.

The fish of choice include salmon, anchovies, herring, shad, sardines, Pacific oysters, trout, and Atlantic and Pacific mackerel. Children and women who are of child-bearing age, pregnant, or nursing should avoid *all* King mackerel, shark, swordfish, and tile fish, species widely acknowledged to be highly contaminated. And these two groups should eat no more than 12 ounces of fish a week, including no more than 6 ounces of canned albacore tuna. (See Chapter 24 for a list of fish and their mercury levels.)

Bring on the veggies

In 1980, the first *Guidelines* directed consumers to "Eat foods with adequate starch and fiber." By 1990, that had become, "Choose a diet with plenty of vegetables, fruits, and grain products." Today, the new, direct directive is to make half of your plate vegetables and fruits. Maybe the whole plate: The *Guidelines* say right out, no mincing words here, that vegetable-rich diets promise a variety of health benefits, including lower weight, a lower risk of heart disease, and — best of all — a longer life.

Get up and go

Regular physical activity is one of the simplest — and most important — things you can do on your own to improve your health.

Clearly, the first thing that comes to mind when you think "exercise" is "lose the pounds." Which makes perfect sense because when you take in more calories (energy) from food than you use up running your body systems (heart, lungs, brain, and so on) and doing a day's physical work, you end up storing the extra calories as body fat. In other words, you gain weight. The reverse also is true. When you spend more energy in a day than you take in as food, you pull the extra energy you need out of stored body fat, and you lose weight.

You don't have to be a mathematician to reduce this principle to two simple equations in which E stands for energy (in calories), > stands for greater than, < stands for less than, and W stands for the change in weight:

If E in > E out: E total = +W

If E in < E out: E total = –W

It's not Einstein's theory of relativity, but you get the picture. For real-life examples of how the energy-in, energy-out theory works, stick your bookmark in this page and go to Chapter 3 to find out how to calculate the number of calories a person can consume each day without pushing up the poundage. Even being mildly active increases the number of calories you can wolf down without gaining weight. The more strenuous the activity, the more plentiful the calorie allowance. Suppose that you're a 25-year-old man who weighs 140 pounds. The formula in Chapter 3 shows that you require 1,652 calories a day to run your body systems. Clearly, you need more calories for doing your daily physical work, simply moving around, or exercising.

Of course, weight control isn't the only benefit you get by moving your body. In 2018, the Department of Health and Human Services released a whole new set of data points on how and why to exercise for every age from preschool tots straight on through senior citizens.

First, the new rules define three types of exercise:

>> **Aerobic activity** increases heart rate and breathing. Moderate aerobic activity includes walking briskly, bicycling on a level path, and dancing. Intense aerobic activity includes jogging, playing tennis, or bicycling uphill.

>> **Muscle-strengthening activity,** such as resistance training, increases the mass and strength of skeletal muscles — that is, your arms, legs, back, and so on.

>> **Bone-building activity** is any exercise, such as running or lifting weights, that makes an impact on your bones.

Then, having set the standards, they move on to specifics:

>> **Exercise increases muscles.** When you exercise regularly, you end up with more muscle tissue than the average bear. Because muscle tissue weighs more than fat tissue, athletes (even weekend-warrior types) may end up weighing more than they did before they started exercising to lose weight. But a higher muscle-to-fat ratio is healthier and more important in the long run than actual weight in pounds. Exercise that changes your body's ratio of muscle to fat gives you a leg up in the longevity race.

>> **Exercise reduces the amount of fat stored in your body.** People who are fat around the middle as opposed to the hips (in other words an apple shape versus a pear shape) are at higher risk of weight-related illness. Exercise helps reduce abdominal fat and thus lowers your risk of weight-related diseases. Use a tape measure to identify your own body type by comparing your waistline to your hips (around the buttocks). If your waist (abdomen) is bigger, you're an apple. If your hips are bigger, you're a pear.

>> **Exercise strengthens your bones.** Osteoporosis (thinning of the bones that leads to repeated fractures) doesn't happen only to little old ladies. True, on average, a woman's bones thin faster and more dramatically than a man's, but after the mid-30s, everybody — male and female — begins losing bone density. Exercise can slow, halt, or in some cases even reverse the process. In addition, being physically active develops muscles that help support bones. Stronger bones equal less risk of fracture, which, in turn, equals less risk of potentially fatal complications.

>> **Exercise increases brainpower.** You know that aerobic exercise increases the flow of oxygen to the heart, but did you also know that it increases the flow of oxygen to the brain? When a rush job (or a rush of anxiety) keeps you up all night, a judicious exercise break can keep you bright until dawn. According to nutrition research scientist Judith J. Wurtman, PhD, when you're awake and working during hours that you'd normally be asleep, your internal body rhythms tell your body to cool down, even though your brain is racing along. Simply standing up and stretching, walking around the room, or doing a couple of sit-ups every hour or so speeds up your metabolism, warms up your muscles, increases your ability to stay awake, and, in Dr. Wurtman's words, "prolongs your ability to work smart into the night." Eureka!

WARNING

Not everybody can — or should — run right out and start chopping down trees or throwing touchdown passes to control their weight. In fact, if you've gained a lot of weight recently, have been overweight for a long time, haven't exercised in a while, or have a chronic medical condition, you need to check with your doctor before starting any new regimen. (*Caution:* Check out of any health club that puts you right on the floor without first checking your vital signs — heartbeat, respiration, and so on.)

Finally, having laid out the ground rules, the new advice makes it clear that all activity counts. The idea that you have to move for a specific number of minutes at one time is yesterday's news.

TECHNICAL STUFF

Those are the basics. Want even more details? You can find the entire report at `health.gov/sites/default/files/2019-10/PAG_ExecutiveSummary.pdf`

NORTHERN NUTRITION NOTES

In 2019, Canada released the latest version of its own dietary guidelines, The Food Guide. The guidelines don't focus on set food groups or serving sizes but rather emphasize replacing most animal proteins and fats with plant-based sources and avoiding most beverages except for water.

The guidelines are arranged in three sections—foundations for healthy eating, foods and beverages that undermine healthy eating, and the importance of food skills.

The first section emphasizes the virtues of plant foods, advising Canadians to replace animal sources of protein and fat with nutrients from plants.

In the second section, like their American cousins, the Canadians advise avoiding processed and prepared foods and beverages, products usually high in sodium, added sugar, or saturated fat (or, sometimes, all three) which may increase the risk for obesity and chronic disease.

The third section doesn't lay out rules for what to eat or what to stay away from but instead emphasizes "food skills" such as cooking, which are important for healthier eating, preventing food waste, and knowing exactly what ingredients go into your food. As an extra bonus, the guide encourages creating and enjoying meals with others, as eating alone can lead to bad dietary habits.

For ten important points from the Canadian Food Guide, check out Chapter 28.

Do the Guidelines Work?

Yes. No. Maybe. And who knows?

On the plus side, the *Guidelines* offer a template for building a healthful diet.

On the down side, not many people take the time to do the building. It is impossible to prove a negative, so there is no way to say whether there would be even more overweight Americans without the *Guidelines*. What we know for sure is that obesity exploded in America while the *Guidelines* were available.

As a result, the release of the latest *Guidelines*, like the publication of the previous seven editions, is likely to trigger specific criticisms from various corners of the food and nutrition world. In general, the critiques may echo broad complaints such as the following:

>> These are nice rules, but nobody follows them. After all, since 2005, the *Guidelines* have said to eat at least 2.5 cups of fruits and veggies a day, but studies show that only 4 percent — 4 out of every 100 Americans — do that.

>> The continuing emphasis on food components, such as fats, carbs, vitamins, and minerals, contradicts the fact that real people eat food, not nutrients. People who espouse this point of view want the guidelines to recommend specific foods — maybe even specific menus — not theoretical nutrition concepts.

>> The *Guidelines* ignore the question of *sustainability*. Producing some foods, such as meat, requires more energy and more natural resources than do others, such as fruits and vegetables. In the years leading up to the release of the new *Guidelines*, there was much discussion about including a section on protecting the planet as well as the humans on it by promoting the consumption of foods that further the sustainability goal.

Nonetheless, the *Guidelines*, imperfect though they may be, do offer *guidelines* on how to eat smart.

To encourage that, the authors want people to work together toward a common goal: to create partnerships with food producers, suppliers, and retailers to convince them to increase access to foods that align with the *Dietary Guidelines*, and to continue to promote the availability of healthful food and food products in restaurants, as well as promote participation in physical activity programs offered in various settings.

WHERE TO FIND THE GUIDELINES

To read and/or download the 2020-2025 *Dietary Guidelines for Americans* or the Executive Summary, go to www.dietaryguidelines.gov and download a PDF from there.

Prefer print? Hard copies of the *Dietary Guidelines for Americans* will eventually be available from the U.S. Government Printing Office either by phone at (866) 512-1800 or from bookstore.gpo.gov/.

The more or less final word.

Life is not a test. No one loses points for failing to follow the USDA/HHS advice every single day of the year.

So this may be the real rule: Let the good times roll every once in a while. Then, after the party's over, compensate. For the rest of the week, go back to your exercise regimen and back to your healthful menu emphasizing lots of the nutritious, delicious foods that should make up most of your regular diet.

In the end, you're likely to have averaged out to a desirable amount with no fuss and no muss and be right in line with that headline from the first page of the 2000 *Guidelines* that I mention at the beginning of this chapter: "Eating is one of life's greatest pleasures."

Chapter **17**

Choosing Wisely with Pyramids, Plates, and Patterns

This chapter is devoted to pictures of pyramids, plates, and patterns, all designed to serve as a kind of set of building blocks for grown-ups, a tool for arranging foods in various ways to create the structure of a healthful diet.

Choose one, take notes, follow directions, and then choose another, create a different healthful menu, and so on. Any way you play, your reward is likely to be a better body.

Checking Out Basic Diet Pictures

The essential message of all good guides to healthful food choices is that no one food is either good or bad — how much and how often you eat a food is what counts. The food pictures, therefore, come with three important messages:

» **Variety:** The fact that each contains or describes several different foods tells you that no single food gives you all the nutrients you need.

>> **Moderation:** Having one group drawn smaller than others on a food pyramid or dinner plate or showing clearly that there is less of one group recommended, as on the Nutrition Facts Label, tells you that although every food is valuable, some — such as fats and sweets — are best consumed in small amounts.

>> **Balance:** You can't build a diet with a set of identical blocks. Blocks of different sizes show that a healthful diet is balanced: the right amount from each food group.

Clearly, food pyramids, plate pictures, and patterns make it possible for you to eat practically everything you like — as long as you follow the recommendations on how much and how frequently (or infrequently) to eat it.

The original USDA Food Guide Pyramid

The first food pyramid was created by the U.S. Department of Agriculture (USDA) in 1992 in response to criticism that the previous government guide to food choices — the Four Food Group Plan (vegetables and fruits, breads and cereals, milk and milk products, meat and meat alternatives) — was too heavily weighted toward high-fat, high-cholesterol foods from animals.

Figure 17-1 depicts the original USDA Food Guide Pyramid. As you can see, this pyramid is based on daily food choices, showing you which foods are in what groups. Unlike the Four Food Group Plan, the pyramid separates fruits and vegetables into two distinct groups and lists the number of servings from each food group that you should have each day. (The number of servings is provided in ranges. The lower end is for people who consume about 1,600 calories a day, and the upper end is for people whose daily dietary intake nears 3,000 calories.)

From pyramid to plate: The evolution of the Food Guide

You may think that after the government came up with this apparently sensible way to decide what's good to eat, everyone in the nutrition establishment would stand up as one to shout, "Huzzah!" You'd be wrong. The complaints began practically the minute the pyramid hit the street, so to speak.

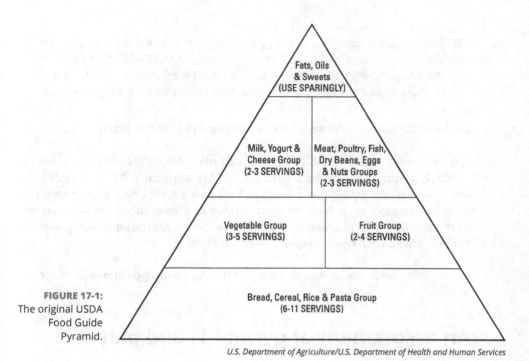

FIGURE 17-1:
The original USDA
Food Guide
Pyramid.

Fats, Oils
& Sweets
(USE SPARINGLY)

Milk, Yogurt &
Cheese Group
(2-3 SERVINGS)

Meat, Poultry, Fish,
Dry Beans, Eggs
& Nuts Groups
(2-3 SERVINGS)

Vegetable Group
(3-5 SERVINGS)

Fruit Group
(2-4 SERVINGS)

Bread, Cereal, Rice & Pasta Group
(6-11 SERVINGS)

U.S. Department of Agriculture/U.S. Department of Health and Human Services

On the one hand, critics said the pyramid was indecisive, lumping all fats — good, bad, and in between — into one category and failing to distinguish between whole grains (good) and refined grains (not great). On the other hand, critics said the advice was decisive but in the wrong direction — for example, by allowing more red meat than considered optimal by the real (or at least the emerging) science. And everybody asked, "How come there's no picture or sentence to tell us to exercise every day to control our weight?"

What to do? Nutritional acrobatics. In 2005, the USDA released a new Food Guide Pyramid, which was actually the first pyramid turned sideways. This version of the pyramid had the following:

>> Unlabeled sections representing the foods in your daily diet, each identified by color: orange for grains, green for vegetables, red for fruits, yellow for oils, blue for milk, and purple for meat and beans

>> An admonition to eat "lots of different kinds of foods to build a better diet" but no specific servings-per-day recommendations for any food group

>> Directions on how to key certain data into a form to find out how many servings of each food group you should eat based on your age, sex, and level of activity but not — to everyone's surprise — your height and weight

>> Steps, actual steps, with a teensy gender-neutral human being climbing up the side of the pyramid to signify (1) physical activity, and (2) the fact that you don't have to leap tall buildings in a single bound like Superman (or woman) to improve your nutrition because even small steps can make a big difference

All these things may have been new — but improved? Not so much.

Call me foolish. Call me old-fashioned. Call me a fan of the simplest solution, which, it seems, is no longer a pyramid. In May 2011, the USDA introduced the *newest* new thing, a plate that shows (sort of) how much of each type of food you should be consuming. It includes more veggies and fewer meats. So now you can go to the USDA website at www.choosemyplate.gov to see the latest version of the Totally Official Food Guide Pyramid — sorry, Plate.

Or you can check one of the diagrams from the loyal oppositions in the next section.

An assortment of pyramids and plates

Government documents, including food guides, are often one-size-fits-all — meaning they may not fit you.

Are you a fan of Asian food? Do you like your menu with a Central or South American accent? Does meat turn you off? If you answer yes to any of these questions, there's a special food pyramid waiting for you. The Oldways Preservation trust, a Boston-based internationally known nonprofit organization devoted to improving people's diet with "positive programs grounded in science, traditions, and delicious foods and drink," has created a number of pyramids based on ethnic food plans, perhaps the best known being the Mediterranean Diet Pyramid. The following Oldways pyramids are a guide to good food in various languages. To see them, go to oldwayspt.org/traditional-diets and choose what pleases you.

Note that if you prefer plates to pyramids, the Oldways website is pleased to offer various adaptations just for your dinner table.

The Asian Diet Pyramid and Plate

Oldways's partners for this pyramid, introduced at the International Conference on the Diets of Asia in San Francisco in 1995, were the Cornell-China-Oxford Project on Nutrition, Health, and Environment and the Harvard School of Public Health. This pyramid codifies a primarily vegetarian diet historically linked to the generally low incidence of cardiovascular disease in Asian countries.

The Vegetarian Diet Pyramid and Plate

This pyramid, created by Oldways and the Harvard School of Public Health, was released at the International Conference on Vegetarian Diets in Austin, Texas, in 1997. It's a traditional vegetarian plan with fruits, vegetables, grains, and dairy products but no meat, fish, or poultry. It's described as promoting "agricultural sustainability." Translation: Producing these foods takes up and thus wastes less use of natural resources — land, fuel, and water — than modern industrial food production. Good for you; good for the planet.

The Traditional Mediterranean Diet Pyramid and Plate

Oldways and the Harvard School of Public Health released the first Mediterranean Diet Pyramid in 1993; this updated version appeared in 2009. As you can see, it has lots of fruits and veggies, poultry and *lean* red meat, olive oil, cheese, and yogurt — all accompanied by moderate amounts of wine. In short, the traditional diet of, yes, the Mediterranean countries circa 1960 when, Oldways explains, "The rates of chronic disease were among the lowest in the world, and adult life expectancy was among the highest, even though medical services were limited." Tastes good, too.

The Latin American Diet Pyramid and Plate

Oldways introduced this pyramid in 1996 at the Latin American Diet Conference in El Paso, Texas; the updated version appeared in 2009. The food plan in this pyramid is based on the traditional and modern-day diet of Central and South America, which Oldways describes as a melding of three distinct cultures: the indigenous Aztecs, Incas, and Maya; the 16th century Spanish explorer; and the Africans brought in first as slaves. The mixture produced a rich blend of local fruit (agave, avocado), vegetables (cassava, chayote), grains (amaranth, maize, quinoa), poultry, and meat (goat), once again accompanied by moderate amounts of alcohol. Plus exercise, of course.

African Heritage Diet Pyramid and Plate

In 2012, Oldways debuted the latest addition to its list of diet pyramids and plates, this one based on the fresh plant foods, healthy oils, homemade sauces and marinades of herbs and spices, fish, eggs, poultry, yogurt, and minimal consumption of meats and sweets common to the diets of African origin now common in places ranging from North and South America to the Caribbean and, of course, in Africa itself.

Tracking Food Patterns

In 2015, along with introducing the Plate, the experts writing the Dietary Guidelines began to approach a new idea: Food Patterns. They describe Food Patterns as "the quantities, proportions, variety, or combinations of different foods, drinks, and nutrients in them, and the frequency with which they are habitually consumed." That's one big verbal mouthful, so here's the simpler description: What you usually eat every day and how much of each food and beverage you consume.

REMEMBER

Food Patterns come in two varieties:

>> *Index-based patterns* are defined by a single numerical score based on the healthful nature of its components. Two familiar examples are the DASH diet (more about that in Chapter 26) and the Mediterranean diet listed (more in Chapter 24).

>> *Exploratory patterns* are based on the content of specific groups of foods with labels such as "sweets" and "healthy" and "Western." The more high-nutrition foods, the better — and vice versa.

TIP

To find out more about dietary patterns, including how dietary patterns are linked to important health outcomes, check out the following PDF online at www. dietaryguidelines.gov/sites/default/files/2020-07/PartD_Ch8_ DietaryPatterns_first-print.pdf.

THE INDULGENT VEGETARIAN

The University of Michigan Integrative Medicine, a program that brings together both traditional and complementary medical practices, introduced this pyramid in 2010 (www.canr.msu.edu/foodsystems/uploads/files/TheHealingFoodsPyramid. pdf). They call it the Healing Foods Pyramid, but you might call it the Semi-Vegetarian Indulgence Pyramid. Yes, it features daily servings of legumes, soy foods, healthy fats (avocados, nuts, seeds, nut butters, and unsaturated oils), an ounce of dark chocolate, and 2 to 4 cups of tea (lower caffeine white or green preferred), plus moderate amounts of alcohol. But it also allows lean meat or poultry in 3-ounce servings, up to three times a week each.

Understanding the Nutrition Facts Label

Once upon a time, the only reliable consumer information on a food label was the name of the food inside. The 1990 Nutrition Labeling and Education Act changed that forever with a spiffy new set of consumer-friendly food labels that include

>> A mini-nutrition guide that shows the food's nutrient content and evaluates its place in a balanced diet

>> Accurate ingredient listings, with all ingredients listed in order of their weight in the original recipe — for example, the most prominent ingredient in a loaf of bread is flour

>> Clear identification of ingredients previously listed simply as *colorings* and *sweeteners*

>> Scientifically reliable information about the relationship between specific foods and specific chronic health conditions, such as heart disease and cancer

The Nutrition Facts Label is *required by law* for more than 90 percent of all processed, packaged foods — everything from canned soup to fresh pasteurized orange juice. Food sold in really small packages — a pack of gum, for example — can omit the Nutrition Facts Label but must carry a telephone number or address so an inquisitive consumer (you) can call or write for the information.

Just about the only processed foods exempted from the nutrition labeling regulations are those with no appreciable amounts of nutrients or those whose content varies from batch to batch or those from very small food processors, such as the following items:

>> Plain (unflavored) coffee and tea

>> Some spices and flavorings

>> Deli and bakery items prepared fresh in the store where they're sold directly to the consumer

>> Food produced by small companies

>> Food sold in restaurants, unless it makes a nutrition content or health claim (Want to know how to eat well when eating out? Check out Chapter 18.)

Labels are voluntary for fresh raw meat, fish, or poultry and fresh fruits and vegetables, but many markets — perhaps under pressure from customers — have put posters or brochures with generic nutrition information near the meat counter or produce bins.

Getting the facts

The star of the Nutrition Facts Label is the Nutrition Facts Panel on the back (or side) of the package. This panel features three important elements: serving sizes, amounts of nutrients per serving, and Percent Daily Value.

In recent years, with the rising concern about obesity often believed to be triggered by the overconsumption of sugary foods, a new Nutrition Facts Label has been evolving. This new one, shown in Figure 17-2, breaks the sugar component into two categories: The sugar that occurs naturally in foods (for example, the natural sugars in an apple) and the sugars added to a food (for example, the sugars added to packaged apple sauce). In addition, instead of showing simply the percentage of the RDA (Recommended Dietary Allowance) for vitamins and minerals and requiring you to guess what the total figure is, the new labels show the exact amount (for example, 260 milligrams calcium) plus the percentage of the RDA (20 percent). Note that these values are required only for certain vitamins and minerals — others are voluntary.

Nutrition Facts

8 servings per container

Serving size	2/3 cup (55g)

Amount per 2/3 cup

Calories	**230**

% DV*	
12%	**Total Fat** 8g
5%	Saturated Fat 1g
	Trans Fat 0g
0%	**Cholesterol** 0mg
7%	**Sodium** 160mg
12%	**Total Carbs** 37g
14%	Dietary Fiber 4g
	Sugars 1g
	Added Sugars 0g
	Protein 3g
10%	Vitamin D 2mcg
20%	Calcium 260mg
45%	Iron 8mg
5%	Potassium 235mg

* Footnote on Daily Values (DV) and calories reference to be inserted here.

©John Wiley & Sons, Inc.

FIGURE 17-2: The current Nutrition Facts Label.

Serving size

No need to stretch your brain trying to translate gram-servings or ounce-servings into real servings. This label does it for you, listing the servings in comprehensible kitchen terms, such as 1 cup or 1 waffle or 2 pieces or 1 teaspoon. It also tells you how many servings are in the package.

The serving size is exactly the same for all products in a category. In other words, the Nutrition Facts Panel enables you to compare at a glance the nutrient content for two different brands of yogurt, cheddar cheese, string beans, soft drinks, and so on.

When checking the labels, you may think the suggested serving sizes seem small (especially with so-called low-fat items). Think of these serving sizes as useful guides, which have become more realistic over time as the FDA brought them into line with what people really eat, which is to say, not one or two fries per serving, more like ten — with the resulting calories and such.

Amount per serving

The Nutrition Facts Panel tells you the amount (per serving) for several important factors:

>> Calories in a new VERY BIG TYPE

>> Total fat (in grams)

>> Saturated fat (in grams)

>> Trans fats (in grams)

>> Cholesterol (in milligrams)

>> Total carbohydrate (in grams)

>> Dietary fiber (in grams)

>> Sugars, total amount and the amount of sugar added during preparation (in grams)

>> Protein (in grams)

Percent Daily Value

The Percent Daily Value enables you to judge whether a specific food is high, medium, or low in fat, cholesterol, sodium, carbohydrates, dietary fiber, sugar, protein, vitamin A, vitamin C, calcium, and iron based on a set of recommendations called the *Reference Daily Intakes (RDI)*, which are similar (but not identical) to the Recommended Dietary Allowances (RDAs) for vitamins and minerals discussed in Chapters 10 and 11.

IS ANYBODY LISTENING?

It may depend on how hungry you are. In 2010, the American Dietetic Association (now renamed the Academy of Nutrition and Dietetics) published a Columbia University report showing that nearly 62 percent of food shoppers read the Nutrition Facts Label, and those who read it consume fewer calories, total fat, saturated fat, and sugar overall. But in 2011, three years after New York City became the first in the country to require calorie labeling in fast-food restaurants, a New York University School of Medicine (NYU SOM) study showed that although nearly as many people saw the calorie information as read the Nutrition Facts Label, fewer than 10 percent said it influenced their food choices. Seven years after that the *Journal of the Academy of Nutrition and Dietetics* narrowed the field, naming six groups most likely to read the label: women, people with advanced degrees and high income, people who regularly prepare food, people who are physically active, people who are overweight, and those trying to lose or gain weight.

Possible conclusion: People who are hungry *right now* pay less attention to nutrition information than people who are buying food to eat when they get hungry later on. And those interested in actual nutrition facts are the ones most likely to check the Nutrition Facts Label. Sounds real.

RDIs are based on allowances set in 1973, so some RDIs now may not apply to all groups of people. For example, the Daily Value for calcium is 1,000 milligrams, but many studies — and two National Institutes of Health Conferences — suggest that postmenopausal women who are not using hormone replacement therapy need to consume 1,500 milligrams of calcium a day to reduce their risk of osteoporosis.

The Percent Daily Values for fats, carbohydrates, protein, sodium, and potassium are based on the *Daily Reference Values (DRV)*. DRVs are standards for nutrients, such as fat and fiber, known to raise or lower the risk of certain health conditions, such as heart disease and cancer.

Relying on labels: Health claims

Ever since man (and woman) came out of the caves, people have been making health claims for certain foods. These folk remedies may be comforting, but the evidence to support them is mostly anecdotal: "I had a cold. My mom gave me chicken soup, and here I am, all bright-eyed and bushy-tailed. Of course, it did take a week to get rid of the cold."

On the other hand, health claims approved by the USDA and the Food and Drug Administration (FDA) for inclusion on the new food labels are another matter entirely. If you see a statement suggesting that a particular food or nutrient plays a role in reducing your risk of a specific medical condition, you can be absolutely 100 percent sure that a real relationship exists between the food and the medical condition. You can also be sure that scientific evidence from well-designed studies supports the claim.

In other words, USDA/FDA-approved health claims are medically sound and scientifically specific. They highlight the known relationships between

>> **Calcium and bone density:** A label describing a food as "high in calcium" may truthfully say: "A diet high in calcium helps women maintain healthy bones and may reduce the risk of osteoporosis later in life."

>> **A diet high in fat, saturated fat, and cholesterol and a higher risk of heart disease:** A label describing a food as "low fat, low cholesterol," or "no fat, no cholesterol" may truthfully say: "This food follows the recommendations of the American Heart Association's diet to lower the risk of heart disease."

>> **A high-fiber diet and a lower risk of some kinds of cancer:** A label describing a food as "high-fiber" may truthfully say: "Foods high in dietary fiber may reduce the risk of certain types of cancer."

>> **A high-fiber diet and a lower risk of heart attack:** A label describing a food as "high-fiber" may truthfully say: "Foods high in dietary fiber may help reduce the risk of coronary heart disease."

>> **Sodium and hypertension (high blood pressure):** A label describing a food as "low-sodium" may truthfully say: "A diet low in sodium may reduce the risk of high blood pressure."

>> **A fruit-and-vegetable-rich diet and a low risk of some kinds of cancer:** Labels on fruits and vegetables may truthfully say: "A diet high in fruits and vegetables may lower your risk of some kinds of cancer."

>> **Folic acid (folate) and a lower risk of neural tube (spinal cord) birth defects such as spina bifida:** Labels on folate-rich foods may truthfully say: "A diet rich in folates during pregnancy lowers the risk of neural tube defects in the fetus."

Navigating the highs and lows

Today, savvy consumers reach almost automatically for packages labeled "low-fat" or "high-fiber." But it's a dollars-to-doughnuts sure bet that hardly one shopper in a thousand knows what "low" and "high" actually mean.

TIP

Because these are potent terms that promise real health benefits, the new labeling law has created strict, science-based definitions:

» *High* means that one serving provides 20 percent or more of the Daily Value for a particular nutrient. Other ways to say "high" are "rich in" or "excellent source," as in "milk is an excellent source of calcium."

» *Good source* means one serving gives you 10 to 19 percent of the Daily Value for a particular nutrient.

» *Light* (sometimes written *lite*) is used in connection with calories, fat, or sodium. It means the product has one-third fewer calories or 50 percent less fat or 50 percent less sodium than usually is found in a particular type of product.

» *Low* means that the food contains an amount of a nutrient that enables you to eat several servings without going over the Daily Value for that nutrient.

  ● *Low calorie* means 40 calories or fewer per serving.

  ● *Low fat* means 3 grams of fat or less.

  ● *Low saturated fat* means less than 0.5 grams trans fat per serving and 1 gram (or less) saturated fat.

  ● *Low cholesterol* means 20 milligrams or less.

  ● *Low sodium* means 140 milligrams sodium or less per serving; a diet plan with less than 1,000 milligrams of sodium per day is considered a low-sodium diet.

» *Reduced saturated fat* means that the amount of saturated fat plus trans fat has been reduced more than 25 percent from what's normal in the given food product.

» *Free* means "negligible" — not "none." In short, this is what counts as "free" preserving:

  ● *Calorie-free* means fewer than 5 calories.

  ● *Fat-free* means less than 0.5 grams of fat.

  ● *Trans fat-free* means the food has less than 0.5 grams trans fat and 0.5 grams saturated fat per serving.

- *Cholesterol-free* means less than 2 milligrams of cholesterol or 2 grams or less saturated fat.

- *Sodium-free* or *salt-free* means less than 5 milligrams of sodium.

- *Sugar-free* means less than 0.5 grams of sugar.

- *Gluten-free,* a term finalized by the FDA in 2019 and 2020, means a food does not contain wheat, rye, barley, or crossbreeds of these grains; does not contain an ingredient derived from these grains; or does not contain an ingredient processed to remove gluten that still contains 20 or more parts gluten per million.

And if that isn't enough to occupy your food brain, consider this: The FDA continues to work on how to define the word *natural* on food labels. The agency explains that "[f]rom a food science perspective, it is difficult to define a food product that is 'natural' because the food has probably been processed and is no longer the product of the earth. That said, FDA has not developed a definition for use of the term natural or its derivatives. However, the agency has not objected to the use of the term if the food does not contain added color, artificial flavors, or synthetic substances." Pass the "natural, organic" aspirin, please!

ORGANIC: THE EVOLUTION OF A LABEL TERM

Organic (as in organic food) is a highly charged food word. To a chemist, *organic* means a substance that contains carbon, hydrogen, and oxygen. By this chemical standard, all foods — and all human beings — are organic.

Of course, the word *organic* has been adopted to describe plant foods grown without pesticides or synthetic chemicals and the poultry, fish, beef, and lamb from animals raised on a diet with no antibiotics or other meds.

But these descriptions were not originally standards recognized by any federal agency. So the USDA set out to create regulations that legally define the term. Here's a timeline of those regulations:

- In December 1997, the USDA National Organic Program released its first proposal on new standards for organic foods.

- In May 1998, the agency announced that although bioengineered and irradiated foods are safe, they're not permitted to carry the organic label.

(continued)

(continued)

- In October 1998, the USDA issued proposals on how animals yielding organic food are to be treated and how the agency would certify producers of organic foods.

- In October 2002, the USDA ruled that "organic" plant foods must be grown without pesticides and "organic" animals raised on organic feed.

- In February 2003, Congress passed legislation allowing organic livestock to be given non-organic feed at any time the price of organic feed reaches two times that of the regular stuff and requiring that organic livestock must be kept in humane conditions.

- In 2004, an amendment to an appropriations bill allowed "organic" foods to contain some synthetic ingredients and refined the terms used for organic foods as follows:

- "100 percent organic" — single ingredient such as a fruit, vegetable, meat, milk and cheese (excludes water and salt).

- "Organic" — multiple ingredient foods that are 95 to 100 percent organic.

- "Made with organic ingredients" — 70 percent of the ingredients are organic. (This note can appear on the front of package, naming the specific ingredients.)

- "Contains organic ingredients" — contains less than 70 percent organic ingredients.

- In 2015, the USDA website listed these rules for labeling organic products:

- "100 percent organic" means a product in which all ingredients are certified organic with the name of the certifying agent listed on the label and any processing must be with organic ingredients or methods.

- "Organic" means a product in which all agricultural ingredients are certified organic (with the name of the certifying agent) except where specified on the National List of Allowed and Prohibited Substances; non-organic ingredients may account for a combined total of 5 percent of non-organic content (excluding water and salt).

- "Made with organic" ingredients means a product in which at least 70 percent — other than water and salt — is certified ingredients (with the agent's name) identified with an asterisk or similar mark; the rest may not have been organically produced but must be produced with organic methods.

- Foods labeled "100 percent organic" or "organic" may carry the USDA organic seal; products may not carry the USDA "organic" seal. Foods labeled "made with organic ingredients" may not.

Will this change again? Probably. For the latest, check out The National Organic Program's "Organic Labeling and Marketing Information" at www.ams.usda.gov/sites/default/files/media/OrganicLabelsExplained.png.

Listing other stuff

The extra added attraction on the Nutrition Facts Label is the complete ingredient listing, in which every single ingredient is listed in order of its weight in the product, heaviest first, lightest last. In addition, the label must spell out the true identity of some classes of ingredients known to cause allergic reactions:

>> Vegetable proteins (*hydrolyzed corn protein* rather than the old-fashioned *hydrolyzed vegetable protein*)

>> Milk products (*nondairy* products, such as coffee whiteners, may contain the milk protein caseinate, which comes from milk)

>> FD&C yellow No. 5, a full, formal chemical name instead of *coloring*

Naming the precise source of sweeteners (*corn sugar monohydrate* rather than just *sugar monohydrate*) is still voluntary, but as is true of information about raw meat, fish, and poultry, manufacturers and stores just may respond to consumer pressure.

Using Pyramids, Plates, Patterns, and Labels to Choose Healthful Foods

The Food Guide Pyramids, Plates, and Patterns are designed to help you balance meals and snacks. For example, although you know that fruits and veggies are good snacks, that doesn't mean you're stuck with boring carrot sticks or an apple. The pyramid says "fruits and vegetables," not "totally raw fruits and raw vegetables." Yes, a fresh apple's fine. But so is a baked apple (100 calories), fragrant with cinnamon and decorated with no-fat sour cream (30 to 45 calories for 2 tablespoons). Carrot sticks are okay. So are vegetarian baked beans — yes, baked beans, which are considered both veggies *and* a member of the high-protein meat/beans group at 140 calories plus 26 grams of carbohydrates, 7 grams of protein, 7 grams of dietary fiber, and 2 grams of fat per ½ cup serving. As for the Nutrition Facts Label, you can use that to eat your cake and have it nutritiously by comparing products to choose the best alternatives.

Here's a good example: You find yourself irresistibly drawn to double dark chocolate ice cream (lots of fat, saturated fat, cholesterol, and a whopping 230 calories per ½ cup serving). But then, just as your hand is opening the freezer door, ready to reach for the ice cream, suddenly out of the corner of your eye, you see the Nutrition Facts Panel on the label of the no-fat but equally irresistible chocolate sorbet. It says, "No fat, no saturated fat, no cholesterol, and only 90 to 130 calories per serving." When you put the labels side by side, do you need to ask which one comes out the winner?

Because you get to indulge while protecting your nutrition status, you opt for the irresistible chocolate sorbet. Who could ask for anything more?

Chapter **18**

Eating Smart When Eating Out

E ating out is pure pleasure: You don't have to cook, and somebody else washes the dishes. The challenge? To avoid letting luxury lull you into ceding responsibility for your food choices to some chef whose heart belongs to butter.

This chapter lays out strategies for making your adventure nutritionally sound. One trick is to edit a menu in a white-tablecloth restaurant (the food professional's description of an upscale eatery), balancing gustatory pleasure with common-sense nutrition. A second is to juggle fast-food choices to fit them into a healthful diet. And the third is to manage the ubiquitous vending machines that are so often the source of last resort.

In all three cases, no cooking, no dishes, no guilt. Who could ask for more?

Reading a Restaurant Menu

Restaurants are businesses; they respond to consumer demand. Unfortunately, what consumers have demanded for years are rich foods and big portions. Does that mean you should stop eating out? No. But it does mean you need to use caution when ordering from the menu.

Apportion the portions

Restaurants don't make friends by serving up teensy little portions. In fact, tiny servings probably sank *nouvelle cuisine*, the 1980s fad that put one string bean, three garden peas, half an artichoke heart, and one sliced cherry tomato on a lettuce leaf and called it the salad course.

TIP

Reality dictates that the portions on most restaurant plates rarely come within striking distance of the official serving sizes issued by the U.S. Department of Agriculture. To protect yourself from humongous servings, you need to fix a picture of real-life versions of the recommended portions firmly in your mind.

The task requires an 8-ounce measuring cup, a kitchen scale, and some basic foods.

>> **Meat, fish, and poultry:** Broil a small steak or roast a chicken breast. Use a kitchen scale to weigh a 3-ounce portion. Does the steak look like a deck of cards? How about a small calculator? That's one serving.

>> **Rice and pasta:** Boil some rice or pasta. When it's done, fill the measuring cup to the halfway mark. Take out the rice or pasta and roll it into a ball, about the size of a tennis ball or a billiard ball. That's one serving.

>> **Salads:** Shred, tear, or chop some greens, such as lettuce, spinach, or kale. Fill the measuring cup to the 8-ounce mark. Turn the greens out onto a salad plate. That's one serving.

>> **Fruits and veggies:** Dice some fresh apples or carrots or open one can of beets or fruit cocktail. Fill the measuring cup to the halfway mark. Spoon the fruit or vegetables onto a plate. That's one serving.

>> **Beverages:** Open a can of soda or a box of juice. Pour the liquid into the measuring cup, right up to the 8-ounce mark. Pour that into a glass. It's probably more than you get in an upscale restaurant, less than you get at the burger barn. No matter: It's still one serving.

Now that you know what a serving looks like, you can slice away the extra from your restaurant plate and take it home for lunch or dinner the next day. That's what *doggie bags* are for. (Cat owners will know that doggie bags are called doggie bags because cats are too smart — or too finicky — to eat someone else's leftovers.)

Ask for proof

When the menu says, "Eat me! I'm healthy," you want proof. The people who make and market processed foods are required by law to provide detailed ingredient labels on their packages.

Legislators have been moving to pass laws that regulate healthful eating in restaurants. For example, chain restaurants must now post the calorie counts and ingredients in their dishes online or at the store. Now the open listing wave is lapping at the doors of those chic, white-tablecloth establishments. But very gently.

True, glorious establishments, such as Per Se in New York, Vetri Ristorante in Philadelphia, or the Mansion in Dallas, each with the symbol $$$$$ after its name in dining guides, still don't have to tell you exactly what's in the truffled gnocchi or the *foie gras* (well, okay, that one's obvious). But if there's a health claim such as "low-fat" or "heart-healthy" next to an item on the menu, the Nutrition Education and Labeling Act says the restaurant has to back up that claim. The law doesn't require an ingredient listing on the menu. The restaurant can comply by keeping a notebook available at the front desk that shows the healthful dish was made according to a recipe from an authoritative professional association or dietary group, such as the ten reliable organizations whose websites are listed in Chapter 27.

Editing Your Menu Choices

From a nutritional point of view, after you get past the serving size, restaurant dining has two other basic pitfalls:

>> Garnishes and side dishes are too rich.

>> Meals have too many courses.

Not to worry. The following tricks solve these two problems.

Start simple

Set the nutritional tone of dinner right off the bat with your choice of appetizer. Your first alternative is to opt for a really rich, high-density food, such as a cream soup, and then coast downward, calorie-fat-and-cholesterol-wise, for the rest of the meal.

Your second alternative is to go the other way, choosing a tasty but low-calorie, low-fat appetizer, such as clear soup, a salad with lemon juice dressing, or shellfish — shrimp cocktail comes in a cost of just 10 to 30 calories per shrimp — with no-fat (catsup/horseradish) sauce, thus allowing yourself richer choices later in the meal.

Is there a nutrition advantage to either choice? No. The plus lies in pleasing your taste buds since you get to choose the menu you like best.

Elevate appetizers to entrees

For smaller portion sizes or to skip the calorie-laden sides that come with most entrees, order an appetizer as your main course. For example, many restaurants serve an appetizer consisting of a really big bowl of maybe 30 steamed mussels in their shells in a low-oil, fresh tomato sauce with perhaps one crusty piece of French bread underneath to sop it up. Add a glass of dry white wine plus one more piece of bread, and this appetizer becomes a meal in itself with fewer calories and less fat than most any entree on the menu. It's often less expensive, too.

Skip the fat on the bread

Don't butter your bread. Don't oil it, either. True, that little bowl of olive oil serves up less saturated fat than butter, but ounce for ounce the calorie count is exactly the same. All fats and oils (butter, margarine, vegetable oils) give you about 100 calories a tablespoon. And you may get even more calories from the oil if you do a lot of dipping.

TIP

Don't assume that your bread is low fat just because you didn't butter it. Many types of bread, such as savory focaccia or deceptively plain popovers, come already buttered (or oiled). To test your bread, pick up a piece or put it on your napkin. If your hand feels greasy or the bread leaves an oily spot on your napkin, you have your answer.

Undress the veggies

Victorians boiled vegetables practically into oblivion — no color, no texture, no taste. Then came 20th-century butter, cheese, and cream sauces, often burnished to a browned crust by the broiler.

Then *natural* became the watchword, often translated as *raw*, a trend not favorable to veggies, such as uncooked cauliflower with all the gustatory charm of cardboard. That brought on *steamed*, a good thing because the difference between raw cauliflower and cauliflower that's been steamed and dusted with, say, dill is so vast that people who insist on passing out the stuff cold should be charged with vegetable abuse.

Now smart restaurant cooks rely on herbs and spices, *reduced* (boiled down and thickened) fat-free bouillons, unusual salad combinations, and imaginative treatments, such as purees and kabobs, to make their vegetables tasty but trim. The result? Food heaven and nutrition joy as the vegetable flavors come through, and the calories stay very, very, very low.

To reap the rewards, avoid veggie dishes labeled

>> *Au beurre* (with butter)

>> *Au gratin* (with cheese sauce)

>> Batter-dipped (eggs, oil, fried)

>> Breaded (breadcrumbs, oil, fried)

>> Fritters (fried)

>> Fritto (fried)

>> Tempura (battered and fried)

Minimize the main dish

From a nutritionist's point of view, the most sensible dinner choice may be something broiled, baked, or roasted — without added fat, and with the drippings siphoned off. But you can also lower the fat content of any main dish simply by wielding a mean knife and fork to cut away the vestiges of visible fat on your chops or steak or the skin on poultry.

TIP

Another approach is to order a main course meat dish without the "main" part. That is, order your meat, fish, or poultry as a small-serving appetizer and then ask your waiter for a veggie entree. Or opt for an assortment of the side dishes that usually accompany the meat course instead of a veggie entree.

Demand tiny boiled onions, baby peas with mint, pickled beets and red cabbage, sugared carrots, sautéed spinach, or darling little boiled or baked potatoes with a crust of paprika or cumin — the more, the merrier. The result: fewer calories, more dietary fiber, and a wider variety of nutrients than plain meat or poultry.

Sideline sauces

Dining out is a treat, so treat yourself — within reason. Have your *béarnaise* (egg yolks, butter), *béchamel* (butter, flour, heavy cream), brown sauce (beef drippings, flour), and hollandaise (butter, egg yolks), as long as you have them in reasonable amounts.

Ask the waiter to bring the sauce on the side, take a tablespoonful (about a soup spoonful), and hand back the rest.

TIP

When ordering from an Italian menu, the general rule is to avoid the olive-oil-based sauces and choose the tomato-based red sauce because many restaurants now make their red sauces skinny — all tomato, with little or no oil.

Satisfy your sweet tooth

After a heavy meal, your body often craves something sweet. To satisfy that sweet tooth but lower your calories and fat totals, split a dessert with your dinner partner. Or pick a rich but fat-free sweetened coffee, such as espresso or a Greek or Turkish brew, or tea, or a diet cola, or, on special occasions, a small after-dinner wine or liqueur, about 100 to 200 fat-free calories per ounce.

THE CLEAN RESTAURANT ABCs

In 1997, the CBS affiliate KCBS-TV in Los Angeles ran a segment called "Behind The Kitchen Door," using hidden cameras to catch the staff in some of the city's spiffiest establishments doing icky things like picking up food from the floor and putting it back on the plate. Then the station noted that reports on restaurant inspections were public but that citizens could get them only by going in person to the Health Department and asking for a copy.

Suitably red-faced at being caught red-handed, the Los Angeles County Board of Supervisors quickly decided to adopt the ABC system already in place in San Diego, made the report easily available to the public, and ordered the restaurants to post a poster with the letter grade in the window.

At first, restaurants objected, but soon there was peace. Restaurants with good grades saw their revenues rise, and restaurants of all makes and models began to improve their sanitary practices in an attempt to do the same. Today, restaurants across the country sport A-B-C rating posters.

The ratings are based on a point system. In New York, for example, a *public health hazard,* such as failing to keep food at the proper temperature, is 7 points; a *critical violation,* such as serving raw food without washing or cleaning it first, is 5 points; and a *general violation,* such as not properly sanitizing pots and pans and dishes and other tools, is at least 2 points. Multiple instances of a violation mean multiple points added on, as in 7 points for one contaminated food item, 10 points for four. The points are then toted up to produce a score that produces a letter grade. In the Big Apple, the Department of Health does the inspecting and awards the following grades:

- A = 0–13 points

- B = 14–27 points

- C = 28 or more points

A fourth poster, the "Grade Pending" sign (translation: "We're working on it, and maybe you should eat somewhere else while we figure out what to do with this place") goes up when

- The restaurant is new and has not yet opened.

- The restaurant scored 14 or higher on a first inspection.

- The restaurant has scored poorly in the past and must score below 28 lest it be closed for continuing violations.

- The restaurant was closed and is seeking to reopen.

- There have been consumer complaints about the restaurant.

Want to see restaurant grades in your city, county, or state? Go to www.foodsafetynews.com/restaurant-inspections-in-your-area and run down the list until you find the area you're looking for. Be warned: Not every place listed will show you a restaurant inspection guide. For example, Connecticut lists three sites but only one, the City of Norwalk, has the info you're looking for. And just to make it more confusing, the actual system of stars and letters varies from place to place.

Writing Rules for Chain Restaurants

According to the U.S. Food and Drug Administration, Americans eat and drink about one-third of their calories away from home, lots and lots of them in *chain restaurants* (a company with more than 20 outlets doing business under the same name and selling pretty much the same products) and what FDA calls "similar retail food establishments," such as the corner deli that makes your ham-and-Swiss sandwich at lunch or the movie theater, sports venue, or amusement park that sells "made on the premises" items such as popcorn.

The latest rules require these restaurants and stores to post calorie counts, calories from fat, total fat, saturated fat, trans fat, cholesterol, sodium, total carbohydrates, fiber, sugars, and protein — everything you expect to see on an ordinary package Nutrition Facts Label (more about that in Chapter 17), menus, and on menu boards. Consumer nutrition alert: You will find more about the Nutrition Facts Label in Chapter 17, including the fact that you may soon see one figure for the sugar that occurs naturally in the food and a second for added sugar.

The covered foods include

>> Meals from sit-down restaurants

>> Foods purchased at drive-through windows

>> Take-out food, such as pizza

>> Foods such as made-to-order sandwiches ordered from a menu or menu board at a grocery store or delicatessen

>> Foods you serve yourself from a salad or hot food bar

>> Muffins at a bakery or coffee shop

>> Popcorn purchased at a movie theater or amusement park

>> A scoop of ice cream, milkshake, or sundae from an ice-cream store

>> Hot dogs or frozen drinks prepared on site in a convenience or warehouse store

>> Certain alcohol beverages, such as coolers

What's not on the list? "Certain foods purchased in grocery stores or other similar retail food establishments that are typically intended for more than one person to eat and require additional preparation before consuming, such as pounds of deli meats, cheeses, or large-size deli salads." In other words, the meat-and-cheese platter for your office bash is nutrient-label free. You can either approach it with a calorie and nutrient guide in hand or just forgo nutrition perfection for one moment of unbridled gorging.

FDA expected these rules to become effective in January 2020, but the implementation dates for federal rules can be, to put it mildly, elastic. Stay tuned. Or better yet, check out the next section to find food facts on your own.

Exploring the Healthful Side of Fast Food

Fast food can be good food. By choosing carefully, you can enjoy burgers and sandwiches and pizza while still meeting recommended dietary allowances for all important nutrients plus vitamins and minerals.

Choosing wisely at the drive-through

The greatest problem with fast food, as with all restaurant food, is *very* big servings with *very* high calorie counts and *very* scary fat content. Case in point: At one point, McDonald's Bacon ClubHouse burger clocked in at 760 calories, 40 grams of fat (15 of them artery-clogging saturated fat) and Papa John's Pizza for One with the same 760 calories per whole pie plus 28 grams of total fat and 12 grams of saturated fat.

On the other hand, who says you have to choose that burger or that pie? As you can plainly see in Table 18-1, both chains and the fat-and-calorie conscious Subway offer servings to meet anybody's nutrition standards.

TABLE 18-1 ## Nutritious Fast-Food Meals? Yes!

Nutrient	McDonald's Hamburger	Subway 6-inch Oven Roasted Chicken Sandwich	Pizza Hut medium original cheese slice
Calories	250	320	210
Fat	8g	5g	10g
Saturated fat	3.5g	2.0g	4.5g
Protein	13g	23g	11 g
Cholesterol	30 mg	25 mg	20 mg
Dietary fiber	2 g	5 g	2 g
Sodium	480 mg	640 mg	460 mg

Sources: Company websites as of June 2020

TECHNICAL STUFF

In the past several years, McDonald's, once the undisputed fast-food champion, has lost ground as a customer favorite with new contenders, such as Chipotle and Panera, filling in former blanks in the fast-food experience. So why is it included in Table 18-1? Because McDonald's, along with Subway, had more stores in the United States and around the globe than their competitors. That means they are the places you're most likely to find when you're hungry anywhere in the world.

Finding a guilt-free, 300-calorie snack solution

As Chapter 14 explains, each time you eat, your pancreas secretes insulin, the hormone than enables your body to turn food into glucose, the sugar fuel on which you run. The insulin temporarily tames your appetite, but over the next three or four hours, the insulin level falls and — bingo! — you're hungry again.

Even before the science of why you're hungry was identified, the rest of the world scheduled an afternoon tea-type snack to cope with the mid-afternoon hungries. Americans, however, were left on their own to grab whatever's close at hand. In other words, the lunch to dinner stretch can be a diet disaster.

It doesn't have to be because guilt-free, 300-calorie-and-under snacks abound to break the hunger without breaking the diet budget. For example, say you're on the road heading from one meeting to the next and what you crave is meat, plain and simple. Head for Burger King where the plain flame-broiled burger is a measly 240 calories or Wendy's where the Jr. Hamburger is the same. Want chicken? Wendy and Burger King score again with 4-nugget servings at 170 calories each.

If sweet's your treat, Dunkin' Donuts is your guide. The basic no-frills Dunkin' glazed donut is a measly 240 calories; the glazed jelly is 280 calories, still 20 calories under the 300-calorie limit. The fruit donuts, though, are definitely not. And, no, the glazed blueberry (350 calories) and the apple stick (470) don't count as one daily serving of fruit. But one apple or one banana, sometimes found at a fast-food parlor, do. One medium banana has about 105 calories; one medium apple has about 80. You can have both plus a 1-ounce box of raisins (85 calories) and still beat the 300-calorie benchmark.

Managing the Mechanical Menu

When it comes to gracious dining, vending machines are so low on the list that they're practically sliding off the bottom of the page. Nonetheless, they do sell food, which means the FDA isn't about to ignore them.

Much of the snack food sold in vending machines is prepackaged and already labeled with nutrition information. And many items do fit into the 300-calorie snack class. For example, a 1-ounce bag of Lay's Oven-Baked Potato Chips is just 120 saturated-fat-and-cholesterol-free calories. You can have two bags and still stay under 300 calories. But you can't read that on the label while the bag is still in the machine, and other foods in packages behind the glass may come with an unpleasant calorie surprise. To prevent that, the FDA has been writing rules that require vending machine operators with more than a certain number of machines to post the nutrient labels next to the machine or show the nutrient listings on a "front label" you can read through the glass window.

In the end. the guiding principle for fast food, as for every other item on your menu is the catchy catchphrase from the 2020–2025 *Dietary Guidelines for Americans:* "Make Every Bite Count."

4
Food Processing

Chapter **19**

Praising Food Processing

S ay "processed food," and most people think "cheese spread." They're right, of course. Cheese spread is, in fact, a processed food. But so are baked pota- toes, canned tuna, frozen peas, skim milk, pasteurized orange juice, and scrambled eggs. In broad terms, food processing is any technique that alters the natural state of food — cooking, freezing, pickling, drying, and so on.

This chapter describes how each form of processing changes food from a living thing (animal or vegetable) into a component of a healthful diet — and at the same time

>> Lengthens shelf life

>> Reduces the risk of foodborne illnesses

>> Maintains or improves a food's texture and flavor

>> Upgrades the nutritional value of foods

Preserving Food: Five Methods of Processing

When you're talking about food, the term *natural* doesn't necessarily translate as "safe" or "good to eat." Food spoils (naturally) when microbes living (naturally) on the surface of meat, a carrot, a peach, or whatever reproduce (naturally) to a population level that overwhelms the food (naturally).

Sometimes you can see, feel, or smell this happening. You can *see* mold growing on cheese, *feel* how meat or chicken turns slippery, and *smell* when the milk turns sour. The mold on cheese, the slippery slickness on the surface of the meat or chicken, and the odor of the milk are caused by exploding populations of micro-organisms. Don't even argue with them; just throw out the food.

Food processing reduces or limits the growth of food's natural microbe popula-tion, thus lengthening the shelf life of food and lowering the risk of foodborne illnesses.

For simplicity's sake, here's a list of the methods used to extend the shelf life of food:

>> Temperature methods

- Cooking

- Canning

- Refrigeration

- Freezing

>> Air control

- Canning

- Vacuum-packaging

- MAP (Modified Atmosphere Packaging) and CAP (Controlled Atmosphere Packaging), processes that remove or lower the amount of oxygen in the package and replace it with nitrogen, carbon dioxide (to inhibit bacterial growth) and, if the package contains meat, carbon monoxide to maintain the meat's red coloring

>> Moisture control

- Dehydration

- Freeze-drying (a method that combines methods of controlling the temperature, air, and moisture)

>> Chemical methods

- Acidification

- Mold/bacteria inhibition

- Salting (dry salt or brine)

>> Irradiation

>> High-pressure processing

For the record, two or more of these methods may be used at the same time, such as vacuum or reduced atmosphere packaged items may be refrigerated to further reduce the rate at which the food inside the package spoils.

Temperature control

Exposing food to high heat for a sufficiently long period of time reduces the growth of the naturally occurring population of bacterial spoilers. For example, *pasteurization* (heating milk or other liquids such as fruit juice to 145 to 154.4 degrees Fahrenheit for 30 minutes) kills nearly all pathogens (disease-causing microorganisms) and most other bacteria, as does high-temperature, short-time pasteurization (161 degrees Fahrenheit for 15 seconds).

HOT AND COLD

Surprise, there's no such thing as "cold." There's only the absence of heat. For example, when you put a pot of "cold" water on to boil, the heat from the stove stirs up the molecules in the water so that they move faster, releasing energy as they bump into each other. They eventually move so fast and release so much energy that the water bubbles into a boil. Add a pinch of salt, and the water will boil even faster and hotter as the molecules spend the extra energy required to push the salt particles out of the way. In other words, the "cold" water felt cold only because its molecules were sitting quiet, a state which is, yes, the absence of heat. The same sort of thing happens in the air around you, which is also full of infinitesimal particles bumping into each other. Reduce the number of particles, and the air feels cooler. That, in the simplest terms, is what happens when you turn on your air-conditioner, which pulls in air from the room, captures some of the particles, and returns the less excited air which now feels cooler but is only less hot. Physicists explore these phenomena in a branch of science *called thermodynamics,* which you can read about in *Physics I For Dummies,* by Steven Holzner (Wiley).

Chilling also protects food by slowing the rate of microbial reproduction. For example, milk refrigerated at 50 degrees Fahrenheit or lower may stay fresh for almost a week because the cold prevents any organisms that survived pasteurization from reproducing.

Removing the water

Like all living things, the microbes on food need water to reproduce. Dehydrate the food, and the bugs won't reproduce, which means the food stays edible longer. That's the rationale behind raisins, prunes, and *pemmican*, a dried mix of meat, fat, and berries adapted from East Coast Native Americans and served to 18th- and 19th-century sailors of every national stripe. Natural dehydration (loss of water) occurs when food is

>> Exposed to air and sunlight

>> Heated for several hours in a very low (250 degrees Fahrenheit) oven or smoked (the smokehouse acts as a very low oven)

Freeze-drying is a modern way to achieve the same result. This process freezes the food so its water turns to ice and then "sublimes" the ice (translation: quickly evaporates it so that it floats as a gas), leaving behind a food far less susceptible to spoilage.

Controlling the air flow

Just as microbes need water, most also need air. Reducing the air supply almost always reduces the bacterial population.

Foods are protected from air by vacuum-packaging. A *vacuum* — from *vacuus*, the Latin word for "empty" — is a space with virtually no air. Vacuum-packaging employs a container (generally a plastic bag or a glass jar) from which the air is removed before it's sealed. When you open a vacuum-packed container, the sudden little pop you hear is the vacuum being broken.

TANTALIZING TIDBIT OF FOOD NOMENCLATURE

Central American Indians dried meat to produce *chaqui,* a name carried north by Spanish explorers who used it to describe the dried meats of the Southwestern Indians, which eventually became jerky (you saw that coming, right?).

WARNING

If there's no popping sound, the seal has already been broken, allowing air inside, and that means the food inside may be spoiled or may have been tampered with. Do not taste-test; throw out the entire package, food and all.

Chemical warfare

Preservatives have had bad press, blamed (inaccurately) for a range of problems they never caused. In fact, the chemicals used as *food additives* or *food preservatives* keep your food and you safe by slowing or preventing spoilage. The most-common preservatives used in food are

» **Acidifiers:** Most microbes don't thrive in highly acidic settings, so a chemical that makes a food more acidic prevents spoilage. Wine and vinegar are acidifying chemicals, and so are *citric acid,* the natural preservative in citrus fruits, and *lactic acid,* the natural acid in yogurt.

» **Mold inhibitors:** Sodium benzoate, sodium propionate, and calcium propionate slow (but do not entirely stop) the growth of mold on bread. Sodium benzoate also is used to prevent the growth of molds in cheese, margarine, and syrups.

» **Bacteria-busters:** Salt is *hydrophilic* (*hydro* = water; *phil* = loving). So is sugar. When you cover fresh meat with salt (or sugar), the salt (or sugar) draws water up and out of the meat — and up and out of the cells of bacteria living on the meat. The bacteria die; the meat dries. And you get to enjoy sugar-cured ham or corned beef (which gets its name from the fact that large grains of salt were once called "corns").

Irradiation

Irradiation is a technique that exposes food to electron beams or to *gamma radiation,* a high-energy light stronger than the X-rays your doctor uses to make a picture of your insides. *Gamma rays* are ionizing radiation, the kind that kills living cells. As a result, irradiation prolongs the shelf life of food by destroying microbes and insects on plants (which also make food safer longer) and slowing the rate at which some plants ripen. For more about the history and effects of food irradiation, check out Chapter 21.

Improving Food's Appeal and Nutritional Value

Some food processing really does make your food taste better. For example, although steak *tartare* (chopped fresh steak) does have its devotees, most people consider a steak processed by heat — cooked — even tastier. Processing also improvers your diet by allowing you to sample a wide variety of seasonal foods (mostly fruits and vegetables) transported from grower to you by refrigerated trains or trucks all year long. And processing enables food producers to improve the nutritional status of many basic foods, such as grains and milk, by enriching or altering them to meet optimal nutrition needs.

Intensifying flavor and aroma

One advantage of food processing is that it can intensify aroma and flavor, almost always for the better. Here's how:

>> **Drying concentrates flavor.** A practically water-free prune has a different, darker, more intensely sweet flavor than a juicy fresh plum.

>> **Heating heightens aroma by quickening the movement of aroma molecules.** In fact, your first tantalizing hint of dinner usually is the scent of cooking food. Chilling has the opposite effect: It slows the movement of the molecules. To sense the difference, sniff a plate of cold roast beef versus hot roast beef straight from the oven. Or sniff two glasses of vodka, one warm, one icy from the freezer. One comes up scent-free; the other has the olfactory allure of pure gasoline. Guess which is which.

>> **Warming foods intensifies flavors.** This development is sometimes beneficial (warm roast beef is somehow more savory than cold roast beef), sometimes not (warm milk is definitely not as popular as the icy-cold version).

>> **Changing the temperature changes texture.** Heating softens some foods (butternut squash is a good example) and solidifies others (think eggs). Chilling keeps the fats in pâté firm so the stuff doesn't melt down into a puddle on the plate. Ditto for the gelatin that keeps dessert molds and dinner aspics standing upright.

Adding nutrients

The addition of vitamins and minerals to basic foods has helped eliminate many once-common nutritional deficiency diseases. For example, goiter (an enlarged thyroid gland) was pretty much eliminated after the early 1900s with the addition of iodine in your common everyday table salt. Today, the practice of improving natural nutrition is so common that you take the following for granted:

>> Breads, cereals, and grains are given extra B vitamins to replace the vitamins lost when whole grains are stripped of their nutrient-rich covering to produce white flour or white rice or degermed cornmeal. The vitamin enrichment reduces the risk of the B vitamin–deficiency diseases beriberi and pellagra.

>> Breads, cereals, and grains are also fortified with iron to replace what's lost in milling.

>> All milk sold in the United States contains added vitamin D to reduce the risk of the bone-deforming vitamin D–deficiency diseases rickets (among children) and osteomalacia (among adults).

>> Added fat-free milk proteins turn *skim milk* — milk from which the fat has been removed — into a creamier liquid with more calcium but less fat and cholesterol than whole milk.

Combining benefits

Adding genes from one food (such as corn) to another food (such as tomatoes) may make the second food taste better and stay fresh longer. You can bet that this is one hot topic; for more about genetic engineering at the dinner table, check out Chapter 22.

Faking It: Food Substitutes

In addition to its many other benefits, food processing offers up some totally fake but widely appreciated substitute fats and sweeteners. Actually, these may be just the tip of the iceberg, so to speak. In 1985, the Brits introduced Quorn, a brand-name meat substitute made from mushrooms that had become the number-1 meat substitute worldwide when it was first brought to the United States in 2002. Unfortunately, a number of consumers reacted badly — think nausea, vomiting, and possibly life-threatening allergic reactions — to the fungal proteins in the dish, so Quorn seems to have slipped back into the nutritional netherworld in the United States. Butt as processing becomes more adventurous, who knows what strange and wonderful dishes lie just beyond the entrance to this Nutritional Twilight Zone.

Alternative foods No. 1: Fat replacers

Dietary fat (the fat found naturally in food) carries flavors and makes food taste and feel "rich." But it's also high in calories, and some fats (the saturated and trans fats described in Chapter 7) can clog your arteries. One way to deal with this problem is to eliminate the fat from food, as in skim milk. Another way is to head for the food lab and create a heart-safe no- or low-calorie substitute.

Classifying fat replacers

Over the years, food technologists have created three types of fat replacers:

>> **Carbohydrate-based fat replacers** comprise complex carbohydrates that thicken food but aren't absorbed by the body. (For more on the different types of carbohydrates in plant foods, see Chapter 8.) Examples include carrageenan (a seaweed extract), guar gum (from guar beans), cellulose (insoluble dietary fiber), inulin (from the chicory root), and food starches (dextrins and maltodextrins) that may be treated chemically to change the texture or make the starch easier to dissolve and digest.

>> **Protein-based fat replacers** are commonly made by heating and blending proteins from egg whites, milk, or corn into tiny balls (technical term: *microparticulated* protein) that form a substance that feels and tastes like fat. *Simplesse* is a protein-based fat substitute. ***Note:*** These products don't provide significant amounts of dietary protein.

>> **Fat-based fat replacers** are made from fatty acids derived from *triglycerides,* the primary constituents of body fat, or from *emulsifiers,* naturally occurring compounds in foods that enable fats and water to mix. For use as fat replacers, they have been modified so they are indigestible and block the body's absorption of other fats.

Table 19-1 lists several examples of fat replacers currently found in various foods.

Evaluating fat replacers

Regardless of their source, the three important nutrition questions about fat replacers are

>> Do these additives contribute to weigh loss?

>> Do these additives enhance the nutrient value of food?

>> Are these additives safe?

TABLE 19-1   **Finding the Fake Fats**

Fat Replacer	Calories/gram	Used in
Carbohydrate-based (Brand names)		
Cellulose (Avicek, Methocel, Solka-Floc)	0	Dairy products (such as imitation sour cream and frozen desserts and salad dressings)
Dextrins (Amylum, N-oil)	4	Dairy products, salad dressings, and spreads
Dietary fiber (Opta, Oat Fiber, Snowite, Ultacel, Z-Trim)	0	Baked products and meat products
Gums (Kelcogel, Keltrol, Slendid)	0	Reduced-calorie food products, such as fat-free dressings
Inulin (Raftiline, Fruitfit, Fibruline)	1–1.2	Baked goods (including fillings and icings), dairy products (including cheese, whipped cream, and yogurt), and meat products
Maltodextrins (Crystalean, Lorelite, Maltrin, Pascelli D-Lite, Pascelli EXCEL, Paselli SA2, Star-Dri)	4	Baked goods, dairy products, salad dressings, and various dessert products
Starch and Modified food starch (Amalean I & II, Fairnex VA15 & VA 20, Instant Stellar, N-Lite, OptaGrade, Perfectamyl AC, Pure-Gel, STA-SLIM)	1–4	Baked goods, dairy products, frozen desserts, salad dressings, and sauces
Oat flour (Beta-Trim, TrimChoice)	<1	Baked goods, nonfat milks (such as non-fat whipped cream)
Polydextrose (Litesse, Stal-Lite)	1	Baked goods, dandies, chewing gum, salad dressing, gelatins, puddings, frozen desserts
Starch and modified food starch (Amalean I & II, Fairnex VA15 & VA20, Instant Stellar, N-Lite, OptaGrade, Perfectamyl AC, AX-1 & AX-2, PURE-GEL, STA-SLIM)	1	Baked goods, margarines, salad dressing, commercial soups, and processed cheese products
Oat, pea, rice, soybean hulls (Z-Trim)	0	Baked goods, salad dressings, sauces, soups, and meat products
Protein-based		
Microparticulated protein (Simplesse), Whey protein concentrate (Dairy-Lo), Others, made from a variety of proteins from eggs milk, and corn (K=Blazer, Ultra Bake, Ultra-Freeze, Lita)	1–2	Dairy products including milk, cheese, yogurt, and ice cream, milk products (ice cream, yogurt), mayonnaise-type and salad dressings, frozen desserts and baked goods

(continued)

TABLE 19-1 *(continued)*

Fat Replacer	Calories/gram	Used in
Fat-based		
Emulsifiers (natural) (Dur-Lo, ECT-25)	9	Cakes, cookies, and icings
Fatty acids and alcohol/sorbitol (Sorbestrin)	1.5	Vegetable oil substitute
Sucrose and edible fats (Olean)	0	Snack foods and baked goods
Triglycerides (Salatrim/Benefat)	5	Baked goods and "filled" milk products

Note: All brand names in this chart are trademarked.

Source: www.caloriecontrol.org/glossary-of-fat-replacers *as of June 2020*

DO FAT REPLACERS HELP PEOPLE LOSE WEIGHT?

Maybe. Fat replacers are designed to reduce the amount of fat and therefore the number of calories in ordinarily high-calorie foods such as cakes, cookies, and potato chips. But lowering the fat content may mean increasing calories from other ingredients such as sugar. In the end, the calorie count of the low-fat food may not be much lower than that of the regular product, and beause it sounds like a diet food, you may eat a lot more and increase your calorie count overall.

On the other hand, even if the calorie count stays the same, simply adding the fat replacer may alter, in a good way, how the food affects your body. In 2008, a team of nutrition researchers from the University of Copenhagen published a report in the *American Journal of Clinical Nutrition* showing that when volunteers were given one of two meals — the first with foods with their normal fats in place, the second with foods whose fats had been replaced with a fat substitute — those who got the second meal were less hungry for a longer period of time after eating. Why? The authors explain that the substitute isn't absorbed by the body and inhibits the body's absorption of other fats in food. As a result, more food fat stays in the intestines longer, creating the feeling of fullness that decreases appetite. Nonetheless, in 2019, a team of Chinese and Canadian researchers noted that there is limited evidence of how and whether starch-based fat replacers actually reduce the risk of heart disease and/or control obesity, thus concluding that, yes, more research is indeed required.

In short. calorie control, a balanced diet, and a reasonable amount of exercise remain the most healthful tools for weight loss.

ARE FAT REPLACERS NUTRITIOUS?

Carbohydrate-based fat replacers do add carbs to food in the form of soluble or insoluble dietary fiber (see Chapter 8). But neither protein-based fat replacers nor fat-based fat replacers contribute anything but infinitesimal amounts of nutrients. In addition, because natural food fats help your body dissolve and absorb fat-soluble nutrients (see Chapter 10), foods made with these substitute fats commonly contain added vitamin A, vitamin D, vitamin E, and vitamin K.

ARE FAT REPLACERS SAFE?

The adverse effects of carb-based fat replacers are usually limited to minor gastro discomfort such as flatulence (intestinal gas) due to an increase in dietary fiber.

The poster child for fat-replacer problems was Olestra (brand name: Olean), a sucrose and fatty acid compound approved by the FDA in 1996. But along with the approval, the FDA required a warning on the label that olestra may cause abdominal cramping and loose stools. In 1998, an 18-member FDA food advisory committee reaffirmed the agency's original decision that olestra is safe for use in snack foods and concluded that the fat alternative's gastrointestinal effects didn't significantly affect public health. Five years later, following a review of several studies conducted after foods with olestra went on sale, the FDA concluded that the statement was no longer required. But the fact is that eating excess amounts of foods containing olestra may lead to uncomfortable results. Be smart: Read labels and limit the chips.

A second class of fat-based fat replacers is made of milk and egg proteins, which means it may be trouble for people who are sensitive to these foods.

Conclusion? As the American Heart Association has written, while "fat replacers on the market are considered safe by the U.S. Food and Drug Administration (FDA), their long-term benefits and safety are not known. The cumulative impact of using multiple fat replacers as they increase in the marketplace is unknown. Still, within the context of a healthy diet that meets dietary recommendations, fat replacers used appropriately can provide flexibility with diet planning."

Alternative foods No. 2: Substitute sweeteners

Most substitute sweeteners were discovered by accident in laboratories where researchers touched a paper or a pencil and then stuck their fingers in their mouths to discover, "Eureka! It's sweet." As Harold McGee wrote in the first edition of his wonderful *On Food and Cooking* (Collier Books, 1988), "These stories make one wonder about the standards of laboratory hygiene." Alas, when Mr. McGee updated and expanded his book for the second edition, he took out most of the entertainingly arch observations such as this one. Get the second edition for the details; keep the first or check out McGee's website www.curiouscook.com for the fun.

Because substitute sweeteners aren't absorbed by your body and don't provide any nutrients, scientists call them by their proper name: *non-nutritive sweeteners*. As with fat replacers, there is serious doubt as to whether these ingredients actually promote weigh loss. In 2019, a team of Korean and Australian scientists cited a seven-year survey of more than 5,000 American adults showing that those who consumed large quantities of artificial sweeteners actually gained more weight than those who just ate plain sweetened foods because rather than cutting back on sugary foods, they simply added the artificially-sweetened ones to their daily diets. More worrying was the fact that the artificial sweeteners seem to alter natural bacteria in the intestinal tract, which may not only lead to weight gain but also increase the risk of Type 2 diabetes. Once again, more studies are needed to reach a solid conclusion.

In the meantime, these are the best known and most widely used sweeteners, listed in order of their discovery and/or FDA approval.

>> **Saccharin (Sweet 'N Low):** This synthetic sweetener was discovered by accident (the fingers-in-the-mouth syndrome) at Johns Hopkins in 1879. A ban on saccharin was proposed in 1977, after it was linked to bladder cancer in rats; however, it's still on the market, and diabetics who have used saccharin for years show no excess levels of bladder cancer. In 1998, the executive committee of the National Toxicology Program (NTP) recommended that saccharin be taken off the list of suspected human carcinogens; in 2010, it was. ***Note:*** Most people think saccharin is very sweet, but if you hate broccoli, you're likely to think saccharin's bitter. Check out Chapter 15 to see why.

>> **Cyclamates:** These sweeteners, created in 1937 at the University of Illinois, were subsequently linked to cancer in laboratory animals and banned (1969) in the United States. Since then, the FDA says that more than 20 years' worth of follow-up studies show no such link. In 2013, the ban was lifted.

>> **Aspartame (Equal, NutraSweet):** Another accidental discovery (1965), *aspartame* is a combination of two amino acids, aspartic acid and phenylalanine. Aspartame is safe for most healthy people; the exception is those born with *phenylketonuria (PKU),* a metabolic defect characterized by a lack of the enzyme needed to digest phenylalanine. In the body (or when it is exposed to heat), aspartame breaks down into its constituent ingredients, and if you lack the required enzyme, the excess phenylalanine can pile up in brain and nerve tissue. Newborns are usually tested for PKU because for them the excess phenylalanine may lead to mental retardation, epilepsy, and retarded growth.

>> **Sucralose (Splenda):** *Sucralose,* discovered in 1976, is a no-calorie sweetener made from sugar. But the body doesn't recognize sucralose as a carbohydrate or a sugar, so it zips through the intestinal tract unchanged. More than 100 scientific studies conducted during a 20-year period attest to its safety, and

the FDA has approved its use in a variety of foods, including baked goods, candies, substitute dairy products, and frozen desserts.

>> **Acesulfame-K (Sunett, Sweet One):** This one is also known as Ace-K; in both cases the K is the chemical symbol for potassium. This artificial sweetener, with a chemical structure similar to saccharin, is found in baked goods, chewing gum, and other food products. In 1998, the FDA approved its use to prolong the shelf life of soft drinks.

>> **Neotame:** Neotame is a modified version of aspartame. In 2002, the FDA approved Neotame for use as a tabletop sweetener as well as for use in jams and jellies, syrups, puddings and gels, fruits, fruit juices, and non-alcohol beverages.

>> **Stevia (Truvia):** In 2008, the FDA ruled that Truvia, a sweetener made from stevia (a South American plant member of the sunflower family) can be designated GRAS ("generally regarded as safe"). Stevia (Truvia), used to sweeten some carb-free soft drinks, is estimated to be 200 to 300 times sweeter than sugar.

Table 19–2 compares the calorie content and sweetening power of sugar versus the substitute sweeteners. For comparison, sugar has 4 calories per gram.

TABLE 19-2   **Comparing Substitute Sweeteners to Sugar**

Sweetener	Calories Per Gram	Sweetness Relative to Sugar*
Sugar (sucrose)	4	
Tagatose	1.5**	Similar
Cyclamates	0	30–50 times sweeter than sugar
Acesulfame-K	0	200 times sweeter than sugar
Aspartame	4**	160–200 times sweeter than sugar
Stevia (Truvia)	0	350–450 times sweeter than sugar
Saccharin	0	300--500 times sweeter than sugar
Sucralose	0	600 times sweeter than sugar
Neotame	0	7,000–13,000 times sweeter than sugar

*The range of sweetness reflects estimates from several sources.

**Aspartame has 4 calories per gram, but you need so little to get a sweet flavor that you can count the calorie content as 0.

SWEET ALCOHOLS

Polyols — sometimes known as sugar alcohols — are naturally occurring, sweet, sugar-free carbohydrate/alcohol compounds with fewer calories per gram than sucrose (sugar).

Eight polyols — erythritol, hydrogenated starch hydrolysates (including maltitol syrups), isomalt, lactitol, maltitol, mannitol, sorbitol, and xylitol — are currently used in foods such as baked goods, sugar-free candy, and chewing gum as well as drugs such as toothpaste (polyols do not contribute to tooth decay), mouthwash, and cough syrup.

The polyols are absorbed and converted to energy with little or no insulin, so these sweeteners are most useful for people with diabetes or those on a low-carbohydrate, sugar-free diet. However, because they're not completely absorbed in the intestines, if consumed in large amounts, polyols may have laxative effects.

A Last Word: Follow That Bird

You can sum up the essence of food processing by following the trail of one chicken from the farm to your table. (Vegetarians and vegans are excused from this section.)

A chicken's first brush with processing is, ugh, slaughtering, after which it's plucked and shipped off to the food processor (in some instances the company doing the slaughtering also processes the chicken into other products) or the supermarket, packed in ice to slow the natural bacterial decomposition. In the food factory, your chicken may be boiled and canned whole, or boiled and cut up and canned in small portions like tuna fish, or boiled into chicken soup to be canned or dehydrated into bouillon cubes, or cooked with veggies and canned as chicken à la king, or fried and frozen in whole pieces, or roasted, sliced, and frozen into a chicken dinner, or you get the picture.

If destined for the supermarket, a raw chicken will be packed and dated. When you buy it and bring it home, you'll do your own processing. First, the chicken goes to the refrigerator (or freezer), then onto your kitchen counter to be designed into whatever dish you are cooking, then into the pan or pot and onto the stove or into the oven. Because raw chicken is sometimes contaminated with salmonella bacteria, at this point, you clean your counter and wash your hands and any knives, forks, spoons, or dishes the raw chicken touched. Then you wait until the chicken is thoroughly done, using a meat thermometer to check the temperature, which should read at least 165 degrees Fahrenheit to make sure that no stray bacteria survive to make their way to your dinner table (or you).

When dinner's done, it's back to the fridge or into the freezer with the leftovers. The chicken's been processed. And you have eaten. That's the point of this story.

Chapter **20**

Healthful and Delicious Heat

You can bet that the first cooked dinner was an accident involving some poor wandering animal and a bolt of lightning that charred the beast into medium rare sirloin. Then a caveman attracted by the aroma tore off a sizzled hunk and forthwith offered up the first restaurant rating: "Yum."

After that, it was but a hop, a skip, and a jump, anthropologically speaking, to gas ranges, electric broilers, and microwave ovens. This chapter explains how these technologies affect the safety, nutritional value, appearance, flavor, and aroma of the foods that you heat.

For more pragmatic details on what and how to cook, check out *Cooking Basics For Dummies*, 5th Edition, by Bryan Miller and Marie Rama, (Wiley), and then fire up the stove.

Exploring Different Methods of Cooking

The dictionary defines cooking as preparing food by heating it. In your kitchen, that means exposing food to the energy created either by a gas fire, an electric heating plate, or the radio waves in your microwave.

Cooking with fire

Ever since man discovered fire and how to control cooking — rather than having to wait for that passing lightning flash — the human race has generally relied on three simple ways to heat food:

>> **An open flame:** You hold the food directly over — or under — the flame or put the food on a griddle on top of the flame. (The electric heating coil is a 20th-century variation on the open flame.)

>> **Hot air:** You put the food in a closed box (an oven) and heat the air in the oven to create high-temperature dry heat.

>> **Hot liquid:** You submerge the food in hot liquid or suspend the food over the liquid so it cooks in the steam escaping from the surface.

Sophisticated cooks may combine two or more of these methods. For example, cooking food in a wrapper, such as aluminum foil or a papaya leaf (see Chapter 31), combines two methods: open fire (the grill) or hot air (the oven) plus the steam from the food's own juices (hot liquid).

The basic methods for cooking with heat generated by fire or an electric coil are

Open Flame	Hot Air	Hot Liquid
Broiling	Baking	Boiling
Grilling	Roasting	Deep-frying
Toasting		Poaching
		Simmering
		Steaming
		Stewing

Cooking with electromagnetic waves

A microwave oven generates electromagnetic energy (microwaves) produced by a device called a magnetron.

The energy transmitted from the magnetron excites water molecules in food. The water molecules leap about like hyperactive 3-year-olds, producing friction, which produces the heat that cooks the food sometimes twice as fast as plain fire.

WARNING

Because the dish on which food sits in a microwave oven has very few water molecules, it generally stays cool. But some dishes or containers do heat up. To be safe, use a potholder when taking a dish out of the microwave.

Understanding How Cooking Alters Food

Cooking changes the way food looks, smells, feels, and tastes, producing more appetizing texture, rich color, intense flavor, and fragrant aroma all due to exposure to heat.

Changing food's texture

Exposure to heat alters the structures of proteins, fats, and carbohydrates, changing their *texture* (the way food particles are linked to make the food feel hard or soft). In other words, cooking can turn crisp carrots soft and tough meat tender.

Protein

Proteins are made of very long molecules that sometimes fold over into accordion-like structures (see Chapter 6 for details about proteins). Although heating food doesn't lower its protein value, it does

>> Break protein molecules into smaller fragments

>> Cause protein molecules to unfold and form new bonds to other protein molecules

GRAINS: SPLIT PERSONALITY PERFORMERS

When grains are cooked, they exhibit split personalities — part protein, part complex carbohydrates. For example, boil an ear of corn and the protein molecules inside the kernels will do the break-unfold-network dance (the molecules break their links, the proteins unfold, and their molecules form new links). At the same time, carbohydrate starch granules begin to absorb moisture and soften.

Want to see this happen? Boil an ear of corn. The trick to doing it right is to take the corn out of the water when starch granules have absorbed enough moisture to soften the kernels but before the protein network has tightened. On the other hand, if you're a person who likes corn chewy, just let it boil away — 15 minutes, 30 minutes, whatever.

Need an example? Consider the egg. When you cook one, the long protein molecules in the white unfold, form new connections to other protein molecules, and link up in a network that tightens to squeeze out moisture so the egg white hardens and turns opaque. The same unfold-link-squeeze reaction turns translucent poultry firm and makes gelatin set. The longer you heat proteins, the stronger the network becomes, and the tougher, or more solid, the food will be. The inevitable exception to this rule is that connective tissue — the tissue that connects, supports, and holds other tissues and organ — softens when exposed to heat, which is why meat becomes more tender when cooked even though it is protein-rich.

To see this work, scramble two eggs — one beaten and cooked plain and one beaten with milk and then cooked. Adding liquid (milk) makes it more difficult for the protein network to squeeze out all the moisture, so the egg with the added milk cooks up softer than the plain egg.

Fat

Heat melts fat, allowing it to run off, which lowers the calorie count. In addition, heat breaks down connective tissue, the body's supporting framework of the body, which includes some *adipose* (fatty) tissue. Thus, the food softens and becomes more pliable. You can see this most clearly when cooking fish, which flakes when it's done because its connective tissue has been destroyed.

When meat and poultry are stored after cooking, their fats continue to change, picking up oxygen from the air. Oxidized fats have a slightly rancid taste, more politely known as *warmed-over flavor.*

TIP

You can slow — but not entirely prevent — this reaction by cooking and storing meat, fish, and poultry under a blanket of food rich in natural *antioxidants*, chemicals that prevent other chemicals from reacting with oxygen. Vitamin C is a natural antioxidant, so gravies and marinades made with tomatoes, citrus fruits, or tart cherries slow the natural oxidation of fats in cooked or stored foods.

Carbohydrates

Cooking has different effects on simple carbohydrates and complex ones (more about them in Chapter 8). When heated

>> Simple sugars — such as sucrose or the sugars on the surface of meat and poultry — caramelize, or melt and turn brown. (Think of the top of a *crème caramel*.)

>> Starch, a complex carbohydrate, becomes more absorbent, which is why pasta expands and softens in boiling water (see the sidebar "Grains: Split personality performers").

>> Some dietary fibers (gums, pectins, hemicellulose) dissolve, which is why vegetables and fruits soften when cooked.

The last two reactions have the added benefit of making nutrients inside previously fiber-stiffened cells more available to your body.

A less beneficial effect of heat on carbs surfaced early in 2002 when Swedish researchers announced that exposing starchy carbohydrate foods — such as potatoes and bread — to the high heat of baking or frying produces *acrylamides*, a family of chemicals known to cause cancer in rats. Then things got worse when scientists at the City of Hope Cancer Research Center (Los Angeles) said that acrylamides could trigger cell changes leading to cancer in human beings.

However, a 2003 analysis of data from a study of 987 cancer patients and 538 healthy "controls" conducted by researchers at Harvard School of Public Health and the Departments of Oncology–Pathology and Medical Epidemiology at Karolinska Institutet in Stockholm showed no evidence of an increased risk of bowel, bladder, or kidney cancer among fans of fries and toast. (Acrylamide also forms in coffee when coffee beans are roasted, not when coffee is brewed at home or in a restaurant. So far, scientists have not found good ways to reduce acrylamide formation in coffee.)

By 2010, the official FDA position on acrylamides was, essentially, no big deal. Nonetheless, the FDA does offer a list of ways to reduce acrylamide formation in potatoes and bread. In the words of the experts:

>> **Frying causes the highest acrylamide formation.** Roasting potato pieces causes less acrylamide formation, followed by baking whole potatoes. Boiling potatoes and microwaving whole potatoes with skin on to make "microwaved baked potatoes" does not produce acrylamide.

>> **Soaking raw potato slices in water for 15-30 minutes before frying or roasting helps reduce acrylamide formation during cooking.** (Soaked potatoes should be drained and blotted dry before cooking to prevent splattering or fires.)

>> **Storing potatoes in the refrigerator can result in increased acrylamide during cooking.** Therefore, store potatoes outside the refrigerator, preferably in a dark, cool place, such as a closet or a pantry, to prevent sprouting.

>> **Generally, more acrylamide accumulates when cooking is done for longer periods or at higher temperatures.** Cooking cut potato products, such as frozen fries or potato slices, to a golden yellow color rather than a brown color helps reduce acrylamide formation.

>> Toasting bread to a light brown color, rather than a dark brown color, lowers the amount of acrylamide.

For even more information on acrylamides, check Acrylamide Questions and Answers at www.fda.gov/food/chemicals/acrylamide-questions-and-answers.

Enhancing flavor and aroma

Heat degrades (breaks apart) flavor and aroma chemicals, allowing the molecules to float off into space and into your nose. As a result, most cooked food has a more intense flavor and aroma than raw food.

A good example is what happens when you cook cruciferous vegetables, such as cabbage and cauliflower. These vegetables get their distinctive flavor and aroma from mustard oils, whose sensory signals grow more intense the longer the vegetables are cooked. But every rule has an exception: Heat destroys *diallyl disulfide*, the chemical that gives raw garlic, onions, and leeks their bite and bark; cooked garlic tastes and smells milder than raw.

By the way, if you, like President George Herbert Walker Bush, absolutely hate the taste of cruciferous veggies, you are a person who is sensitive to phenylthiocarbamide (PTC), a bitter chemical in these plants. The theory is that disliking bitter tastes helped protect early man (and woman) from poisonous plants. Today, nutritionists know that in some cases — like broccoli, Brussels sprouts, and their relatives — bitter is better.

Shading the color palette

Carotenoids — the natural red and yellow pigments that make carrots and sweet potatoes orange and tomatoes red — are practically impervious to heat and the acidity or alkalinity of cooking liquids. No matter how you cook them or how long, these particular pigments stay bright and sunny.

That's not the case for the other pigments that make other foods naturally red, green, or white. These pigments react — usually for the worse — to heat, acids (such as wine, vinegar, or tomato juice), and basic (alkaline) chemicals (such as mineral water or baking soda and water). Here's a brief rundown on the color changes that you can expect when you cook food:

» Red beets and red cabbage get their colors from pigments called *anthocyanins.* Acids make these pigments redder. Alkaline solutions fade anthocyanins from red to bluish purple.

» Potatoes, cauliflower, rice, and white onions are whitened by pigments called *anthoxanthins.* When anthoxanthins are exposed to alkaline chemicals (mineralized water or baking soda), they turn yellow or brownish. Acids prevent this reaction. Boil cauliflower florets in water, and they darken slightly. Boil them in tomato juice, rinse off the juice, and you'll see — white cauliflower.

» Green veggies are colored by *chlorophyll,* a pigment that reacts with acids in cooking water (or in the vegetable itself) to form *pheophytin,* a brown pigment. The only way to short-circuit this reaction is to protect the vegetables from acids. Old-time cooks added alkaline baking soda, but that increases the loss of certain vitamins (see the section "Protecting the Nutrients in Cooked Foods," later in this chapter) and softens the vegetables. Fast cooking at high heat or cooking in lots of water (which dilutes acids) lessens these color changes.

» The natural red color of fresh meat comes from *myoglobin* in the muscle tissue and *hemoglobin* in blood. When meat is heated, the pigment molecules are *denatured,* or broken into fragments. They lose oxygen and turn brown or — after long cooking — turn the really unappetizing gray characteristic of steam-table meats. This inevitable change is more noticeable in beef than in pork or veal because beef, which contains more myoglobin, starts out naturally redder.

RED TO BLUE AND BACK AGAIN

The following experiment lets you see colors change right before your very eyes. You will need

- 1 small can sliced beets
- 1 saucepan
- 3 small glass bowls
- 1 cup water
- 1 teaspoon baking soda
- 3 tablespoons white vinegar

Line up the glass bowls on your kitchen counter. Open the can of beets. Remove six slices of beets. Put two slices in the first glass bowl and four slices in the saucepan. Put the rest in a small container and refrigerate for dinner. No sense wasting good beets!

Mix the baking soda into the water and add this alkaline solution to the saucepan. Warm over low heat for 4 minutes; don't heat too high because this solution foams. Turn off the heat. Remove the beets from the pan. Put two slices each in the second and third glass bowls.

Ignore the second bowl. Add the vinegar (an acid) to the third bowl. Wait two minutes. Now look: The beets in the first bowl (straight from the can) should still be bright red. Alkaline compounds darken colors, so the beets in the second bowl, straight from the baking soda bath, should be almost navy blue. Acids reverse the reaction, so beets in the third bowl, with added vinegar, should be heading back to bright red. Not yet? Add another tablespoon of vinegar and watch chemistry do its magic.

Picking the Right Cooking Materials

The pot you choose may affect the nutritional value of food by

» Adding nutrients to the food

» Slowing the natural loss of nutrients during cooking

» Actively increasing the loss of nutrients during cooking

In addition, some pots make the food's natural flavors and aromas more intense, which, in turn, can make the food more — or less — appetizing. The following sections describe the effects different pots and materials have on your food.

Aluminum

Aluminum is lightweight and conducts heat well. That's good. But the metal makes some aroma chemicals, such as those in the cruciferous veggies, much smellier and releases microscopic flakes that can turn white foods, such as cauliflower or potatoes, yellow or brownish.

TECHNICAL STUFF

Yes, that old chestnut about aluminum being hazardous to your health is f-a-l-s-e. True, cooking salty or acidic foods (wine, tomatoes) in aluminum pots increases the flaking, but even then, the amount of aluminum you get from the pot is less than you get naturally every day from plain food and water.

Copper

Copper pots heat steadily and evenly. To take advantage of this property, many aluminum or stainless steel pots are made with a layer of copper sandwiched into the bottom. But naked copper is a potentially poisonous metal, so copper pots are lined with tin or stainless steel. To be safe, check the lining of your copper pots from time to time. If it's damaged — meaning that you can see the orange copper through the silvery surface — have the pot relined or throw it out.

COPPER AND EGG WHITES: A CHEMICAL TEAM

When you whip an egg white, its proteins unfold, form new bonds, and create a network that holds air in. That's why the runny white turns into stable foam.

You can certainly whip egg whites successfully in a glass or ceramic bowl that is chilled, and absolutely free of any fat, including egg yolk, which would prevent the proteins from linking tightly. But the best choice is copper: The ions (particles) flaking off the surface bind with and stabilize the foam. (Aluminum ions stabilize but darken the whites.)

But wait. Isn't copper toxic? Yes, but the amount you get in an occasional batch of whites is so small it's insignificant, safety-wise.

Ceramics

The chief virtue of plain terra cotta (the orange clay that looks like red bricks) is its *porosity*, the fact that it contains millions of tiny pores that allow excess steam to escape while holding in just enough moisture to make food tender.

Decorated ceramic vessels are another matter. For one thing, the glaze makes the pot much less porous so meat or poultry cooked in a covered painted ceramic pan steams instead of roasts, producing a soggy surface rather than a crisp one.

More importantly, some pigments used to paint or glaze the pots may contain lead. To seal the decoration and prevent lead from leaching into food, the painted pots are *fired* (baked in an oven). If the pots are fired in an oven that isn't hot enough or if they aren't fired for a long enough period of time, lead will leach from ceramics when in contact with acidic foods, such as fruit juices or foods marinated in wine or vinegar.

Ceramics made in the United States, Japan, and Great Britain generally are considered safe, but for maximum protection, hedge your bets. Unless the pot comes with a tag or brochure that specifically says it's acid-safe, don't use it for cooking or storing foods. And always wash decorated ceramics by hand; repeated passes through the dishwasher can wear down the surface.

Enamelware

Enameled pots are made of metal covered with *porcelain*, a fine translucent china. Enamelware heats more slowly and less evenly than plain metal. A good-quality enameled surface resists discoloration and doesn't react with food, but it can chip, and it's easily marked or scratched by cooking utensils other than wood or hard plastic. If the surface chips and you can see the metal underneath, discard the pot lest metals flake into your food.

Glass

Glass is a neutral material that doesn't react with food. However, two cautions apply:

>> If your glass pot or dish has a metal band or handle, don't stick it in the microwave oven. Not only does the metal block microwaves, it also causes *arcing* — a sudden electrical flare that may damage the oven and scare you out of your wits.

>> Glass breaks, sometimes all over the floor. Are you a person who often drops things? Pass on the glass.

Iron

Iron conducts heat well and stays hot significantly longer than other pots. It's easy to clean. It lasts forever, and it releases iron ions into food, which may improve the nutritional value of dinner.

In 1985, nutrition researchers at Texas Tech University (Lubbock) conducted a classic experiment to measure the iron content of foods cooked in iron pots. Among their conclusions: Beef stew (0.7 milligrams of iron per 100 grams/ 3.5 ounces, raw) can end up with as much as 3.4 milligrams of iron per 100 grams after cooking slightly longer than an hour in an iron pot.

The downside? "Pumping iron" isn't a bad way to describe the experience of cooking with iron pots. They're really, really heavy.

Nonstick

Nonstick surfaces are made of plastic (polytetrafluoroethylene — PTFE for short) plus *hardeners* — chemicals that harden and seal the surface. As long as the surface is unscratched and intact, it won't react with food.

To avoid surface scratches, stick to wooden or plastic spoons when using these pots. Otherwise, your pot may end up looking like chickens have been stomping on the surface. Scratched nonstick pots and pans are not a health hazard. If you swallow tiny pieces of the nonstick coating, they pass through your body undigested.

However, when nonstick surfaces get very hot, they may

>> Separate from the metal to which they're bound (the sides and bottom of the pot).

>> Emit odorless fumes. If the cooking area isn't properly ventilated, you may experience *polymer fume fever* — flulike symptoms with no known long-term effect. To prevent this, keep the stove flame moderate. And you may as well open a window.

Stainless steel

Stainless steel is an *alloy*, a substance composed of two or more metals. Its virtues are hardness and durability; its drawback is poor heat conduction. In addition, stainless steel isn't *really* stainless. When exposed to high heat, stainless steel develops a characteristic multi-hued "rainbow" discoloration. Starchy foods, such as pasta and potatoes, may darken the pot, and undissolved salt can pit the surface. If your stainless steel pot is scratched deeply enough to expose the inner layer under the shiny surface, the metals in the alloy may flake into your food. Toss the pot.

Plastic and paper

Plastic melts and paper burns, so you obviously can't use plastic or paper containers in a stove with an open flame (gas) or heat source (electric). But you can use them in the microwave so long as you pick a proper plastic.

When plastic dishes or plastic wrap are heated in a microwave oven, they may emit potentially carcinogenic compounds that can migrate into your food. Because the Food and Drug Administration (FDA) requires microwave-safe plastics to meet strict safety standards, repeated studies show no ill effects from their minimal leakage.

The U.S. Department of Agriculture's Food Safety and Inspection Service (FSIS) offers these rules for safe microwave cooking with plastics:

>> Choose only copper and plastic cookware specially manufactured and labeled for microwave oven use.

>> Plastic storage containers such as margarine tubs, take-out containers, whipped topping bowls, and other one-time use containers should not be used in microwave ovens. These containers can warp or melt, possibly causing harmful chemicals to migrate into the food.

>> Microwave plastic wraps, wax paper, cooking bags, parchment paper, and white microwave-safe paper towels should be safe to use. Do not let plastic wrap touch foods during microwaving.

>> Never use thin plastic storage bags, brown paper or plastic grocery bags, newspapers, or aluminum foil in the microwave oven.

Protecting the Nutrients in Cooked Foods

Myth: All raw foods are more nutritious than cooked ones.

Fact #1: Some foods (such as meat, poultry, and eggs) are positively dangerous when consumed raw (or undercooked). Other foods are less nutritious raw because they contain substances that destroy or disarm other nutrients. For example, raw dried beans contain enzyme inhibitors that interfere with your body's ability to digest protein. Heating disarms the enzyme inhibitor.

Fact #2: That said, there's no denying that some nutrients are lost when foods are cooked. Simple strategies such as steaming vegetables quickly rather than boiling, or broiling rather than frying, can significantly reduce the loss of nutrients.

Maintaining minerals

Virtually all minerals are unaffected by heat. Cooked or raw, food has the same amount of calcium, phosphorus, magnesium, iron, zinc, iodine, selenium, copper, manganese, chromium, and sodium. However, potassium, like the B vitamins (see Table 20-1), does leech from foods into the cooking liquid.

TABLE 20-1   ## What Takes Vitamins Out of Food?

Vitamin	Heat	Air	Water	Fat
Vitamin A	X			X
Vitamin D				X
Vitamin E	X	X		X
Vitamin C	X	X	X	
Thiamin	X		X	
Riboflavin			X	
Vitamin B6	X	X	X	
Folate	X	X		
Vitamin B12	X		X	
Biotin			X	
Pantothenic acid	X			
Potassium			X	

Keeping those volatile vitamins

Many vitamins are sensitive to and easily destroyed by heat, air, water, or fats (cooking oils). Table 20-1 shows which vitamins are sensitive to these influences.

TIP

To avoid specific types of vitamin loss, keep in mind the following tips for the different vitamins:

>> **Vitamins A, E, and D:** To reduce the loss of fat-soluble vitamins, cook with very little oil. For example, bake or broil liver, which is rich in vitamin A, with very little oil. Ditto for fatty fish (salmon, tuna, and mackerel), one of the few natural food sources of vitamin D.

>> **B vitamins:** Conserve the B vitamins that leak out of meat and poultry into cooking liquid or drippings by using the liquid in soup or sauce.

Caution: Don't shorten cooking times or use lower temperatures to lessen the loss of heat-sensitive vitamin B12 from meat, fish, or poultry. These foods and their drippings must be thoroughly cooked to ensure that they're safe to eat.

To preserve the B vitamins in grains, don't rinse the grains before cooking unless the package advises you to do so. Some rice, such as basmati, does need to be rinsed and/or soaked to release its nutrients when cooked, but rinsing other rices even once may wash away as much as 25 percent of their thiamin (vitamin B1).

>> **Vitamin C:** To reduce the loss of water-soluble, oxygen-sensitive vitamin C, cook fruits and vegetables in the least possible amount of water. A series of experiments at Cornell University demonstrated that when you cook 1 cup of cabbage in 4 cups of water, the leaves lose as much as 90 percent of their vitamin C. Reverse the ratio — 1 cup water to 4 cups cabbage — and you hold on to more than 50 percent of the vitamin C.

Another vitamin C–saver is to bake or boil root vegetables (carrots, potatoes, and sweet potatoes) whole, in their well-washed skins. This trick retains about 65 percent of the vitamin C.

Serve cooked vegetables quickly: After 24 hours in the fridge, most vegetables lose one-fourth of their vitamin C; after two days, nearly half.

Keeping Food Safe by Cooking

In 2018, the Food and Drug Administration estimated that each year 48,000,000 Americans, one in every six, falls ill after eating contaminated food. About 128,000 end up in the hospital, and 3,000 die from foodborne illness caused primarily by pathogens (disease-causing organisms).

Should these numbers worry you? Yes. Although pathogens in food are most dangerous for the very young, the very old, and those whose immune systems have been weakened by illness or medication, the truth is that these microorganisms are equal-opportunity troublemakers — anyone who eats food carrying them may get sick.

Naming the bad guys

Many microbes living naturally in food are harmless or even beneficial. For example:

>> *Lactobacilli* (*lacto* = milk; *bacilli* = rod-shaped bacteria) digest sugars in milk and convert the milk to yogurt, acidophilus buttermilk, kefir, koumiss, and Swiss or Ementhal cheese. (For more on friendly *Lactobacilli,* see Chapter 2.)

>> Nontoxic molds convert milk to cheeses such as Brie, Camembert, Gorgonzola, or blue cheese whose blue streaks are safe, edible mold. But molds not part of the cheese-making process can be hazardous. For your convenience, the USDA has put together a Fact Sheet on good versus bad molds at www.fsis.usda.gov/wps/portal/fsis/topics/food-safety-education/get-answers/food-safety-fact-sheets/safe-food-handling/molds-on-food-are-they-dangerous_/ct_index.

Some organisms, however, are decidedly unfriendly. For example:

>> *Clostridium botulinum (C. botulinum)* thrives in the absence of air and acidity to churn out a potentially fatal neurotoxin, which is why it is important to be careful about such low-acid canned foods as string beans. A bulging can means air has gotten in. Don't taste. Don't test. As the saying goes, "When in doubt, throw it out." (***Note:*** Yes, this is the same microbe used in a purified, nontoxic injection to relax facial muscles and reduce wrinkles.)

>> *Campylobacter jejuni (C. jejuni),* which flourishes in raw meat and poultry and unpasteurized milk, has been linked to Guillain-Barré syndrome, a paralytic illness that sometimes follows flu infection.

Table 20-2 lists the most-common food pathogens and the foods in which they're most likely to be found.

TABLE 20-2 **Disease-Causing Organisms in Food**

The Bug	Where You Find It
Campylobacter jejuni	Raw meat and poultry, unpasteurized milk
Clostridium botulinum	Under-processed low-acid canned foods, vacuum-packed smoked fish, herb-infused oils
Clostridium perfringens	Foods made from poultry or meat
E. coli	Raw beef, precut bagged salads, raw sprouts
Listeria monocytogenes	Raw meat and seafood, raw milk, some raw cheeses, ready-to-eat deli meats and hot dogs, refrigerated smoked fish, raw vegetables
Salmonella	Poultry, meat, eggs, dried foods, dairy products, raw sprouts, nuts
Shigella	Salads, raw vegetables, milk and other dairy products, poultry
Staphylococcus aureus	Custards, salads (that is, egg, chicken, and tuna salads)

USDA Meat and Poultry Hotline, Centers for Disease Control

Heating to the appropriate temperature

Cleanliness along the line from field to processing to marketing to dinner table is essential for controlling foodborne illness. Proper cooking is equally important.

Simply heating food to the temperatures shown in Table 20-3 isn't a guaranteed protection against foodborne illness, but cooking food thoroughly and keeping it hot (or chilling it quickly) after it has been cooked will incapacitate many dangerous microbes or slow the rate at which they reproduce, thus reducing the risk.

TIP

Don't rely on instinct to tell you whether a food has reached safe temperature during cooking. *Use a food thermometer.* And because some things are more complicated than they seem, read the directions that come with the thermometer to be sure you're doing it right.

TIP

When cooking a stuffed chicken or turkey, it's smart to heat up the stuffing before stuffing it into the bird. After the chicken or turkey is done, make sure the temperature inside the stuffing as well as in the body of the bird (the wide part of the leg is a good place to test) is safely high, and then remove the stuffing and refrigerate it separately. To be absolutely safe, many experts recommend cooking the stuffing separate from the bird, particularly if the stuffing is not heated prior to putting it in the bird.

TABLE 20-3   **How Hot Is Safe?**

Category	Food	Temperature (°F)
Ground meat and meat mixtures	Beef, pork, veal, lamb	160
	Turkey, chicken	165
Fresh beef, veal, lamb	Steaks, roasts, chops	145
Poultry	Chicken and turkey, whole (all cuts)	165
Pork and ham	Fresh pork	145
	Fresh ham (raw)	145
	Precooked ham (to reheat)	165
Eggs and egg dishes	Eggs	Cook until yolk and white are firm.
	Egg dishes	160
Leftovers and casseroles	Leftovers	165
	Casseroles	165
Seafood	Fin fish	145 or cook until flesh is opaque and separates easily with a fork.
	Shrimp, lobster, and crabs	Cook until flesh is pearly and opaque.
	Clams, oysters, and mussels	Cook until shells open during cooking.
	Scallops	Cook until flesh is milky white or opaque and firm.

Source: www.foodsafety.gov/food-safety-charts/safe-minimum-cooking-temperature

TWO HOURS — AND YOU'RE OUT!

Microorganisms thrive on food at temperatures between 40 and 140 degrees Fahrenheit, the temperature cooked food is likely to reach within two hours after being removed from the oven or taken off the stove and left unrefrigerated. To protect food after cooking, keep it hot or chill it right away.

If you have more questions about food safety, contact the following:

- FDA Center for Food Safety and Applied Nutrition (CFSAN)

  Website: www.fda.gov/about-fda/fda-organization/center-food-safety-and-applied-nutrition-cfsan

  Phone: 1-888-SAFE FOOD (888-723-3366)

- USDA Meat and Poultry Hotline

  Phone: 1-888-MPHotline (1-888-674-6854)

  Email: mphotline.fsis@usda.gov

Chapter **21**

How Freezing, Canning, Drying, and Zapping Protect Your Food

Cold air, hot air, no air, and radioactive rays all can be used to make food safer for longer periods of time by reducing or eliminating damage from exposure to air or to the organisms that live naturally on food.

The methods described in this chapter all have one important thing in common: Used correctly, each process can dramatically lengthen food's shelf life. The downside? Nothing's perfect, so you still have to monitor your food from time to time to make sure that the preservation treatment has preserved it. The following pages tell you how.

Cold Comfort: Chilling and Freezing

Keeping food cold, sometimes very cold, slows or suspends the activity of micro-organisms bent on digesting your food before you do.

Unlike heat, which kills many microorganisms (see Chapter 20), chilling or freezing food may only reduce the population, sidelining them for a while. For example, *mold spores* (hibernating mold organisms) may sleep inside frozen food like so many bears inside a wintry cave. When spring comes, the bears bounce back to life; thaw the food, and the mold spores do the same.

How long things stay safe in the refrigerator or freezer varies from food to food and to some extent on the packaging (better packaging, longer freezing time). Table 21-1 provides a handy guide to the limits of safe cool storage for fresh food in a refrigerator/freezer maintaining a constant temperature. If these conditions aren't met, food may spoil more quickly.

TABLE 21-1   **How Long Foods Generally Stay Safe in Cold Storage**

Food	Type	Refrigerator (40 °F or below)	Freezer (0 °F or below)
Salad	Egg, chicken, ham, tuna and macaroni salads	3 to 4 days	Does not freeze well
Hot dogs	Opened package	1 week	1 to 2 months
	Unopened package	2 weeks	1 to 2 months
Luncheon meat	Opened package or deli sliced	3 to 5 days	1 to 2 months
	Unopened package	2 weeks	1 to 2 months
Bacon and sausage	Bacon	1 week	1 month
	Sausage, raw, from chicken, turkey, pork, or beef	1 to 2 days	1 to 2 months
	Sausage, fully cooked, from chicken, turkey, pork, or beef	1 week	1 to 2 months
Hamburger and other ground meats	Hamburger, ground beef, turkey, veal, pork, lamb, and mixtures of them	1 to 2 days	3 to 4 months
Fresh beef, veal, lamb, and pork	Steaks	3 to 5 days	4 to 12 months
	Chops	3 to 5 days	4 to 12 months
	Roasts	3 to 5 days	4 to 12 months
Ham	Fresh, uncured, uncooked	3 to 5 days	6 months
	Fresh, uncured, cooked	3 to 4 days	3 to 4 months

Food	Type	Refrigerator (40 °F or below)	Freezer (0 °F or below)
	Cured, cook-before-eating or uncooked	5 to 7 days or "use by" date	3 to 4 months
	Fully cooked, vacuum-sealed at plant, unopened	"Use by" date	1 to 2 months
	Cooked, store-wrapped, whole	1 week	1 to 2 months
	Cooked, store-wrapped, slices, half, or spiral cut	3 to 4 days	1 to 2 months
	Country ham, cooked	1 week	1 month
	Canned, labeled "Keep Refrigerated," unopened	6 to 9 months	Do not freeze
	Canned, shelf-stable, opened **Note**: An unopened, shelf-stable, canned ham can be stored at room temperature for 6-9 months.	5 to 14 days	1 to 2 months
	Prosciutto, Parma or Serrano ham, dry Italian or Spanish type, cut	2 to 3 months	1 month
Fresh poultry	Chicken or turkey, whole	1 to 2 days	1 year
	Chicken or turkey, pieces	1 to 2 days	9 months
Fresh fish	Fatty fish (salmon, tuna)	1 to 2 days	2 to 3 months
	Lean fish (cod)	1 to 2 days	6 months
Eggs	Raw eggs in shell	3 to 5 weeks	Do not freeze. Beat yolks and whites together, then freeze.
	Raw egg whites and yolks Note: Yolks do not freeze well	2 to 4 days	12 months
	Raw egg accidentally frozen in shell	Use immediately after thawing	Keep frozen, then refrigerate to thaw
	Hard-cooked eggs	1 week	Do not freeze
	Egg substitutes, liquid unopened	1 week	Do not freeze
	Egg substitutes, liquid opened	3 days	Do not freeze

(continued)

TABLE 21-1 *(continued)*

Food	Type	Refrigerator (40 °F or below)	Freezer (0 °F or below)
	Egg substitutes, frozen, unopened	After thawing, 1 week or refer to "use by" date	12 months
	Egg substitutes, frozen, opened	After cooking, 3 to 4 days or refer to "use by" date	Do not freeze
	Casseroles with eggs	3 to 4 days	After baking, 2 to 3 months
	Eggnog, commercial	3 to 5 days	6 months
	Eggnog, homemade	2 to 4 days	Do not freeze
	Pies: Pumpkin or pecan	3 to 4 days	After baking, 1 to 2 months
	Pies: Custard and chiffon	3 to 4 days	Do not freeze
	Quiche with filling	3 to 5 days	After baking, 2 to 3 months
Soups & Stews	Vegetable or meat added	3 to 4 days	2 to 3 months
Leftovers	Cooked meat or poultry	3 to 4 days	2 to 6 months
	Chicken nuggets or patties	3 to 4 days	1 to 3 months
	Pizza	3 to 4 days	1 to 2 months

https://www.foodsafety.gov/food-safety-charts/cold-food-storage-chartsDate *Last Reviewed, April 12, 2019*

TIP

Use your common sense: If food seems in any way questionable, *throw it out without tasting.* This is extremely important because smell alone can't determine whether a food contains foodborne pathogens. Or as the catchy saying goes: "When in doubt, throw it out." And for more information on the effects of freezing, go to www.usda.gov, type "freezing food FACs" in the search bar, click, and follow the prompts.

How freezing affects the texture of food

When food freezes, the water inside each cell forms tiny crystals that can tear cell walls. As the food is thawed, the liquid inside the cell leaks out, leaving thawed food dryer than fresh food. The method of freezing (slow versus rapid) affects the amount of drip loss on thawing.

WHAT'S THAT BROWN SPOT ON MY BURGER?

Freezer burn is a dry brownish spot left when moisture evaporates from the surface of frozen food. Because freezer burn changes the composition of fats on the surface of foods such as meat and poultry, it will cause some change in flavor as well.

To prevent freezer burn, wrap food securely in freezer paper or aluminum foil and put the item in a plastic bag. The more air you keep out, the fewer brown spots will develop.

Beef that has been frozen, for example, is noticeably dryer than fresh beef. Dry cheeses, such as cheddar, turn crumbly. Bread dries, too. You can reduce the loss of moisture by thawing the food in its freezer wrap so that it has a chance to reabsorb the moisture that's still in the package.

Unfortunately, you can't restore the crispness of vegetables that get their crunch from stiff, high-fiber cell walls. After ice crystals puncture the walls, the vegetable (carrots are a good example) turns mushy. The solution? Remove carrots and other crisp vegetables such as cabbage, before freezing the stew.

Thawing frozen food

To minimize the chance of spoilage, thaw frozen foods in the refrigerator, not on the kitchen cabinet.

Refreezing frozen food

The official word from the U.S. Department of Agriculture is that you can refreeze frozen food — as long as the food still has ice crystals or is at or below 40F (4.4C) on your refrigerator/freezer thermometer.

The exception may be sauced frozen food, such as frozen macaroni and cheese, because there may be hidden pockets of thawed food where the bacteria are whooping it up as we speak. In other words, partial thaw? Out the door.

Canned Food: Keeping Out Contaminants

Canning food (sealing it in a glass jar) is a three-step heat-dependent process. First, the food is heated, usually in the open container. Second, the container is sealed to keep out air (and microbes). Third, the sealed container is reheated.

Like all heated food, canned food is subject to changes in appearance and nutritional content. Heating food often changes its color and texture (see Chapter 20). It also destroys some vitamin C. But canning and jarring effectively destroy a variety of pathogens and deactivate enzymes that might otherwise cause continued deterioration of the food.

A modern variation on canning is the sealed plastic or aluminum bag known as the *retort pouch*. Food sealed in the pouch is heated but for a shorter period than that required for canning. As a result, the pouch method does a better job of preserving flavor, appearance, and heat-sensitive vitamin C.

The sealed can, jar, or pouch also protects food from deterioration caused by light or air, so the seal must remain intact. If the seal is broken, air seeps into the can or pouch, carrying microbes that can begin to spoil the food.

WARNING

A more serious hazard associated with canned food is *botulism,* the potentially fatal form of food poisoning that may result if the food is not heated for a sufficient period of time to a temperature high enough to kill all *Clostridium botulinum* (or *C. botulinum*) spores. *C. botulinum* is an *anaerobic* (*an* = without; *aerobic* = air) organism that thrives in the absence of oxygen, a condition nicely fulfilled by a sealed can. If a low-acid food (such as green beans or peas or potatoes) is incorrectly canned, *botulinum* spores not destroyed by high heat during the canning process may produce a toxin that can kill by paralyzing muscles, including the heart muscle and the muscles that enable you to breathe.

To avoid potentially hazardous canned food, don't buy, store, or use any can that is

>> **Swollen:** The swelling suggests that bacteria are growing inside and producing gas.

>> **Damaged, rusted, or deeply dented along the seam:** A break in the can permits air to enter and may promote the growth of organisms other than *C. botulinum.*

WARNING

Consumer alert: Never, never, *never* taste any food from a swollen or damaged can "just to see if it's all right." *Remember:* When in doubt, throw it out.

TIP

Yes, Botox is a purified form of C. botulinum. Used correctly, it's safe — meaning it won't cause botulinum poisoning.

Dried Food: No Life without Water

Drying protects food by removing the moisture that bacteria, yeasts, and molds need to live.

People have been drying food the low-tech way for centuries by simply putting it out in the sun and waiting for it to dry on its own, the technique used to produce the famous dates of the Arabian desert and the dried meat of the American plains. Drying food the high-tech, modern commercial way means putting food out on racks and employing fans to quick-dry the food at a low temperature under vacuum pressure. At home, a food dehydrator works similar magic.

Spray drying is a method used to dry liquids, such as milk, by blowing the liquids (in very small droplets) into a heated chamber where the droplets dry into a powder that can be reconstituted (made back into a liquid) by adding water. Instant coffee is a spray-dried product. So are instant teas, powdered milk, and all the various instant fruit beverages.

How drying affects food's nutritional value

As always, exposure to heat and/or air (oxygen) reduces a food's vitamin C content, so dried foods have less vitamin C than fresh foods.

One good example is the plum versus the prune (a dried plum):

» One fresh, medium-size plum, weighing 66 grams (a bit more than 2 ounces) without the pit, has 6 milligrams vitamin C, 7 to 8 percent of the Recommended Dietary Allowance (RDA) for a healthy adult.

» An equivalent amount of uncooked dried (low-moisture) prunes (66 grams) has only 1.3 milligrams vitamin C.

But wait! Before you leap to the conclusion that fresh is always more nutritious than dried, consider this: Dried fruit has less water than fresh fruit. That means its weight reflects more solid fruit. Although drying destroys some vitamin C, removing water concentrates what's left, along with other nutrients, jamming more calories, dietary fiber, and/or air-resistant vitamins and minerals into a smaller space.

As a result, dried food often has surprisingly more nutritional bounce to the ounce than fresh food. Once again, consider the plum and the prune:

>> A medium-size, pit-free plum weighing slightly more than 2 ounces provides 35 calories, 0.1 milligrams iron, and 670 IU (67 RE) vitamin A. (What's IU? What's RE? Check out Chapter 3.)

>> Two ounces of uncooked, low-moisture prunes have about 193 calories, 2 milligrams iron, and 952 IU (72 RE) vitamin A. In other words, if you're trying to lose weight, you need to be aware that although dried fruit is low in fat and rich in nutrients, it's also high in calories.

When dried fruit may be hazardous to your health

WARNING

Many fruits, such as apples, contain *polyphenoloxidase*, an enzyme that darkens the flesh when the fruit is exposed to air. To prevent the fruits from darkening when dried, they're treated with sulfur compounds known as *sulfites*. The sulfites — sulfur dioxide, sodium bisulfite, sodium metabisulfite — can cause potentially serious allergic reactions in sensitive individuals. For more about sulfites, see Chapter 22.

IS THAT FOOD STILL GOOD TO EAT?

Understanding the dating terms on food package labels can help you figure out whether the food inside is still safe and tasty — or ready to be discarded. Here's what the words mean:

- **Sell by:** The last date on which the food can be offered for sale. Stored properly, most perishable foods like milk and packaged meats are safe for a few days past the sell-by date.

- **Best if used by or Use by:** Refers to the food's flavor and quality, not its safety; the manufacturer's recommendation of the last date on which the food is likely to taste best.

- **Expires or Do not use after:** The last date on which a product either provides the highest nutritional value or works best (for example, the last date yeast is likely to make bread rise).

- **Packing date:** Used on eggs from USDA; written as a number from 1 (January 1) to 365 (December 31 — except in a leap year, naturally). Eggs from USDA-inspected plants may also carry an expiration date.

Irradiation: A Hot Topic

Irradiation is a technique that exposes food to electron beams or *gamma radiation*, a high-energy light stronger than the X-rays your doctor uses to make a picture of your insides. Gamma rays are *ionizing radiation*, the kind of radiation that kills living cells. Ionizing radiation can sterilize food or at least prolong its shelf life by

>> Killing microbes and insects on plants (wheat, wheat powder, spices, dry vegetable seasonings)

>> Killing disease-causing organisms on pork *(Trichinella)*, poultry *(Salmonella)*, and ground beef (pathogenic *E. coli*)

>> Preventing potatoes from sprouting during storage

>> Slowing the rate at which some fruits ripen

Irradiation doesn't change the way food looks or tastes. It doesn't change food texture. It doesn't make food radioactive. It does, however, alter the structure of some chemicals in foods, breaking molecules apart to form new substances called *radiolytic products* (*radio* = radiation; *lytic* = break).

About 90 percent of all compounds identified as radiolytic products (RP) are also found in raw, heated, and/or stored foods that have not been exposed to ionizing radiation. A few compounds, called *unique radiolytic products* (URPs), are found only in irradiated foods.

TIP

For reliable answers to the most commonly asked questions about food irradiation, check out this U.S. Food and Drug Administration Fact Sheet: www.fsis. usda.gov/wps/portal/fsis/topics/food-safety-education/get-answers/ food-safety-fact-sheets/production-and-inspection/irradiation-and- food-safety/irradiation-food-safety-faq

ARE IRRADIATED FOODS HARMFUL?

Food irradiation has been declared safe and effective in controlling microbial food poisoning and preserving food quality by the United States Department of Health and Human Services, the United States Public Health Service, the American Medical Association, the National Association of State Departments of Agriculture, the American Dietetic Association, and the World Health Organization.

(continued)

(continued)

Around the world, all irradiated food is identified with this international symbol.

Just in case that isn't enough to get the message across, the package must also carry the words "treated by irradiation" or "treated with irradiation." The only exceptions are spices and commercially produced food that contains some irradiated ingredients, such as spices. For example, neither the symbol nor the wording is required on the packaging for a frozen pizza that's seasoned with irradiated oregano. The following table lists the foods approved for irradiation in the United States.

Food	Approval Date
Wheat, wheat flour	1964
White potatoes	1964
Garlic powder, onion powder, dried spices	1983, 1985
Dried enzyme preparations (such as milk protein clotting enzymes used in making cheese)	1985
Pork	1985
Fruit and vegetables (fresh)	1986
Herbs, herbal teas, spices, vegetable seasonings	1986
Poultry (fresh, frozen)	1990 (FDA), 1992 (USDA)*
Beef, lamb, pork, horsemeat & byproducts	1997 (FDA), 2000 (USDA)*
Ready-to-eat, unrefrigerated meat/poultry products	1999
Fresh eggs (in shell)	2000
Seeds for sprouting	2000
Fruit and vegetable juices	2000
Imported fruits and vegetables	2002

Food	Approval Date
Meat for the National School Lunch program	2002
Fresh spinach and iceberg lettuce	2008
Fresh or frozen mollusks (oysters, clams, mussels, scallops)	2009
Fresh or frozen crustacean (shrimp, crabs, lobster)	2014

*: Both the FDA and the USDA must approve treatment of meat and poultry.

Federal Centers for Disease Control; Food and Drug Administration; Food Safety and Inspection Services, U.S. Department of Agriculture, and www.fda.gov/Food/ResourcesForYou/Consumers/ucm261680.htm

Chapter **22**

Better Eating through Chemistry

f the title of this chapter turns you off, you're not alone. Many people think that when you're talking about food, natural is good, and chemical is bad. Period. In fact, every single thing in the world is made of chemicals: your body, the air you breathe, the paper on which this book is printed, and all your food and drink.

This chapter is about the naturally occurring *and* the added natural or synthetic chemicals in your food and the technology that helps make food more nutritious; enhance its appearance, flavor, and texture; and keep it fresh on the shelf longer. Finally, this chapter talks about new and unusual processes, such as genetic engineering, that make it possible to create foods Nature never made.

Nature's Beneficial Chemistry

The same plant foods that yield carbohydrates (see Chapter 8) are also the source of *phytochemicals* — natural compounds other than vitamins manufactured only in plants (*phyto* is the Greek word for plant).

Phytochemicals are the substances that give plants their color, flavor, and odor and — more importantly — produce many of the beneficial effects associated with a diet rich in fruits, vegetables, beans, and grains.

The most interesting phytochemicals in plant foods are antioxidants, hormone-like compounds, and enzyme-activating sulfur compounds most plentiful in plant foods. Each group plays a specific role in maintaining health and reducing your risk of certain illnesses, which is one reason every edition of the *Dietary Guidelines for Americans* urges you to have as many as nine servings of fruits and vegetables and several servings of grains every day.

Antioxidants

Antioxidants are named for their ability to prevent a chemical reaction called *oxidation*, which enables molecular fragments called *free radicals* to join together, forming what appear to be potentially carcinogenic (cancer-causing) compounds in your body.

Hormonelike compounds

Many plants contain compounds that behave like *estrogens*, the female sex hormones. Because only an animal body can produce true hormones, these plant chemicals are called *hormonelike compounds* or *phytoestrogens* (plant estrogen).

The three kinds of phytoestrogens are

>> Isoflavones, in fruits, vegetables, and beans

>> Lignans, in grains

>> Coumestans, in sprouts and alfalfa

The most studied phytoestrogens are the soy isoflavones *daidzein* and *genistein*, two compounds with a chemical structure similar to *estradiol*, the estrogen produced by mammalian ovaries. Like natural or synthetic estrogens, phytoestrogens hook onto sensitive spots in reproductive tissue (breast, ovary, prostate, and so on).

These plant estrogen-like compounds are weaker, so researchers once suggested that they might provide postmenopausal women with the benefits of estrogen (stronger bones and relief from hot flashes) without the higher risk of reproductive cancers associated with hormone replacement therapy (HRT). But repeated animal and human studies suggested that, like natural and synthetic hormones, the plant compounds may stimulate tumor growth while having little effect on menopausal symptoms such as hot flashes. For more on soy's unique proteins, check out Chapter 6.

Sulfur compounds

Slide an apple pie in the oven, and soon the kitchen fills with an aroma that makes your mouth water and your digestive juices flow. But boil some cabbage and — what is that awful smell? It's sulfur, the same chemical you smell in rotten eggs.

Cruciferous vegetables (the name comes from *crux*, the Latin word meaning *cross*, a reference to their *x*-shape blossoms), such as broccoli, Brussels sprouts, cauliflower, kale, kohlrabi, mustard seed, radishes, rutabaga, turnips, and watercress, all contain stinky sulfur compounds such as *sulforaphane glucosinolate (SGSD)*, *glucobrassicin, gluconapin, gluconasturtin, neoglucobrassicin,* and *sinigrin* whose aromas are liberated when the food is heated.

TIP

Many researchers previously believed that these natural chemicals could tell your body to rev up to fight cancer, but the evidence from multiple studies in the early 2000s, when the cruciferous veggies movement was at its height, were conflicting. There is no proof that they are anticarcinogens.

However, in 2005, a trial conducted in China by researchers from Johns Hopkins Medical School, the University of Minnesota Cancer Institute, and the Qidong Liver Cancer Institute of Jiao Tong University (Shanghai) produced a possible explanation for why cruciferous vegetables might reduce the risk of some forms of cancer. The sulforaphane in Brussels sprouts inactivates *aflatoxins* — toxins released by molds on grains, such as rice, that are known to damage cells and, yes, increase the risk of cancers of the stomach and liver, two diseases more common in China than elsewhere in the world. In 2014, researchers from Johns Hopkins School of Medicine, the University of Pittsburgh, and the Qidong (China) Liver Cancer Institute confirmed that sulforaphane produces a cellular reaction that protects against carcinogenic changes. Clearly, this is a subject of interest.

TIP

What should you do while waiting for a final answer? Enjoy your phytochemicals. Dig into those veggies, fruits, and grains. Then turn to Chapter 12 to find out why you need to wash them down with plenty of cold, clear water.

Exploring the Natural and Synthetic Nature of Food Additives

Food additives may be natural or synthetic. For example, vitamin C is a natural preservative. *Butylated hydroxyanisole* (BHA) and *butylated hydroxytoluene* (BHT) are synthetic preservatives. To ensure your safety, both the natural *and* synthetic food additives used in the United States come only from the group of substances known as the generally recognized as safe (GRAS) list.

All additives on the GRAS list

>> Are approved by the Food and Drug Administration (FDA), meaning that agency is satisfied that the additive is safe and effective

>> Must be used only in specifically limited amounts

>> Must be used to satisfy a specific need in food products, such as protection against molds

>> Must be effective, meaning that they must actually maintain freshness and safety

>> Must be listed accurately on the label

Nutrient additives

Vitamin D, which is added to virtually all milk sold in the United States, is one example of a clearly beneficial food additive. Most U.S. bread and grain products are fortified with added B vitamins, plus iron and other essential minerals to replace what's lost when whole grains are milled into white flour for white bread. Some people say that people would be better off simply sticking to whole grains, but adding vitamins and minerals to white flours enhances a product that many people prefer.

Some nutrients are also useful preservatives. For example, as Chapter 10 explains, vitamin C is an antioxidant that slows food spoilage and prevents destructive chemical reactions, which is why American food packagers must add a form of vitamin C (*isoascorbic acid* or *sodium ascorbate*) to bacon and other luncheon meats to prevent the formation of potentially cancer-causing compounds.

Color additives

Colors, flavoring agents, and flavor enhancers make food look and taste better. Like other food additives, these three may be either natural or synthetic.

Natural colors

The natural coloring agents in food are also antioxidants that slow the normal wear and tear on body cells, which may be why so many studies suggest that a diet rich in plant foods (fruits, vegetables, grains, and beans) is likely to reduce the risk of chronic conditions, such as heart disease. But you gotta get the plants to get the benefit: Stuffing yourself with antioxidant vitamin supplements shows absolutely no effects on heart health.

One good example of a natural coloring agent is *beta carotene*, the yellow pigment extracted from many fruits and vegetables and used to turn naturally white margarine to buttery yellow.

Some other natural coloring agents are *annatto*, a yellow-to-pink pigment from a tropical tree; *chlorophyll*, the green pigment in green plants; *carmine*, a reddish extract of *cochineal* (a pigment from crushed beetles); *saffron*, a yellow herb; and *turmeric*, a yellow spice.

See Table 22-1 for the antioxidant coloring agents found naturally in common foods.

TABLE 22-1

Natural Antioxidant Coloring Agents in Food

Coloring Agent	Color	Found in
Anthocyanins	Red, blue, purple	Berries, plums
Betaine	Red	Beets
Carotenoids	Red, yellow, orange	Carrots, oranges
Chlorophylls	Green	Leafy vegetables

TIP

Want to see more? Check out en.wikipedia.org/wiki/List_of_antioxidants_in_food.

NEW COLORS FOR CLASSIC VEGGIES

What color is your cauliflower? Once upon a time, the only answer was "white." Today, as every serious foodie knows, cauliflower also comes in green, purple, and a smashing orange that first bloomed by accident among the crops grown by a Toronto, Canada, vegetable producer, the result of a completely natural and completely unexpected cross pollination between a carrot and a cauliflower. After that, the scientists at the New York State Agricultural Experiment Station in Geneva (NY) and various European food labs stepped in with carefully conducted cross-breeding to brighten up the cauliflower's white florets.

Whether orange cauliflower is prettier than the white is a personal decision, but there's no question that it's more nutritious. The color comes from beta carotene, a natural pigment your body converts to vitamin A, and an orange cauliflower has about 25 times more convertible carotenoids than a white one. A purple cauliflower has red and blue anthocyanins, pigments found naturally in blueberries, beets, red cabbage, and strawberries. As for lime green, that's a cauliflower crossed with broccoli, which contributes green chlorophyll along with yellow carotenoids.

Carotenoids, anthocyanins, and chlorophyll are all antioxidants that protect a plant from changes due to exposure to oxygen. They may also do something similar for human beings. The theory is that when we eat foods with antioxidant plant pigments, the pigments become *chemo preventers,* substances thought to stop trouble before it starts by keeping molecular fragments, called free radicals, from hooking up to form compounds that can damage cells, causing changes that may lead to heart disease, cancer, and other age-related degenerative diseases.

Notice the carefully chosen words *theory, may,* and *thought to* because science is still waiting for positive proof. Nonetheless, this health benefit is potentially so valuable that from time to time people have tried to take the pigments out of the plants and put them and their benefits into a pill. That doesn't seem to work. In one famous incident in the late 1980s, people who took beta carotene supplements to lower their risk of various kinds of cancer turned out to raise their risk instead.

To get the goods, you have to eat the food, so another benefit of cross-breeding veggies is making food look more inviting. On the other hand, some colors that aren't natural to food can be definite turn-offs. In psychological studies, the classic "yuck" food has always been mashed potatoes tinted blue with food coloring. But when JetBlue cabin attendants handed out bags of blue (get it?) potato chips made from the airline's very own naturally blue variety of potatoes grown right on the grounds of JFK airport, they went like hotcakes. Go figure.

THE COLOR ALPHABET

When you read the label on a food, drug, or cosmetic product containing artificial colors, you may see the letters *F, D,* and *C* — as in FD&C Yellow No. 5. The *F* stands for food. The *D* stands for drugs. The *C* stands for cosmetics. An additive whose name includes all three letters can be used in food, drugs, and cosmetics. An additive without the *F* is restricted to use in drugs and cosmetics or is for external use only (*translation:* You don't take them by mouth). For example, D&C Green No. 6 is a blue-green coloring agent used in hair oils and pomades. FD&C Blue No. 2 is a bright blue coloring agent used in hair rinses, as well as mint jellies, candies, and cereals.

Synthetic colors

An example of a synthetic coloring agent is FD&C Blue No. 1, a bright blue pigment made from coal tar and used in soft drinks, gelatin, hair dyes, and face powders, among other things.

And, yes, as scientists have discovered more about the effects of coal-tar dyes, including the fact that some are carcinogenic, many of these coloring agents have been banned from use in food in one country or another but are still allowed in cosmetics.

Flavor additives

Every cook worth his or her spice cabinet knows about natural flavor ingredients, especially salt, sugar, vinegar, wine, and fruit juices.

Artificial flavoring agents reproduce natural flavors. For example, a teaspoon of fresh lemon juice in the batter lends cheesecake a certain *je ne sais quoi* (French for "I don't know what" — a little something special), but artificial lemon flavoring works just as well. You can sweeten your morning coffee with natural sugar or with the artificial sweetener saccharin. (For more about substitute sweeteners, see Chapter 19.)

Flavor enhancers are a slightly different kettle of fish. They intensify a food's natural flavor instead of adding a new one. The best-known flavor enhancer is *monosodium glutamate (MSG),* widely used in Asian foods.

WARNING

Although it improves flavor, MSG may also trigger short-term, generally mild reactions, such as headaches, flushing, sweating, facial numbness and tingling, and rapid heartbeat in people sensitive to the seasoning.

Preservatives

Food spoilage is a totally natural phenomenon. Milk sours. Bread molds. Meat and poultry rot. Vegetables wilt. Fats turn rancid. The first three kinds of spoilage are caused by *microbes* (bacteria, mold, and yeasts). The last two happen when food is exposed to *oxygen* (air).

All the preservative techniques explained in Chapters 20 and 21— cooking, chilling, canning, freezing, and drying — prevent spoilage either by slowing the growth of the organisms that live on food or by protecting the food from the effects of oxygen. Chemical preservatives do essentially the same thing:

>> *Antimicrobials* are natural or synthetic preservatives that protect food by slowing the growth of bacteria, molds, and yeasts.

>> *Antioxidants* are natural or synthetic preservatives that protect food by preventing food molecules from combining with oxygen (air).

Table 22-2 is a representative list of some common preservative chemicals and the foods in which they're found.

TABLE 22-2

Preservatives in Food

Preservative	Found in . . .
Ascorbic acid*	Sausages, luncheon meats
Benzoic acid	Beverages (soft drinks), ice cream, baked goods
BHA (butylated hydroxyanisole)	Potato chips and other foods
BHT (butylated hydroxytoluene)	Potato chips and other foods
Calcium propionate	Breads, processed cheese
Isoascorbate*	Luncheon meats and other foods
Sodium ascorbate*	Luncheon meats and other foods
Sodium benzoate	Margarine, soft drinks

*A form of vitamin C

Other additives in food

Food chemists use a variety of the following types of natural and chemical additives to improve the texture of food or prevent mixtures from separating:

>> *Emulsifiers,* such as lecithin and polysorbate, keep liquid-plus-solids, such as chocolate pudding, from separating into liquid and solids. They can also keep two unfriendly liquids, such as oil and water, from divorcing so that your salad dressing stays smooth.

>> *Stabilizers,* such as the alginates (alginic acid) derived from seaweed, make food such as ice cream feel smoother, richer, or creamier in your mouth.

>> *Thickeners* are natural gums and starches, such as apple pectin or cornstarch, that add body to foods.

>> *Texturizers,* such as calcium chloride, keep foods such as canned apples, tomatoes, or potatoes from turning mushy.

Although many of these additives are derived from foods, their benefit is aesthetic (the food looks better and tastes better), not nutritional.

Determining the Safety of Food Additives

The safety of any chemical approved for use as a food additive is determined by evaluating its potential as a toxin, carcinogen, or allergen, each of which I define in the following sections.

Defining toxins

A toxin is a poison. Some chemicals, such as cyanide, are toxic (poisonous) in very small doses. Others, such as sodium ascorbate (a form of vitamin C), are nontoxic even in very large doses. All chemicals on the generally recognized as safe (GRAS) list are considered nontoxic in the amounts that are permitted in food.

By the way, both vitamin C and cyanide are *natural* chemicals — one beneficial, the other not so much.

Explaining carcinogens

A carcinogen is a substance that causes cancer. Some natural chemicals, such as *aflatoxins* (poisons produced by molds that grow on peanuts and grains), are carcinogens. Some synthetic chemicals, such as specific dyes, are also potentially carcinogenic.

In 1958, driven by a fear of potentially carcinogenic pesticide residues in food, New York Congressman James Delaney proposed, and Congress enacted into law, an amendment to the Food, Drug, and Cosmetic Act that banned from food any synthetic chemical known to cause cancer (in animals or human beings) when ingested in *any* amount, no matter how small. (The Delaney clause didn't apply to natural chemicals, even those known to cause cancer.)

For a time, the only exception to the Delaney clause was saccharin, which was exempted in 1970. Although ingesting very large amounts of the artificial sweetener is known to cause bladder cancer in animals, no similar link was ever found to human cancers. Nonetheless, in 1977, Congress required all products containing saccharin to carry a warning statement: "Use of this product may be hazardous to your health. This product contains saccharin, which has been determined to cause cancer in laboratory animals."

When the Delaney clause was introduced, ingredients such as additives were measured in parts (of the additive) per thousand parts (of the product). Today, scientists have the ability to measure an ingredient in parts per trillionths. As a result, the zero-risk standard of the Delaney clause in regard to pesticide residue in food was repealed and replaced with a standard of "reasonable risk." The saccharin warning was lifted in 2000.

THE NITRATE/NITRITE CONUNDRUM

Some preservatives are double-edged — good and not-so-good at the same time. For example, nitrates and nitrites are effective preservatives that prevent the growth of disease-bearing organisms in cured meat. But when they reach your stomach, nitrates and nitrites react with natural ammonia compounds called *amines* to form *nitrosamines,* substances known to cause cancer in animals fed amounts of nitrosamines much higher than found in any human food.

But avoiding foods with added nitrates and nitrites won't prevent your having to cope with nitrosamines. Beets, celery, eggplant, lettuce, radishes, spinach, and turnip greens all contain naturally occurring nitrates and nitrites, sometimes at higher levels than in cured meat products. When their nitrates and nitrates shake hands in your stomach, they make — you got it! — nitrosamines.

To take the sting out of added nitrates and nitrites in processed foods such as cured meats, the USDA, which regulates meat, fish, and poultry, sensibly requires manufacturers to add an antioxidant vitamin C compound, such as sodium ascorbate, or an antioxidant vitamin E compound (a tocopherol). The antioxidant vitamins prevent the formation of nitrosamines while boosting the antimicrobial powers of the nitrates and nitrites.

Listing allergens

Allergens are substances that trigger allergic reactions. Some foods, such as peanuts, contain natural allergens that can provoke the fatal allergic reaction known as anaphylaxis.

The best-known example of an allergenic food additive is the sulfites, a group of preservatives that

>> Keep light-colored fruits and vegetables (apples, potatoes) from browning when exposed to air

>> Prevent shellfish (shrimp and lobster) from developing black spots

>> Reduce the growth of bacteria in fermenting wine and beer

>> Bleach food starches

>> Make dough easier to handle

Sulfites are safe for most people but not for all. In fact, the FDA estimates that 1 out of every 100 people is sensitive to these chemicals; among people with asthma, the number rises to 5 out of every 100. For people sensitive to sulfites, even infinitesimally small amounts may trigger a serious allergic reaction, and asthmatics may develop breathing problems by simply inhaling fumes from sulfite-treated foods.

In 1986, the FDA tried banning sulfites from food but lost in a court case brought by food manufacturers, so two years later the agency wrote rules to protect sulfite-sensitive people.

Today, sulfites are not considered GRAS for use in

>> Meats

>> Foods that are an important source of vitamin B1 (thiamin), a nutrient sulfites destroy

>> Fruits and veggies served raw (think salad bars), or described as "fresh" (think fruit salad)

Sulfites are permitted in some foods, such as dried fruit, but the package must list sulfites if the additives account for more than ten parts sulfites to every million parts food (10 ppm). These rules, plus plenty of press information about the risks of sulfites, have led to a dramatic decrease in the number of sulfite reactions.

For more on allergens in food, check out Chapter 23.

Beyond Additives: Foods Nature Never Made

Genetically engineered foods, also known as *GMO*s or *bioengineered foods,* are foods with extra genes added artificially through special laboratory processes. Like preservatives, flavor enhancers, and other chemical boosters, the genes — which may come from plants, animals, or microorganisms such as bacteria — are used to make foods more resistant to disease and insects, more nutritious, and better tasting.

Genetic engineering may also help plants and animals grow faster and larger, thus increasing the food supply. The Big Question is, "Are genetically engineered foods safe?"

Many consumers have doubts. To enable them to make a clear choice — "Yes, I'll take that biotech food" or "No, I won't" — the European Union requires food labels to specifically state the presence of any genetically altered ingredients. In the United States, the FDA currently requires wording on labels to alert consumers to genetic engineering only when it results in an unexpected added allergen (such as corn genes in tomatoes) or changes the nutritional content of a food.

Does the wording on the label matter to consumers? Are most willing to accept genetically altered foods? The answer depends on who you ask and how you ask.

The International Food Information Council (IFIC), a trade group for the food industry, accepts the current label-wording rules. The Center for Science in the Public Interest (CSPI), a Washington-based consumer advocacy group, wants to see the words *genetically altered* on all foods that have been, well, genetically altered. In 2005, each organization conducted a survey that seemed designed to bolster its point of view.

For example, IFIC's survey says that nearly two-thirds (61 percent) of Americans expect food technology to serve up better-quality, better-tasting food. CSPI's competing survey says, "Not so fast." The difference may lie in the questions. IFIC's emphasizes the benefits of biotech; CSPI's leans more heavily on the drawbacks. For example:

>> **CSPI Version:** Would you buy food labeled "genetically engineered"? Forty-three percent said yes.

>> **IFIC Version:** Would you buy a food if it had been modified by biotechnology to taste better or fresher? Or stay fresher? Fifty-four percent said yes.

Twenty-one years after the introduction of the first genetically modified food (a tomato approved as safe as those traditionally grown and bred) went on sale, little had changed. In 2015, when the Neilsen company conducted an online poll of 30,000 people in 60 countries about which health benefits they considered "very important" when buying food, the two top answers were "all-natural" and "GMO-free."

In the end, despite a slight wariness about exploring new nutritional ground, Americans are intrigued by the promise of food innovations and willing to give the whole idea a try. Only 32 percent of them considered "GMO-free" very important versus 47 percent in Europe and 46 percent in Latin America.

Eventually, the proof of GMOs' promise will be in the (genetically engineered) labeled sales pudding — which should happen by 2022 when all GMO foods are mandated to carry an identifying label.

TIP

Check out www.watchusgrow.org/2019/01/08/everything-you-need-to-know-about-gmo-labeling-in-2019 for a picture of the proposed label.

5

Food and Medicine

Chapter 23

When Food Fights Back

I n 2019, the *Journal of the American Medical Association* (JAMA) reported that while nearly 1 in 5 adults believe themselves to be food allergic, actually only 1 in 20 are estimated to have a food allergy diagnosed by a physician. In fact, according to the U.S. National Institutes of Health, 5 percent of all American adults and 4 percent of children have a true *food allergy* (also known as *food hypersensitivity*).

Many childhood allergies seem to fade with age. But food allergies that don't disappear can trigger reactions ranging from the trivial (a stuffy nose the day after you eat the food) to the truly dangerous (immediate respiratory failure) sending more than 400,000 of us to the emergency room each year. To complicate matters, a person with food allergies is likely to be allergic to other things, such as dust, pollen, or the family cat. So forewarned (about food allergies) is forearmed (against the rest).

TIP

A word to the allergy-wise: You can stay current with allergy news by checking out the American Academy of Allergy, Asthma & Immunology (www.aaaai.org) and FARE (Food Allergy Research and Education) Network (www.foodallergy.org).

Diagnosing Food Allergies

Your immune system is designed to protect your body from harmful invaders, such as bacteria. Sometimes, however, the system responds to substances normally considered harmless. The substance that provokes the attack is called an *allergen*; the substances that attack the allergen are called *antibodies*.

A food allergy can provoke such a response as your body releases antibodies to attack specific proteins in food. When this happens, some of the physical reactions include

>> Hives

>> Itching

>> Swelling of the face, tongue, lips, eyelids, hands, and feet

>> Rashes

>> Headaches, migraines

>> Nausea and/or vomiting

>> Diarrhea, sometimes bloody

>> Sneezing, coughing

>> Asthma

>> Breathing difficulties caused by *tightening* (swelling) of tissues in the throat

>> Loss of consciousness (from anaphylactic shock)

WARNING

If you're sensitive to a specific food, you may not have to eat the food to have the reaction. For example, people sensitive to peanuts may break out in hives just from touching a peanut or peanut butter and may suffer a potentially fatal reaction after tasting chocolate that has touched factory machinery that previously touched peanuts. People sensitive to seafood — fin fish and shellfish — have been known to develop breathing problems after simply inhaling the vapors or steam produced by cooking the fish.

Understanding how an allergic reaction occurs

When you eat a food containing a protein to which you're sensitive, the protein reaches antibodies on the surface of white blood cells called *basophils* and immune system cells called *mast cells* either in your gastrointestinal tract or by circulating through the bloodstream.

The basophils and mast cells produce, store, and release *histamine*, a natural body chemical that causes the symptoms — itching, swelling, hives — associated with allergic reactions (some allergy pills designed to counter this are called *antihistamines*). When the antibodies on the surface of the basophils and mast cells come in contact with food allergens, the cells release histamine, and the result is an *allergic reaction*.

ALLERGY GLOSSARY

allergen: Any substance that sets off an allergic reaction (see *antigen* in this sidebar).

anaphylaxis: A potentially life-threatening allergic reaction that involves many body systems, creating a cascade of adverse effects beginning with sudden, severe itching and moving on to tissue swelling in the air passages that can lead to breathing difficulties, falling blood pressure, unconsciousness, and death.

antibody: A protein in your blood that reacts to an antigen and tries to render it harmless.

antigen: A substance that stimulates a response from the immune system; an allergen is a specific type of antigen.

basophil: A white blood cell that carries IgE and releases histamine.

ELISA: Short for *enzyme-linked immunosorbent assay,* a test used to determine the presence of antibodies in your blood, including antibodies to specific allergens.

epinephrine: Also known as adrenaline, β,3,4-trihydroxy-N- methylphenethylamine, a naturally occurring hormone used as medicine to treat severe allergic reactions.

histamine: The substance released by the immune system (specifically by the white blood cells known as basophils and by basophil-filled mast cells) that produces the symptoms of an allergic reaction, such as itching and swelling.

IgE: An abbreviation for *immunoglobulin E,* the antibody that reacts to allergens.

intolerance: A non-allergic adverse reaction to food.

mast cell: A cell in body tissue that releases histamine.

RAST: An abbreviation for *radioallergosorbent test,* a blood test used to determine whether you're allergic to certain foods.

urticaria: The medical name for hives.

Investigating two kinds of allergic reactions

Your body may react to an allergen in one of two ways — immediately or later on:

>> **Immediate reactions** are more dangerous because they involve a fast swelling of tissue, sometimes within seconds after contact with the offending food.

>> **Delayed reactions,** which may occur as long as 24 to 48 hours after you've been exposed to the offending food, are usually much milder, perhaps a slight cough or nasal congestion caused by swollen tissues.

Most allergic reactions to food are unpleasant but essentially mild. However, as many as 150 or more people die every year in the United States from a severe reaction to a food allergen.

WARNING

Call 911 immediately if you or a friend or relative show any signs of an allergic reaction — including an allergic reaction to food — that affects breathing.

Identifying food allergies

A tendency toward allergies (although not necessarily the specific allergy itself) is inherited. If one of your parents has an allergy, your risk of having one is two times higher than it would be if neither of your parents had a history of allergic disease. If both your mother and your father have allergies, your risk is four times higher.

To identify the culprit causing your food allergy, your doctor may suggest an *elimination diet.* This regimen removes from your diet foods — most commonly milk, egg, soy, wheat, peanuts — known to cause allergic reactions in many people. Then, one at a time, the foods are added back. If you react to one, bingo! That's a clue to what triggers your immune response.

To be absolutely certain, your doctor may challenge your immune system by introducing foods in a form (maybe a capsule) that neither you nor he can identify as a specific food. Doing so rules out any possibility that your reaction has been triggered by emotional stimuli — that is, seeing, tasting, or smelling the food.

Other tests that can identify allergens to specific foods include skin tests and two types of blood tests — *ELISA* (enzyme-linked immunosorbent assay) and *RAST* (radioallergosorbent test) — that can identify antibodies to specific allergens in your blood. But these two tests are rarely required.

Coping with Food Allergies

To keep yourself or your allergic friends and family safe in a world practically teeming with allergens, know what's in your food, check out unusual allergenic couplings, work with others to make rules that work, and practice simple protection.

Reading the food ingredient label

According to FARE, more than 90 percent of all allergic reactions to foods are caused by just eight foods: eggs, fish, milk, peanuts, shellfish, soy, tree nuts, and wheat.

TIP

If you're sensitive to one of these foods, the best way to avoid an allergic reaction is to avoid the food. And you can do that by reading the label to ferret out hidden ingredients — peanuts in the chili or caviar (fish eggs) in the dip.

In the past, a hidden allergen might be hidden in plain sight on a food label that used alternative or chemical code names, such as whey or casein or lactoglobulin for milk. But in 2004, Congress passed and the president signed into law the Food Allergen Labeling and Consumer Protection Act. As of January 1, 2006, all food labels must use plain English words for the eight most-common food allergens.

Table 23-1 lists and describes The Allergy Eight, with special attention to those unexpected appearances on the menu (also see Figure 23-1).

TABLE 23-1	The Allergy Eight	
Food	**People Affected[1]**	**Where This Food May Hide in Commercial Products**
Eggs	1–2% of young children; most outgrow this allergy	Foam/topping on coffee drinks; egg substitutes; pasta in prepared foods (like soups); pretzels/bread (egg wash on crust)
Fish	2.3% of all Americans (children and adults)	Dressings and sauces (Worcestershire sauce); Asian and Mexican dishes; prepared meat products (like meatloaf)
Milk	2.3% of children under 3; most outgrow this allergy	Canned tuna, meat, and nondairy products (as casein, the protein in milk)
Peanuts[2]	1% of American children and adults; recent studies suggest that up to 20% of allergic children may outgrow this allergy	Dressings and sauces; marinades; pizza; Asian and Mexican dishes; meat substitutes

(continued)

TABLE 23-1 *(continued)*

Food	People Affected[1]	Where This Food May Hide in Commercial Products
Shellfish	2.3% of all Americans	Sauces (like fish sauce); Asian dishes
Soy	NA[3]; many children outgrow this allergy	Baked products including cereals and snacks; margarines; meat substitutes (textured vegetable protein); nut butters; sauces; prepared soups
Tree nuts[4]	0.5% of American children and adults	Salad dressings; sauces (barbecue sauce); breaded foods; meat substitutes (vegetarian burgers); pastas
Wheat[5]	>1% of children younger than 3; most outgrow this allergy	Various foods including ice cream; chips; meat, fish, and poultry products (prepared burgers, hot dogs, imitation crab meat [surimi])

(1) Estimates.

(2) Peanuts, sometimes known as ground nuts, are legumes, a vegetable class that includes peas and beans.

(3) Depending on the source, estimates range from a low of 0.3% of young children to a high of 20% of all children and adults.

(4) Including, among others, almonds, Brazil nuts, cashews, chestnuts, coconuts, hazelnuts, Macadamia nuts, pecans, pistachios, walnuts.

(5) Wheat allergy has no relationship with celiac disease, a genetic malabsorption disorder in which the body reacts to gluten, a protein in some grains (primarily wheat, barley, oats, and rye). Celiac disease is a lifelong condition.

About.com, http://foodallergies.about.com/od/soyallergies/p/soyallergy.htm, FARE, www.foodallergy.org; Mayo Clinic, www.mayoclinic.com/health/soy-allergy/DS00970; "Is Soy Allergy Overestimated?" Luisa Businco. Pediatric Asthma, Allergy & Immunology, Summer 1993, 7(2): 73-76

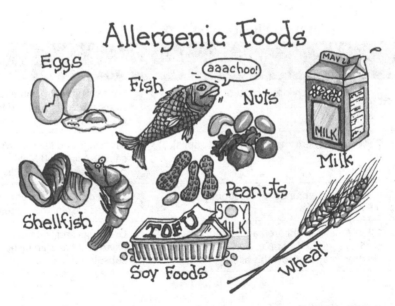

FIGURE 23-1: These foods can set off an allergic reaction.

Avoiding unusual interactions

Sometimes a food label doesn't list an allergen because the allergen is simply (surprise!) a natural component of the food.

Salicylates are a perfect example. These natural chemicals occur in many plants, including some plants that end up on the dinner table. The salicylates protect the plants by destroying mold and other microorganisms. For human beings, salicylates act as analgesics (pain killers), the most famous of which is *acetylsalicylic acid*, better known as *aspirin*. People who are sensitive to salicylates may experience an allergic reaction (wheezing and difficulty breathing, headache, hives, rash or itchy skin, and swollen hands, feet, or face) when exposed even to very small amounts, including the salicylates in otherwise highly nutritious plant foods such as fruits and vegetables.

TIP

If you or someone you know is sensitive to salicylates, you'll be pleased to know that the allergy experts at the Wegeningen University in the Netherlands have put together a nifty little list of foods grouped into five categories according to the amount of salicylates they contain. The following list, adapted from the Wegeningen chart shown at `http://www.food-info.net/uk/qa/qa-fi27.htm`, is a basic guide to the salicylate content of common foods. For comparison, one regular aspirin contains 365 milligrams of acetylsalicylic acid; one low-dose aspirin, the medicine prescribed to reduce the risk of heart disease, has 81 milligrams.

>> **Foods with negligible amounts of salicylates:** Bananas, cabbage, cashews, celery, chives, garlic, green beans, pears, peas, and lentils

>> **Foods low in salicylates (0.1–0.25 milligrams per 3.5 ounces/100 grams):** Apples (golden, delicious [red]), asparagus (fresh), cauliflower, cherries (sour), grapes (green), hazel nuts, lemon, mango, mushrooms (fresh), onions, passion fruit, pecans, peanut butter, tamarillo, saffron, sesame seeds, soy sauce, and vinegar

>> **Foods moderate in salicylates (0.25–0.49 milligrams per 3.5 ounces/ 100 grams):** Asparagus (canned), Brazil nuts, Chinese vegetables, coconut, fennel, grapefruit juice, loquat, lychee, marrow (the British/European term for zucchini), nectarines, olives (black), plum, pumpkin, snow peas, and watermelon

>> **Foods high in salicylates (0.5–1.0 milligrams per 3.5 ounces/100 grams):** Alfalfa, apples (Granny Smith), avocado, broccoli, cherries (red), cucumber, fava beans, Macadamia nuts, mandarin oranges, pine nuts, pistachios, spinach, sweet potato, tangelo (tangerine/grapefruit or honeybell), and vegemite (a salty food paste made from yeast)

>> **Foods very high in salicylates (>1 milligram per 3.5 ounces/100 grams):** Almonds, apricots, blackberries, blueberries, canella (a cinnamon-like seasoning), cantaloupe, chicory, cumin, curry powder, dates, dill (dried), green pepper, guava, mushrooms (canned), mustard, olive, oregano, paprika (hot), peanuts, radishes, raisins, rosemary, thyme, tomatoes, and turmeric

WORKING TO CHANGE AN ALLERGENIC ENVIRONMENT

In the real world, having a peanut allergy may affect your ability to enjoy simple pleasures, such as a baseball game where peanuts are sold. So imagine the delight of parents in New Britain, Connecticut, when the local Eastern League team formerly known as the Rock Cats and now named the Hartford Yard Goats after they moved to the capital city, decided to set aside a special 138-seat food-free section during its 2002 season for baseball-crazy but peanut-allergic kids and their families at a game between the Rock Cats and the New Haven Ravens.

The team and the Food Allergy & Anaphylaxis Network, a national consumer advocacy group with 250 members in the Hartford area, cooked up the idea because, as then general manager John Willi said, "No child should be deprived of the Rock Cats experience."

By 2019, the peanut-free theme had moved well into the majors, with teams in 17 American cities and Toronto, Canada designating games with peanut-free areas and some game days completely peanut-free. But as Robert Wood, MD, director of pediatric allergy and immunology at the Johns Hopkins Children's Center in Baltimore, author of *Food Allergies For Dummies* (Wiley), and a person with a peanut allergy himself, has noted, watching a game in an outdoor ballpark is less hazardous than, say, sitting in the cabin in an airplane where the air carries peanut particles and scattered crumbs on the floor or seats. Funny he should mention that. As long ago as 1998, the U.S. Department of Transportation (DOT) considered imposing a ban on peanuts on U.S. carriers. The DOT's proposals included the following options:

- An outright ban on airlines serving peanuts and peanut products

- Banning service of peanuts and peanut products only on a flight where a passenger with a peanut allergy requests a peanut-free flight in advance

- Requiring the airline to provide a peanut-free buffer zone around a passenger with a medically documented severe peanut allergy if the passenger makes a request in advance

While you're waiting to see whether these proposals ever fly, you can click on to Very Well Health's site at https://www.verywellhealth.com/want-a-peanutfree-flight-learn-airline-allergy-rules-1324387 for the low down on allergy rules at some U.S. airlines or call the one you're flying and ask some pertinent questions.

Practicing pragmatic protection

If you're someone with a known potentially life-threatening allergy to food (or another allergen, such as wasp venom), your doctor may suggest that you carry a syringe prefilled with *epinephrine,* the naturally occurring hormone that counteracts the reactions.

You may also decide to wear a tag that identifies you as a person with a serious allergic problem. One company that provides these tags is Medic-Alert Foundation International (www.medicalert.org), a nearly 50-year-old firm located in Turlock, California. Their telephone line (800-432-5378) is open from 8:00 a.m. to 4:00 p.m. PST Monday through Friday. The benefits of membership, beginning at $24.99 a year, include a 24/7 hotline. In January 2020, the U.S. Food and Drug Administration approved a new drug called Palforzia to ameliorate the adverse effects of an allergic person's accidental exposure to peanuts. The drug is not a cure, but, according to the FDA's Peter Marks, it does provide an approved treatment option.

If a group of researchers at the University of South Australia are successful, there may soon be an even better option, a vaccine to immunize against peanut allergy based on a virus "platform" that can "rewrite" the body's immune response to peanut allergens so that they behave in a calm rather than active manner. Stay tuned for much more on this one.

Recognizing Other Body Reactions to Food

Allergic reactions aren't the only way your body registers a protest against certain foods. Other reactions to foods include

>> **A metabolic reaction:** Food intolerance, also known as a non-allergic food hypersensitivity, is an inherited inability to metabolize (digest) certain foods, such as fat or lactose (the naturally occurring sugar in milk). The reaction may include intestinal gas, diarrhea, or other signs of gastric revolt.

>> **A physical reaction to a specific chemical:** Your body may react to things such as the laxative substance in prunes or monosodium glutamate (MSG), the flavor enhancer commonly found in Asian food. Although some people are more sensitive than others to these chemicals, their reaction is a physical one. It doesn't involve the immune system.

>> **A body response to psychological triggers:** When you're very fearful or very anxious or very excited, your body moves into hyper drive, secreting hormones that pump up your heartbeat and respiration, speed the passage of food through your gut, and cause you to empty your bowels and bladder. The entire process, called the *fight-or-flight response,* prepares your body to defend itself by either fighting or running. On a more prosaic level, a strong reaction to your food may cause diarrhea. It isn't an allergy; it's your hormones.

>> **A change in mood and/or behavior.** Some foods, such as coffee, contain chemicals, such as caffeine, that may cause hyperactivity, as well as having a real effect on mood and behavior, the subject of Chapter 24.

IN THIS CHAPTER

» Exploring how what you eat affects your brain

» Matching your brain diet to your age

» Choosing food to change your mood

» Healing food for the injured brain

Chapter **24**

Brain Food

A re you an average adult? Then your average brain weighs an average 3 pounds, about 2 percent of your average (150 pounds) body weight. But that 2 percent uses nearly 20 percent of the calories you consume each day to power more than 100 billion neurons (nerve cells) that, working at top speed, convert those calories into enough energy to turn on a 25-watt incandescent light bulb.

Calories aren't the whole story, of course. *What* you eat and *when* you eat it also matter. This chapter tells you *why* and introduces you to a new, exciting — and constantly evolving — field of investigative science: food and your brain.

Nourishing the Developing Brain

In 1987, pediatricians at North Shore University Hospital in Manhasset, New York, faced an unusual situation. In a thriving middle class community, they were suddenly called to treat seven infants who were definitely *not* thriving, meaning that the babies' bodies and, more disturbing, their brains were not developing as expected.

Failure to thrive is commonly linked to malnutrition. And, in an unusual way, this failure turned out to be the case. After a series of diagnostic exams and questions, the Long Island doctors discovered that seven sets of nutrition-conscious parents had been feeding their children a low-fat, low-cholesterol diet meant to protect adults at risk of heart disease.

Happily, the doctors changed the diet, the infants recovered, and everybody got the point: Not only does a developing brain need plenty of calories, but also a lot of those calories should come from fats, particularly the polyunsaturated omega-3 fatty acid, docosahexanoic acid, better known as DHA.

Fats and the fetal brain

The human body is about 60 percent water. The human brain is about 60 percent fat, and most of that is DHA. This fatty acid is vital for the proper functioning of the adult brain but even more important for the development of the fetal brain and spinal cord. (Consuming foods with DHA also helps reduce the risk of cardiovascular disease, but that's a story for another chapter or another book; perhaps check out *Controlling Cholesterol For Dummies*, which I coauthored with Martin W. Graf, MD [Wiley].)

More than 20 years after the seven fat-deprived babies showed up at North Shore, an entire catalog of well-designed studies has documented the advantages conferred on infants whose mothers get plenty of DHA — the best source is fish oils, fish, and seafood (see Table 24-2, later in this chapter) while pregnant — along with all the normal vitamins, minerals, and other essential components of a healthful diet, of course.

Right from the start, babies delivered by women with higher blood levels of DHA are more attentive to new stimuli. For the next six months, they score higher on tests of cognition (thinking processes) than babies born to women with lower levels of DHA. According to one report from Harvard Medical School, by the time the DHA-enriched babies are 3 years old, they may also score several points higher on vocabulary tests.

But DHA's brain benefit doesn't end with babies.

Fish and the teenage brain

The next time your teen brother, nephew, son, or friend tells you he's a grown-up, smile pleasantly and hand him a tuna sandwich. In fact, the brain of an older teen — think 15, 16, 17, and 18 — is particularly "plastic," meaning particularly able to build the new connections required to learn new things like high school math, science, history, and literature.

In 2009, scientists at Sweden's Gothenburg University reported that 15-year-old boys who eat fish more than once a week score higher on intelligence tests than their non-fish-eating friends.

Not being totally chauvinistic, the Gothenburg researchers soon filed another report, this one on teenage females. Sure enough, those who ate fish did better in school. So when you're serving tuna on rye, make sure your teen brother, nephew, son, or friend shares that tuna sandwich with his sister, niece, or girlfriend. And vice versa.

Determining how much DHA a body needs

In 2002, the National Academy of Science's Food and Nutrition Board set recommendations for daily consumption of omega-3 fatty acids, as shown in Table 24-1. By the way, as I explain in Chapter 3, the Adequate Intake (AI) is a recommendation for nutrients for which there is no Recommended Dietary Allowance (RDA).

TABLE 24-1   Adequate Intakes (AIs) for Omega-3s

Age	Male	Female	Pregnancy	Lactation
Birth to 6 months*	0.5 g	0.5 g		
7–12 months*	0.5 g	0.5 g		
1–3 years**	0.7 g	0.7 g		
4–8 years**	0.9 g	0.9 g		
9–13 years**	1.2 g	1.0 g		
14–18 years**	1.6 g	1.1 g	1.4 g	1.3 g
19-50 years**	1.6 g	1.1 g	1.4 g	1.3 g
51+ years**	1.6 g	1.1 g		

Source: https://ods.od.nih.gov/factsheets/Omega3FattyAcids-HealthProfessional/

Avoiding malicious mercury

Naturally, there is a catch in the day's catch. Some fish contain an unhealthful amount of methylmercury, a compound produced by bacteria that chemically alter the naturally occurring mercury in rock and soil or the mercury released into water through industrial pollution.

Little fish eat mercury-contaminated algae, bigger fish eat the smaller fish, people eat the bigger fish, and the mercury ends up there. The larger the fish and the longer it lives, the higher its mercury content is likely to be. To reduce the risk to fetal development, the *2015–2020 Dietary Guidelines for Americans* advisory committee advises pregnant women to avoid the Mercury Big Four (shark, swordfish, king mackerel, and tilefish) and limit their weekly consumption of seafood to two or less 4-ounce servings of seafood high in omega-3s and low in mercury.

Luckily, you can also get DHA from foods other than fish. For example, many infant formulas now contain DHA derived from fermented algae, and health-food stores sell algae-based DHA supplements for adults. One plain egg yolk contains 20 milligrams/0.02 grams of DHA; an egg yolk from an egg laid by a hen fed a DHA-enriched diet may contain up to 200 milligrams/0.2 grams of DHA. Some nuts and seeds (think walnuts and flaxseed) contain alpha linolenic acid, a precursor converted by our bodies to DHA.

Table 24-2 shows the DHA and mercury content of some popular fish and shellfish.

TABLE 24-2

DHA & Mercury Content of Common Fish & Seafood

Fish	Milligrams (mg) of DHA per 100 g/3.5 oz	Mercury Content*
Catfish	200	Low
Clams	200-500	Not detectible
King mackerel	1,500	High
Salmon, Atlantic, wild	1,500	Low
Salmon, Atlantic, farmed	1,500	Low
Sardine, canned, drained	500–1,000	Low
Scallop	200	Low
Tuna (canned, light)	540	Low
Tuna (canned, albacore)	500–1,000	High

* Low = less than 0.12 ppm; high = more than 0.730 ppm.

USDA, Appendix G2: Original Food Guide Pyramid Patterns and Descriptions of USDA Analyses, Addition A: EPA and DHA Content of Fish Species, 2005; FDA, Mercury Levels in Commercial Fish and Shellfish, 2006; USDA Nationals Nutrient Database for Standard Reference

Protecting the Adult Brain

Once upon a time, people thought that as soon as you and your brain were born, that was the end of making new neurons and that barring illness or injury, what you had, structurally speaking, was pretty much what you would have until "The End." Today, a growing body of evidence suggests that may be partially a fairy tale.

In the last decade, several studies at institutions as diverse as the University of Victoria (Canada), the University of Hong Kong, the University of Cambridge (Great Britain), and the U.S. National Institute on Aging point to the conclusion that important areas of the brain, such as the hippocampus — the site of memory, learning, and emotion — continue to generate new cells. And guess what? The same exercise that tones your abs may tone your brain. In experiments with rats, scientists have found that the little critters who run about the most produce the most new cells.

We all know that a brisk run in the park can clear cobwebs from an overworked brain, but will it also make new cells for our human brains? While we're waiting to find out, you can and certainly should use your full-grown brain to learn new things. And regardless of age, you can strive to protect and preserve your intellectual brain functions: *cognition* (the processes of learning, thinking, and reasoning) and *memory* (the ability to retain and recall past experiences).

REMEMBER THIS

Short-term memory lasts a few minutes. If you are reading a book, and you put it down to answer the phone, short-term memory enables you to go back and recognize where you left off. Or to remember a strange phone number long enough to dial it.

Long-term memory lasts for years. If what you were reading strikes a chord, you may store it in your brain and pull it out from time to time. For example, few people who read Charles Dickens's *A Tale of Two Cities* ever forget the first two lines: "It was the best of times. It was the worst of times." Or, on a more practical level, their own phone numbers.

Amnesia is loss of memory related to an illness or an injury. *Retrograde amnesia* is the inability to remember things that happened before the illness or injury; *anterograde amnesia* is the inability to form new memories afterward. With the former, you can't remember the phone number you had in high school. With the latter, you won't be able to remember the new phone number you might get tomorrow.

Introducing the natural enemies of thought and memory

The old news was that after a certain age, say, 30, your brain begins to shrink until it simply shrivels into nothing. But, as noted earlier, scientists who have actually taken the time to sit down and count brain cells find practically no age-related loss of those hippocampal cells responsible for cognition and memory. However, the cells in your adult brain — like other body cells — do face two natural enemies: oxidative stress and inflammation.

» *Oxidative stress* is damage done by particles called *free radicals* that form during chemical reactions occurring in the body. As you grow older, your cells' sensitivity to this kind of injury goes up while your ability to heal afterward goes down.

» *Inflammation* is your immune system's natural response to injury: swelling, heat, and pain. The American Heart Association regards *C-reactive protein* (CRP), a protein whose presence increases during inflammation, as a risk factor for heart disease and stroke. A natural increase in the level of *tumor necrosis factor alpha* and *interleukin-6,* two inflammatory agents in your brain and spinal cord, appears to play a role in the age-related loss of both cognition and memory.

How do you counter these two enemies? One possibility: nutrition.

ARE VITAMINS VITAL?

Using nutritional supplements to boost brain power is an iffy proposition, long on theory and short on proof.

True, deficiencies of specific nutrients, such as iron, can adversely affect brain development and function. For example, in 1996, researchers at Johns Hopkins Children's Center recruited iron-deficient but not-yet-anemic high school girls from four Baltimore high schools, gave them iron supplements, and watched their test scores rise.

But do supplements increase brain health for healthy people? Yes. No. And maybe — the evidence is far from conclusive. As for herbs, such as ginko biloba, ginseng, and gotu kola — is there something special in plants beginning with the letter *g?* — they come into vogue and then slide out again as scientific studies show a lack of effect.

The best advice on nutrients for your brain is to always stick to that boring but effective varied diet, beating the belly to keep your brain in shape.

Dieting to keep your brain in shape

The human body stores extra fat in several well-defined places, and as the body ages, these fat deposits tend to expand. For women, it's hips and thighs. For men, it's shoulders and the abdomen, the large area between chest and pelvis commonly known as the belly. Simple observation shows that men are more likely than women to have big bellies, particularly as they grow older. But belly fat may be hazardous to brain health for both genders, even when the body with the belly isn't overweight and its BMI (the body mass index described in Chapter 4) is within normal range.

In 2008, data from a Kaiser Permanente study of nearly 7,000 volunteers, age 40 to 45, showed that people with big bellies are more likely than those with flat tummies to develop Alzheimer's later in life. One theory to explain this is that belly fat sends damaging molecules through the bloodstream to the brain, but the true link is still a true mystery. Or as one nutrition researcher elegantly puts it, "An exciting area that needs to be explored." Then, in 2010, researchers enlisted 733 men and women who agreed to a CT-scan of the abdomen and an MRI scan of the brain. What the picture showed was that the more deep fat around the belly, the lower the volume of the brain. Clearly, another exciting area to be explored.

TECHNICAL STUFF

As Chapter 4 explains, healthy bodies come in all sizes and shapes. Holding to a brain-healthy shape definitely doesn't mean dieting to skeleton size. Doing that deprives your brain (and the rest of your body) of essential nutrients. In short, a sensible diet leads to a sensible body and a sensible brain.

Choosing foods that boost the brain

Plants are deceptive. On the outside, they're mostly green and calm. On the inside, they're busy little chemical factories churning out multitudinous compounds, many of which have properties that protect the plant — and various parts of your body, including, of course, your brain.

One class of these natural chemicals is the *polyphenols,* so named because their molecules are built of many *(poly-)* ring-shaped *(phenol)* components. Polyphenols are widely distributed in fruits and vegetables as well as in nuts, seeds, and grains. Some have antioxidant, antiallergic, anti-inflammatory, antiviral, or antiproliferative (prevents cell from irregular reproduction, an anticancer trait) effects.

One group of important antioxidant and anti-inflammatory polyphenols are the *flavonoids* (sometimes incorrectly spelled flavanoids), the pigments that color plants yellow, red, orange, green, or white. Some flavonoids may also be antiviral and antiproliferative. Altogether flavonoids protect plants from oxidative stress, including stress triggered by attacks from insects, fungi, and microbes.

Minding your mind diet

If there is one — no, two — diets on whose virtues every reputable expert agrees, it's the Mediterranean diet and DASH, also known as *Dietary Approaches to Stop Hypertension*. Both diets, built on a base of plant foods plus low-fat, protein-rich foods, such as fish and poultry, are known to reduce the risk of cardiovascular disease.

A team of nutritional epidemiologists at Harvard University and Rush University Medical Center in Chicago put them together to create the MIND diet, short for *Mediterranean-DASH Intervention for Neurodegenerative Delay*, a mouthful in itself ranked among *U.S. News and World Reports'* top five healthful diets in 2018.

The MIND diet has 15 food categories: 10 are brain-healthy; 5, not so much.

The ten "good" foods are

>> Berries

>> Beans

>> Fish

>> Nuts

>> Olive oil

>> Poultry

>> Vegetables (green leafy)

>> Vegetables (everything else)

>> Whole grains

>> Wine

The five "not so good" foods are

>> Butter and stick margarine

>> Cheese

>> Fried or fast food

>> Pastries and sweets

>> Red meats

Overall, the MIND diet provides three servings of whole grains, one salad (those leaves), and one more vegetable a day, beans every other day, poultry and berries at least twice a week, and fish at least once. The recommended snack is nuts. And, yes, a glass of wine to top off every day's delights.

As for those other foods, less than a tablespoon of butter or stick margarine a day, less than one serving of fried or fast food a week (presumably, fast-food salads meet muster).

Does it work? The best proof that the Rush people can offer is the result of their five-year-long study of 960 adults average age 81 and older who were dementia-free at the start. Participants were asked to fill out food questionnaires, listing what they ate and how often they chose various foods. Each year, they were given standardized tests of memory and their ability to interpret and act on visual cues. At the end, according to a report in *Alzheimer's & Dementia*, the journal of the Alzheimer's Association, those who followed the MIND diet to the letter reduced their risk of Alzheimer's by as much as 53 percent; those who sort of followed the diet reduced their risk by about 35 percent.

Altering the Emotional Brain

A *mood* is a feeling, an internal emotional state that can affect how you see the world. If your team wins the World Series, your happiness may last for days, making you feel so mellow that you simply shrug off minor annoyances, such as finding a ticket on your windshield because your parking meter expired while you were having lunch. If you're sad because the project you spent six months setting up didn't work out, your disappointment can linger long enough to make your work seem temporarily unrewarding or your favorite television sitcom totally unfunny.

Most of the time, after shifting one way or the other, your mood swings back to center fairly soon. You come down from your high or recover from your disappointment, and life resumes its normal pace — some good news here, some bad news there, but all in all, a relatively level field.

Occasionally, however, your mood may go haywire. Your happiness over your team's victory escalates to the point where you find yourself rushing from store to store buying things you can't afford, or your sadness over your failure at work deepens into a gloom that steals joy from everything else. This unpleasant state of affairs — a mood out of control — is called a *mood disorder*.

Recognizing mood malfunctions

Approximately one in every four human beings (more frequently a woman than a man) experiences some form of mood disturbance during his or her lifetime. Eight or 9 out of every 100 people will experience a *clinical mood disorder*, a mood disorder serious enough to be diagnosed as a disease.

The two most-common moods are happiness and sadness. The two most-common mood disorders are *clinical depression*, an elongated period of overly intense sadness, and *clinical mania*, an elongated period of overly intense elation. Clinical depression alone is called a *unipolar (one-part) disorder*; clinical depression plus clinical mania is a *bipolar (two-part) disorder*.

Natural chemicals that affect mood

Your body makes a group of substances called *neurotransmitters*, which are chemicals that enable brain cells to send messages back and forth. Three important neurotransmitters are

>> Dopamine (*doe*-pa-meen)

>> Norepinephrine (*nor*-e-pe-*nef*-rin)

>> Serotonin (ser-a-*toe*-nin)

Dopamine and *norepinephrine* are chemicals that make you feel alert and energized. *Serotonin* is a chemical that can make you feel smooth and calm. Some forms of clinical depression appear to be a malfunction of the body's ability to handle these neurotransmitters effectively.

Mood meds

Several medical drugs are useful in making neurotransmitters more available to your brain or enabling your brain to use them more efficiently. These medications include

>> **Tricyclic antidepressants:** These drugs were the first truly effective antidepressants. They're named for their chemical structure: three ring-shaped groups of atoms (*tri* = three; *cyclic* = ring). They relieve symptoms by increasing the availability of serotonin. One well-known tricyclic is amitriptyline (Elavil).

>> **Monoamine oxidase inhibitors (MAO inhibitors):** These drugs interrupt the actions of an enzyme that triggers the natural elimination of dopamine and other neurotransmitters so that they remain available for your brain. Nardil (phenelzine), Parnate (tranylcypromine), Eldepryl and Emsam (selegiline), and moclobemide (brand names Amira, Aurorix, Clobemix, Depnil, Manerix) are MAO inhibitors.

» **Selective serotonin reuptake inhibitors (SSRIs):** These medicines slow the body's natural reabsorption of serotonin, leaving more serotonin available to your brain. Celexa (citalopram), Lexapro (escitalopram oxalate), Luvox (fluvoxamine), Paxil (paroxetine), Prozac (fluoxetine), and Zoloft (sertraline) are SSRIs.

» **Selective serotonin-norepinephrine reuptake inhibitors (SNRIs):** These medicines slow the body's natural reabsorption of both serotonin and norepinephrine. Cymbalta (duloxetine), Effexor (venlafaxine), Fetzima (levomilnacipran), Irenka (duloxetine), Khedzia (desvenlafaxine), and Priztiq (desvenlafaxine) are SNRIs.

» **Norepinephrine and dopamine reuptake inhibitor (NDRI):** This medicine slows the body's natural reabsorption of norepinephrine and dopamine. Wellbutrin (bupropion) is the earliest and best-known NDRI, also marketed as an anti-smoking drug under the brand name Zyban.

Seeing how food can affect your mood

Good morning: Time to wake up, roll out of bed, and sleepwalk into the kitchen for a cup of coffee.

Good afternoon: Time for a moderate glass of whiskey or wine to soothe away the tensions of the day.

Good grief: Your lover has left. Time for chocolate, *lots* of chocolate, to soothe the pain.

Good night: Time for milk and cookies to ease your way to Dreamland.

For centuries, millions of people have used these foods in these situations, secure in the knowledge that each food will work its mood magic. Today, modern science knows why. Having discovered that your emotions are linked to your production or use of neurotransmitters, nutrition scientists have been able to identify the natural chemicals in food that change the way you feel by

» Influencing the production of neurotransmitters

» Hooking onto brain cells and changing the way the cells behave

» Opening pathways to brain cells so that other mood-altering chemicals can come on board

The following sections describe chemicals in food commonly known to affect mood.

Alcohol

Alcohol is man's (and woman's) most widely used natural relaxant. Contrary to common belief, alcohol is a depressant, not a mood elevator. If you feel relaxed or, conversely, exuberant after one drink, the reason isn't that the alcohol is speeding up your brain; it's that alcohol loosens your *controls*, the brain signals that normally tell you not to put a lampshade on your head or take off your clothes in public.

For more about alcohol's effects on virtually every body organ and system, turn to Chapter 9. Right here, it's enough to say that many people find that, taken with food and in moderation — defined as one drink a day for a woman and two for a man — alcohol can comfortably change a mood from tense to mellow.

Anandamide

Anandamide is a *cannabinoid,* a chemical that hooks up to the same brain receptors that catch similar ingredients in marijuana smoke. Your brain produces some anandamide naturally, but you also get very small amounts of the chemical from cocoa bean products — chocolate. In addition, chocolate contains two chemicals similar to anandamide that slow the breakdown of the anandamide produced in your brain, thus intensifying its effects.

Maybe that's why eating chocolate makes you feel so good. And that really does mean *mildly:* You'd have to eat at least 25 pounds of chocolate at one time to get any marijuanalike effect. In 2009, a team of nutrition scientists at the Nestle Research Center in Lausanne (Switzerland) produced the still-classic study of the beneficial calming effects. Their results put the amount required to reduce the body's production of stress hormones at 40 grams (about 1.5 ounces) of dark chocolate a day. The chocolate used in the study was 74 percent cocoa, served in two daily doses, 20 grams in the morning and 20 grams in the afternoon, after which the researchers tested the volunteers' blood to measure levels of stress hormones and found the levels of stress hormones dropping among the chocolate eaters, thus making chocoholics everywhere even happier than usual.

Caffeine

Caffeine is a mild stimulant that

>> Raises your blood pressure

>> Speeds up your heartbeat

>> Makes you burn calories faster

>> Makes you urinate more frequently

>> Causes your intestinal tract to move food more quickly through your body

Although it increases the level of serotonin, the calming neurotransmitter, caffeine also hooks up at specific receptors (sites on the surface of brain cells) normally reserved for another naturally occurring tranquilizer, *adenosine* (a-*den*-o-seen). When caffeine latches on in place of adenosine, brain cells become more reactive to stimulants such as noise and light, making you talk faster and think faster.

But caffeine can be confusing. People react to it in highly individual ways. Some can drink seven cups of regular ("with caffeine") coffee and still stay calm all day and sleep like a baby at night. Others tend to hop about on decaf. Perhaps those who stay calm have enough brain receptors to accommodate both adenosine and caffeine, or perhaps they're more sensitive to the adenosine that manages to hook up to brain cells. Nobody really knows. Either way, caffeine's bouncy effects may last anywhere from one to seven hours. Read even more about that in Chapter 30.

Table 24-3 lists some common food sources of caffeine. The caffeine content listed here is an average for the generic versions of the food or drink — in other words, plain, no-brand products. You can check out the caffeine content of brand-name products such as a Starbucks Espresso Solo (75 mg/oz) or Ben & Jerry's coffee flavored ice cream (34 mg/4 oz) at the Center for Science in the Public Interest website at `www.cspinet.org/new/cafchart.htm`.

TABLE 24-3 ## Foods That Give You Caffeine

Food	Average Amount of Caffeine (mg)
6-ounce cups	
Coffee, regular, drip	71
Coffee, regular, instant	47
Coffee, decaffeinated	1
Tea	36
Tea, instant	20
Cocoa (mix + water)	4
12-ounce can	
Soft drinks, cola	29
8-ounce container	
Chocolate milk (commercial, low-fat)	5

(continued)

TABLE 24-3 *(continued)*

Food	Average Amount of Caffeine (mg)
1-ounce serving	
Milk chocolate	6
Semisweet chocolate	24
Bitter (baker's) chocolate	23

USDA National Nutrient Database for Standard Reference, www.nal.usda.gov/fnic/foodcomp/search

Tryptophan and glucose

Tryptophan is an amino acid, another one of those "building blocks of protein" (see Chapter 6). Glucose, the end product of carbohydrate metabolism, is the sugar that circulates in your blood, the basic fuel on which your body runs (see Chapter 8). Milk and cookies, a classic calming combo, owe their power to the tryptophan/glucose team.

Start with the fact that the neurotransmitters dopamine, norepinephrine, and serotonin are made from the amino acids tyrosine and tryptophan, which are found in protein foods (like milk). *Tyrosine* is the most important ingredient in dopamine and norepinephrine, the alertness neurotransmitters. *Tryptophan* is the most important ingredient in serotonin, the calming neurotransmitter.

All amino acids ride into your brain on chemical pathways, but your brain makes way for the bouncy tyrosine first and the soothing tryptophan last. That's why a high-protein meal heightens your alertness.

To move the tryptophan along faster, you need glucose, and that means carbohydrate foods (like those cookies). When you eat carbs, your pancreas releases *insulin*, a hormone that enables you to metabolize the carbs and produce glucose. The insulin also keeps tyrosine and other amino acids circulating in your blood so that tryptophan travels on plenty of open paths to the brain. With more tryptophan coming in, your brain can increase its production of soothing serotonin. That's why a meal of starchy pasta (starch is composed of chains of glucose molecules, as explained in Chapter 8) makes you feel calm and cool.

The effects of simple sugars, such as sucrose (table sugar), are more complicated. If you eat simple sugars on an empty stomach, the sugars are absorbed rapidly, triggering an equally rapid increase in the secretion of insulin, a hormone needed to digest carbohydrates. The result is a rapid decrease in the amount of sugar circulating in your blood, a condition known as *hypoglycemia* (*hypo* = low; *glycemia* = sugar in the blood) that can make you feel temporarily jumpy rather than calm. However, when eaten on a full stomach — dessert after a full meal — simple sugars are absorbed more slowly and may exert the calming effect usually linked to complex carbohydrates (starchy foods).

Obvious conclusion: Some foods, such as meat, fish, and poultry, make you more alert. Others, such as pasta, bread, potatoes, rice, and other grains, calm you down. The effect of the food depends on its ability to alter the amount of serotonin available to your brain (see Figure 24-1).

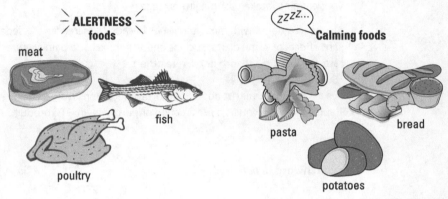

FIGURE 24-1:
Some foods may calm you, and some foods may make you more alert.

© John Wiley & Son, Ltd

Fascinating factoid: Even though turkey is high in protein, it's also high in trypto-phan, the precursor of (that is, the chemical that leads to the creation of) sero-tonin, which may explain why so many people nod off after Thanksgiving dinner.

Phenylethylamine (PEA)

Phenylethylamine — sometimes abbreviated PEA — is a natural chemical that your body releases when you're in love, making you feel, well, good all over. A big splash occurred in the late 1980s when researchers discovered that chocolate, the food of lovers, is a fine source of PEA.

In fact, many people think that PEA has a lot to do with chocolate's reputation as the food of love and consolation. Of course, to be fair about it, chocolate also contains the mood elevator caffeine, the muscle stimulant theobromine, and the cannabinoid anandamide (see the earlier section on anandamide).

Using food to manage mood

No food will change your personality or alter the course of a mood disorder. But some may add a little lift or a small moment of calm to your day, increase your effectiveness at certain tasks, make you more alert, or give you a neat little push over the finish line.

CAUTION! MEDICINE AT WORK

Some of the mood-altering chemicals in food interact with medicines. As you may have guessed, the two most notable examples are caffeine and alcohol.

- Caffeine makes painkillers, such as aspirin and acetaminophen, more effective. On the other hand, many over-the-counter (OTC) painkillers and cold medicines already contain caffeine. If you take the pill with a cup of java, you may increase your caffeine intake past the jitters stage.

- Alcohol is a no-no with most medicines because it increases the sedative or depressant effects of some drugs, such as antihistamines and painkillers, and alters the rate at which you absorb or excrete others.

Always ask your pharmacist about food-drug interactions (you can read more about this in Chapter 25) when you fill a prescription or purchase an OTC product.

The watchword is *balance:*

>> One cup of coffee in the morning is a pleasant push into alertness. Seven cups of coffee a day can make your hands shake.

>> One alcohol drink is generally a safe way to relax. Three may be a disaster.

>> A grilled chicken breast (white meat, no skin) for breakfast on a day when you have to be on your toes before lunch can help make you sharp as a tack.

>> Got an important lunch meeting? Order starches without fats or oils: pasta with fresh tomatoes and basil, no oil, no cheese; rice with veggies; rice with fruit. Your aim is to get the calming carbs without the high-fat food that slows thinking and makes you feel sleepy.

As in other aspects of a healthy life, the point is to make sure that you use the tool (in this case, food), not the other way around.

Healing the Injured Brain

Slice off your finger while chopping wood, and as you're on the way to the emergency room, some helpful passerby can pick up the finger, hopefully stick it into a cup of ice to chill and preserve the tissues, and dawdle his way over to the hospital to meet you. If the finger arrives within a couple of hours, it likely can be successfully reimplanted. New cells will grow to heal the damage. Blood will flow through reattached vessels. Newly stitched nerves and muscles will signal and move. Bones will knit together. And you may well enjoy a working five-fingered hand.

But hit your head hard enough to injure brain cells, suffer a stroke, or have a heart attack that interrupts the flow of oxygenated blood to the brain, and your brain cells begin to die within minutes.

To reduce the loss of brain cells and limit damage to an injured brain, doctors concentrate on ensuring an adequate supply of oxygen and controlling swelling that pushes the soft brain against the inside of the hard skull.

But there may be another weapon in the arsenal: food.

The 5, 7, 2, 4, 100, 200 solution

After any injury, your body goes into a *hypermetabolic state* (*hyper* is the Greek word for "over"), meaning that it suddenly requires more calories than normal to provide the energy and material to rebuild damaged tissues. True, an injured brain won't be producing new cells, but this 2 percent of your weight that consumes 20 percent of your calorie intake will need extra energy to establish the new connections that can enable you to function.

In fact, feeding patients with brain injuries is so important that neurologists at Presbyterian Hospital/Weill Cornell Medical Center in New York have actually put some hard numbers to it: 5, 7, 2, 4, 100, 200.

Translation: Patients with brain injury who are not fed either intravenously or through a tube into the stomach within 5 days after the injury occurs are 2 times more likely to die than are patients who get fed. Patients not fed within 7 days are 4 times more likely to die. And the best menu provides *100* percent of the normal recommended daily calories for that particular patient (see Chapter 3); up to 200 percent is even better.

"There is no miracle drug for patients with severe traumatic brain injury," says Roger Härtl, Professor of Neurological Surgery and Director of Spinal Surgery and Neurotrauma at the Weill Cornell Brain and Spine Center in New York, and the Director of the Weill Cornell Medicine Center for Comprehensive Spine Care (he's also the official neurosurgeon for the New York Giants football team). "But we have been able to reduce the mortality and improve outcome in these patients dramatically by maintaining their blood pressure and supplying the brain early on with oxygen and nutrients. We now start feeding patients with severe brain injuries very aggressively from the moment they first hit the intensive care unit, and early nutrition is now recognized as one of the most important factors improving outcome in these patients." So important, in fact, that the regimen has now been incorporated in the international Guidelines for Management of Severe Traumatic Brain injury.

Protein possibilities

Leucine, isoleucine, and valine are amino acids, the building blocks of protein described in Chapter 6. Because these three particular amino acids share a distinct chemical structure — a long central chain with smaller side chains branching off — they're called *branched chain amino acids* (BCAA, for short).

The body uses BCAA to build neurotransmitters, the naturally occurring chemicals that enable cells to exchange messages: Think! Move! Feel! Unfortunately, an injury to the brain that damages the hippocampus, a part of the brain that helps direct memory and cognition, may reduce brain levels of leucine, isoleucine, and valine.

As long ago as 1983, studies suggested that intravenous doses of BCAA would benefit patients with liver disease by forcing additional amino acids into their brain. Some sports nutritionists think that BCAA supplements can improve muscle performance.

In 2009, neuroscientist Akiva Cohen and his team at The Children's Hospital of Philadelphia saw a more direct application. When they added BCAA to the drinking water of brain-injured mice, Cohen's team observed improvements in both mouse memory and cognition. If future studies with human beings demonstrate the same effect, patients with traumatic brain injuries might be able to avoid the feeding tubes and intravenous needles to improve their thinking and remembering simply by sipping a glass of branched-chain-amino-acid-enriched (building blocks of protein) water. A follow-up study in 2013 showed that the amino acids also improve "wakefulness" — the ability to stay awake and alert — after traumatic brain injury (TBI), thus enhancing recovery.

The (eventual) official word

Because military personnel, especially those in combat zones, face a distinct risk of TBI, in 2009, the Department of Defense (DoD) asked the Institute of Medicine (IOM) to convene an expert committee to review the potential role of nutrition in the treatment of and resilience against TBI.

The IOM is the division of the National Academy of Sciences that sets and publishes the RDAs, RDIs, and other nutritional recommendations listed in Chapter 3. To meet the DoD request, IOM set up a Consensus Study on Nutrition, Trauma, and the Brain to determine "the potential role for nutrition in providing resilience (i.e., protecting), mitigating or treating of primary (i.e., within minutes of insult), secondary (i.e., within 24 hours of insult), and long-term (i.e., more than 24 hours after insult) associated effects of neurotrauma, with a focus on traumatic brain injury."

Two years later, in 2011, IOM issued a first report from the study. The primary message, an echo of Dr. Härtl's (see the earlier section "The 5, 7, 2, 4, 100, 200 solution"): All military personnel suffering from traumatic brain injury should get adequate protein and calories as soon as possible to reduce inflammation and improve their recovery and eventual outcome. This advice, they noted, also applied for non-military people, such as athletes, who were at risk of concussion and other brain injuries.

Eating to Benefit Your Brain and Your Body

While you're waiting for nutrition science to catch up with your brain, make your own medicine with these four simple rules for a diet that benefits your brain and your body, too:

>> **Eat enough food.** Sounds foolish in a country where obesity is a problem, doesn't it? But constant on-and-off dieting or even occasional crash dieting can rob your brain of energy without producing lasting weight control. Get the calories you need. And not a smidgen more. (For your calorie requirements, see Chapter 5.)

>> **Eat smaller portions but more often.** Who says three scheduled large meals a day are right for everybody? Frequent smaller meals provide a continuous flow of energy to your brain. And by allowing them to eat before they are ravenously hungry, these grazing moments may enable some people to keep from overeating. (Want to know why you eat when you eat? See Chapter 14.)

>> **Choose foods that turn to energy slower rather than faster.** Simple carbs, such as table sugar, pep you up fast and then let you down just as quickly. Your body metabolizes complex carbs, such as fruits and vegetables and whole grains, more slowly, so their effect on your brain's energy bank is smoother and lasts longer. (For more about which carbs are which, see Chapter 8.)

>> **Pick the perfect fats.** Protect your brain as well as your heart by emphasizing fats that build you up without blocking arteries, including those in your brain. (What you need to know is in Chapter 7.)

TIP

Be patient. If nutrition is a new science, brain nutrition is the newest of the new. Expect to hear something interesting on Monday, have it discredited on Tuesday, and on Wednesday read about the latest wrinkle in the story. Eventually, we will know exactly what to eat to keep the brain as fit as the body. The key word: *eventually.*

Chapter **25**

Food and Drug Interactions

oods nourish your body. Medicines cure (or relieve) what ails you. The two should work together in perfect harmony. Sometimes they do, but sometimes they fight. In some cases, the medicine prevents your body from absorbing or using the nutrients in food, or the food (or nutrient) incapacitates the medicine.

The medical phrase for this is *adverse interaction.* This chapter describes several adverse interactions and lays out some simple strategies that enable you to short-circuit them.

SIDE EFFECTS VERSUS ADVERSE EFFECTS

Although these terms sound alike, they describe different medical phenomena. A *side effect* is simply something a medicine or chemical does in addition to what it's supposed to do. For example, the common antihistamine diphenhydramine (Benadryl) relieves allergy symptoms but also causes drowsiness and dry mouth. Side effects are usually listed on a drug package and are usually short-lived with no lasting complications. *Adverse effects,* on the other hand, are less common, more serious, and may interfere with the progress of a disease or the success of a treatment. One such example is the severe and potentially lethal allergic reaction called *anaphylaxis,* which may occur when people sensitive to penicillin are given even a normal "safe" dose of this antibiotic or one of its relatives such as amoxicillin.

Following Food and Drug Interactions

When you eat, food moves from your mouth to your stomach to your small intestine, where the nutrients that keep you strong and healthy are absorbed into your bloodstream and distributed throughout your body. Take medicine by mouth, and it follows pretty much the same path from mouth to stomach to the small intestine for absorption. Nothing is unusual about that.

WARNING

A problem may arise when a food or drug brings the process to a halt by behaving in a way that interferes with your ability to digest, absorb, or use either the drug or the food (see Figure 25-1). For example:

>> Some drugs or foods change the natural acidity of your digestive tract so that you absorb nutrients less efficiently. For example, your body absorbs iron best when your stomach is acidic. Taking antacids reduces stomach acidity — and iron absorption.

>> Some drugs or foods change the rate at which food moves through your digestive tract, which means that you absorb more (or less) of a particular nutrient or drug. For example, eating prunes (a laxative food) or taking a laxative drug speeds things up so that medicines, like foods, move more quickly through your body, giving you less time to absorb either the medicine or the nutrients in the food.

>> Some drugs and nutrients *bond* (link up with each other) to form insoluble compounds that your body can't break apart. As a result, you get less of the drug and less of the nutrient. The best-known example: Calcium (in dairy foods) bonds to the antibiotic tetracycline so that both move swiftly out of your body.

>> Some drugs and nutrients have similar chemical structures. Taking them at the same time fools your body into absorbing or using the nutrient rather than the drug. One good example is Coumadin (the generic version of Warfarin, a drug that keeps blood from clotting) and vitamin K (a nutrient that makes blood clot). Eating lots of vitamin K–rich leafy greens while taking Warfarin counteracts the medicine's ability to prevent blood clots.

>> Some foods contain chemicals that either lessen or intensify the natural side effects of certain drugs. For example, the caffeine in coffee, tea, and cola drinks reduces the sedative effects of antihistamines and some antidepressant drugs but increases the nervousness, insomnia, and shakiness common with pills such as cold medications containing caffeine or a *decongestant* (an ingredient that temporarily clears a stuffy nose).

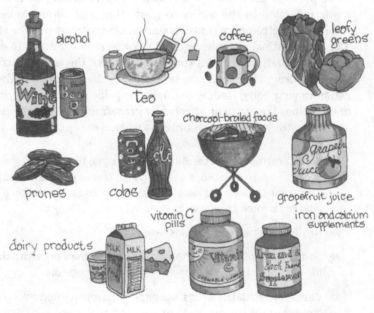

FIGURE 25-1: Some foods may affect the way your body interacts with drugs.

© John Wiley & Sons, Ltd.

Listing the Reactions of Drugs and Certain Foods

Sometimes the combinations of interacting foods and drugs are surprising. Astounding. Or breathtaking.

Everyone knows that people with asthma may find it hard to take a deep breath around the barbecue. The culprit's the smoke, right? Yes. And no. Breathing in smoke does irritate air passages, but — the surprise — eating charcoal-broiled food speeds the body's elimination of *theophylline*, a widely used asthma drug, reducing the drug's ability to protect against wheezing. Take the drug, eat the food, and maybe end up wheezing.

Another potential troublemaker is an acidic beverage, such as fruit juice or soft drinks, which may inactivate the antibiotics erythromycin, ampicillin, and penicillin.

Grapefruit juice is a particularly potent offender.

In the mid-1990s, researchers tracking the effects of alcohol beverages on the blood pressure drug felodipine (Plendil) tripped across the *Grapefruit Effect*, a dramatic reduction in the ability to metabolize and eliminate certain drugs. Why? Because grapefruit juice contains substances that suppress the effectiveness of CYP 3A4, an intestinal enzyme required to convert many drugs to water-soluble substances you can flush out of your body; without the enzyme activity, you can't get rid of the drug. The result may be an equally dramatic rise in the amount of medication in your body, leading to unpleasant side effects. Following is a selected list of medicines known to be affected by grapefruit juice. It is by no means complete, so check with your doctor or druggist whenever you get a new prescription.

>> **Some statins (cholesterol-lowering drugs):** lovastatin (Mevacor), atorvastatin (Lipitor), simvastatin (Zocor). (Other statins, such as fluvastatin (Lescol), pravastatin (Pravachol), and rosuvastatin (Crestor), have little or no interaction with grapefruit juice.)

>> **Antihistamine:** fexofenadine (Allegra)

>> **Some types of calcium channel blockers (blood pressure drugs):** felodipine (Plendil), nifedipine (Adalat, Afeditab CR, Procardia)

>> **Certain psychiatric drugs:** buspirone, triazolam (Halcion), carbamazepine (Tegretol), diazepam (Valium), midazolam (Versed), sertraline (Zoloft)

>> **Some immunosuppressants:** cyclosporine (Neoral), tacrolimus (Prograf)

>> **Pain medication:** methadone

>> **Impotence drug (erectile dysfunction):** sildenafil (Viagra)

>> **HIV medication:** saquinavir (Invirase)

>> **Some antiarrhythmics:** amiodarone (Cordarone, Nexterone, Pacerone)

Source: www.webmd.com/hypertension-high-blood-pressure/guide/grapefruit-juice-and-medication

WARNING

Taking a slow-release medicine along with grapefruit juice may cause the entire dose of medicine in the pill or capsule to be released and metabolized at once.

Discovering Drug Interactions with Nutrients

Like food, individual nutrients — vitamins and minerals — may also interact with medicines. Here are four examples:

>> Antacids containing aluminum compounds bind with the bone-building mineral phosphorous, carrying it right out of your body.

>> Antiulcer drugs cimetidine (Tagamet) and ranitidine (Zantac) can make you positively giddy. These drugs reduce stomach acidity, which means the body absorbs alcohol more efficiently. According to experts at the Mayo Clinic, taking ulcer medication with alcohol leads to twice the wallop. Drink one beer, and you feel as though you've had two.

>> Diuretics, commonly known as water pills, increase urination, which increases your loss of the mineral potassium. To make up what you lose, experts suggest adding potassium-rich bananas, oranges, spinach, corn, and tomatoes to your diet.

>> Oral contraceptives reduce the body's absorption of the B vitamin folate and possibly B12.

Table 25-1 lists some common vitamin/mineral and drug interactions. (For more information on supplements, see Chapter 13.)

TABLE 25-1   **Interactions between Nutrients and Medications**

Vitamin	Medication	Interaction Effects
Vitamin A	Retinoids (isotretinoin, acitretin)	Risk of toxicity, nausea, vomiting, dizziness, blurred vision, poor muscle coordination
Pyridoxine (Vitamin B$_6$)	Levodopa	Decreased efficacy leading to parkinsonian symptoms
	Phenytoin	Risk of seizure
Vitamin E	Warfarin	Risk of bleeding

(continued)

TABLE 25-1 *(continued)*

Vitamin	Medication	Interaction Effects
Vitamin K	Warfarin	Decreased efficacy, risk of thromboembolism
Niacin	HMG-CoA reductase inhibitors	Risk of myopathy or rhabdomyolysis
Folic acid	Methotrexate	Prevents adverse effects or toxicities from methotrexate
Calcium	Fluoroquinolones and tetracyclines	Decreased efficacy, risk of antibiotic failure
	Levothyroxine and bisphosphonates	Decreased efficacy, risk of hypothyroidism
Aluminum and magnesium	Fluoroquinolones, tetracyclines, levothyroxine, and bisphosphonates	Decreased efficacy of affected medication
Iron	Fluoroquinolones, tetracyclines, digoxin, and levothyroxine	Decreased efficacy of affected medication
	Methyldopa	Worsening of hypertension
Potassium	ACE inhibitors, angiotensin receptor blockers, digoxin, indomethacin, prescription potassium supplements, and potassium-sparing diuretics	Hyperkalemia

Source: https://www.uspharmacist.com/article/drug-interactions-with-vitamins-and-minerals

Using Food to Improve a Drug's Performance

Not every food and drug interaction is an adverse one. Sometimes a drug works better or is less likely to cause side effects when you take it on a full stomach. For example, aspirin is less likely to upset your stomach if you take the painkiller with food, and eating stimulates the release of stomach juices that improve your ability to absorb griseofulvin, an antifungal drug.

Table 25-2 lists some drugs that may work better when your stomach is full.

TABLE 25-2

Drugs That Work Better on a Full Stomach

Purpose	Drug
Analgesics (painkillers)	
	Acetaminophen
	Aspirin
	Codeine
	Ibuprofen
	Indomethacin
	Mefenamic acid
	Metronidazole
	Naproxen/naproxen sodium
Antibiotics, antivirals, antifungals	
	Ethambutol
	Griseofulvin
	Isoniazid
	Ketoconazole
	Pyrimethamine
Antidiabetic agents	
	Glipizide
	Glyburide
	Tolazamide
	Tolbutamide
Cholesterol-lowering agents	
	Cholestyramine
	Colestipol
	Lovastatin
	Probucol
Gastric medications	
	Cimetidine
	Ranitidine

James J. Rybacki, The Essential Guide to Prescription Drugs 2002 (New York: Harper Collins, 2001)

WITH THIS MEDICINE, WHO CAN EAT?

Interactions aren't the only drug reactions that keep you from getting nutrients from food. Some drugs have side effects that also reduce the value of food. For example, a drug may

- Sharply reduce your appetite so that you simply don't eat much. The best-known example may be the amphetamine and amphetamine-like drugs such as fenfluramine used (surprise!) as diet pills.

- Make food taste or smell bad or steal away your senses of taste or smell so that eating isn't pleasurable. One example is the antidepressant drug amitriptyline (Elavil), which can leave a peculiar taste in your mouth.

- Cause nausea, vomiting, or diarrhea so that you either can't eat or do not retain nutrients from the food you do eat. Examples include the antibiotic erythromycin and many drugs used to treat cancer.

- Irritate the lining of your intestinal tract so that even if you do eat, your body has a hard time absorbing nutrients from food. The most-common examples of this kind of interaction occur with drugs used in cancer chemotherapy.

The moderately good news is that new medications appear to make some drugs (including anticancer drugs) less likely to cause nausea and vomiting. The best news is that many drugs are less likely to upset your stomach or irritate your gut if you take them with food (refer to Table 25-2). For example, taking aspirin and other nonprescription painkillers, such as ibuprofen, with food or a full glass of water may reduce their natural tendency to irritate the lining of your stomach.

Chapter **26**

Using Food as Medicine

A healthful diet gives you the nutrients you need to keep your body in top-flight condition. In addition, evidence suggests that eating well may prevent or minimize the risk of a long list of serious medical conditions, including heart disease and high blood pressure.

This chapter describes what nutritionists know right now about how to use food to prevent, alleviate, or cure what ails you.

Defining Food as Medicine

TIP

Start with a definition. A food that acts like a medicine is one that increases or reduces your risk of a specific medical condition or cures or alleviates the effects of a medical condition. For example:

» Eating foods, such as wheat bran, that are high in *insoluble dietary fiber* (the kind of fiber that doesn't dissolve in your gut) moves food more quickly through your intestinal tract and produces soft, bulky stool that reduces your risk of constipation.

- » Eating foods, such as beans, that are rich in *soluble dietary fiber* (fiber that dissolves in your intestinal tract) seems to help your body mop up the cholesterol circulating in your bloodstream, preventing it from sticking to the walls of your arteries. This reduces your risk of heart disease.

- » Eating sufficient amounts of calcium-rich foods (accompanied by vitamin D, as noted in Chapter 10) ensures the growth of strong bones early in life.

- » Eating very spicy foods, such as chili, makes the membrane lining your nose and throat weep a watery fluid that makes blowing your nose or coughing up mucus easier when you have a cold.

- » Eating (or drinking) foods (or beverages) with mood-altering substances such as caffeine, alcohol, and phenylethylamine (PEA) may lend a lift when you're feeling down or, conversely, help you chill when you're tense. (For more on food and mood, see Chapter 24.)

The joy of food as medicine is that it's cheaper and much more pleasant than managing illness with drugs. Given the choice, who wouldn't opt to control cholesterol levels with oats or chili (all those yummy beans packed with soluble dietary fiber) than with a list of medicines whose possible side effects include kidney failure and liver damage? Right.

Naming Diets with Absolutely, Positively Beneficial Medical Effects

Some foods and some diet plans are so obviously good for your body that no one questions their ability to keep you healthy or make you feel better when you're ill. For example, if you've ever had abdominal surgery, you know all about liquid diets — the water–gelatin–clear broth regimen your doctor prescribed right after the operation to enable you to take some nourishment by mouth without upsetting your intestines.

Or if you have *Type 1 diabetes* (an inherited inability to produce the insulin needed to process carbohydrates), you know that your ability to balance the carbohydrates, fats, and proteins in your daily diet is important to stabilizing your illness.

Other proven diet regimens include

- » **The high-fiber diet:** A high-fiber diet quickens the passage of food through the digestive tract. This diet is used to prevent constipation. If you have *diverticula* (outpouchings) in the wall of your colon, a high-fiber diet may reduce the possibility of an infection. It can also alleviate the discomfort of irritable bowel syndrome (sometimes called a nervous stomach). Extra bonus: A diet high in soluble fiber also lowers cholesterol (see the preceding section, "Defining Food as Medicine"). A word to the wise: When increasing your dietary fiber intake, be sure to drink enough fluid (see Chapter 12) to prevent the fiber from clumping in and maybe even blocking your digestive tract.

>> **The sodium-restricted diet:** Sodium is hydrophilic (*hydro* = water; *philic* = loving). It increases the amount of water held in body tissues. For people who are sensitive to the effects of sodium, a diet low in salt often lowers water retention, which can be useful in treating high blood pressure, congestive heart failure, and long-term liver disease. By the way, not all the sodium in your diet comes from table salt.

>> **The extra-potassium diet:** People use this diet to counteract the loss of potassium caused by *diuretics* (drugs that make you urinate more frequently and more copiously, causing you to lose excess amounts of potassium in urine). Some evidence also suggests that the high-potassium diet may lower blood pressure a bit.

>> **The low-protein diet:** This diet is prescribed for people with chronic liver or kidney disease or an inherited inability to metabolize amino acids, the building blocks of proteins. The low-protein regimen reduces the amount of protein waste products in body tissues, thus reducing the possibility of tissue damage.

Using Food to Prevent Disease

Using food as a general preventive is an intriguing subject. True, much anecdotal evidence ("I did this, and that happened") suggests that eating some foods and avoiding others can raise or lower your risk of some serious diseases. But anecdotes aren't science. The more important indicator is the evidence from scientific studies tracking groups of people on different diets to see how things such as eating or avoiding fat, fiber, meat, dairy foods, salt, and other foods affects their risk of specific diseases or conditions. One intriguing example is a 2019 report from the University of Buffalo (New York) suggesting that what you eat may affect how well you see. Their data suggests that people who follow a diet high in red or processed meat, fried foods, refined grain, and high-fat dairy are three times more likely to develop late-stage macular degeneration resulting in loss of sight than those who avoid or cut back consumption of these foods.

The general name for foods that deliver a health benefit is *functional foods.* One example of a group of natural functional foods that prevent illness is the vitamin A-rich collection of dark green, yellow, red, and orange fruits and vegetables that protect the ability to see in dim light. An example of a manufactured functional food is margarines made with heart-and-brain protective omega-3 fatty acids, whipped up by food technologists. (See Chapter 7 for more information on specific dietary fats.)

Battling deficiency diseases

The simplest example of food's ability to act as preventive medicine is its ability to ward off a *deficiency disease,* a condition that occurs when you don't get sufficient amounts of a specific nutrient. For example, people deprived of vitamin C develop scurvy, the vitamin C–deficiency disease; or there's pellagra, the deficiency disease due to a lack of the B vitamin niacin. Because flour processing often removes B vitamins found in the germ of the grain, virtually all grain products sold in the United States are enriched with the B vitamins.

Reviewing the evidence on anticancer diets

Is there really an anticancer diet? Probably not. The problem is that cancer isn't one disease; it's many diseases with many causes. Some foods seem to protect against some specific cancers, but none seem to protect against all. For example:

>> **Fruits and vegetables:** Plants contain some potential anticancer substances, such as *antioxidants,* chemicals that appear to prevent molecular fragments called *free radicals* from hooking up to form cancer-causing compounds.

   However, despite early predictions that antioxidant-rich plant foods would reduce the risk of cancer overall, to date, no seriously controlled study has ever shown that belief to be true.

>> **Foods high in dietary fiber:** Human beings can't digest dietary fiber, but friendly bacteria living in your gut can. Chomping away on the fiber, the bacteria excrete fatty acids that appear to keep cells from turning cancerous. In addition, insoluble dietary fiber helps speed food through your body, reducing the formation of carcinogenic compounds.

   For more than 30 years, doctors have assumed that eating lots of dietary fiber reduces the risk of colon cancer, but in 1999, data from the long-running Nurses' Health Study at Boston's Brigham and Women's Hospital and Harvard's School of Public Health threw this assumption into question. Since then, several very large studies — one with more than 350,000 people! — confirmed that dietary fiber probably has no protective effect against colon cancer. But even if dietary fiber doesn't fight cancer, it does prevent constipation. One out of two ain't bad.

FEAST ON FISH

Over several decades, a plethora of studies have suggested a higher risk of colon cancer among meat eaters than among vegetarians. Exactly how beef, pork, and lamb exercise their adverse effect remains a matter of controversy, but in 2015, researchers at Loma Linda University in California added a new twist to the story: Don't just pass up the meat, they said; Pick up the fish.

Their advice is based on an analysis of the daily menus of more than 70,000 men and women. As previously noted, following a vegetarian diet lowered the risk of colon cancer by 22 percent. But adding fish produced an even greater reduction in risk, 43 percent lower than meat eaters.

The beneficial veggie-plus-fish-and-other-seafood diet is not just tasty and maybe protective. It even has a catchy new name: *pescovegetarian* from *piscis*, the Latin word for fish.

>> **Low-fat foods:** Some dietary fat appears to increase the proliferation of various types of body cells, but not all fats appear to be equally guilty. In several studies, fat from meat seems linked to an increased risk of colon cancer, but fat from dairy foods comes up clean.

TIP

The American Cancer Society Advisory Committee on Diet, Nutrition, and Cancer Prevention issued a set of nutrition guidelines that shows how to use food to reduce the risk of cancer. These are the American Cancer Society's recommendations:

>> **Choose most of the foods you eat from plant sources.** Eat five or more servings of fruits and vegetables every day. Eat other foods from plant sources, such as breads, cereals, grain products, rice, pasta, or beans, several times a day.

>> **Limit your intake of high-fat foods, particularly from animal sources.** Choose foods low in fat. Limit consumption of meats, especially high-fat meats.

>> **Be physically active.** Achieve and maintain a healthy weight. Be at least moderately active for 30 minutes or more on most days of the week. Stay within your healthy weight range.

>> **If you drink alcohol, drink in moderation.** Chapter 9 lays it out: Moderate consumption means no more than one drink a day for a woman, two for a man.

THREE DEGREES OF VEGETARIANISM

Vegetarianism isn't one diet; it's four plant-based menu plans, each one distinguished by what's allowed to be on the dinner plate along with the plants.

- Vegetarian variation #1 is a diet for people who don't eat meat but do eat fish and poultry or just fish. (Fairness dictates that I state that many strict vegetarians don't consider people who eat fish or poultry to be vegetarians.)

- Vegetarian variation #2 is a diet for people who don't eat meat, fish, or poultry but do eat other animal products, such as eggs and dairy products. Vegetarians who follow this regimen are called *ovo-lacto vegetarians* (*ovo* = egg; *lacto* = milk).

- Vegetarian variation #3 is a diet for people who eat absolutely no foods of animal origin. Vegetarians who eat only plant foods are called *vegans*.

- Vegetarian variation #4 is a diet comprising only fruit. Naturally, vegetarians who use this diet are called *fruitarians*.

DASHing to healthy blood pressure

More than 50 million Americans have high blood pressure (also referred to as *hypertension*), a major risk factor for heart disease, stroke, and heart or kidney failure.

The DASH diet (Dietary Approaches to Stop Hypertension) is a lifelong approach to healthy eating developed by research sponsored by the National Institutes of Health to help treat or prevent high blood pressure (hypertension) without medication. It often ranks number one on lists of healthy ways for all of us to eat because it is rich in fruits and vegetables, plus low–fat dairy products with controlled sodium levels. No surprise there. But the DASH diet suggests that you get no more than 27 percent of your calories each day from fats, lower than the 35 percent considered standard by several other diets.

The difference does seem to make a difference. Your blood pressure is measured in two numbers that look something like this: 130/80. The first number is your *systolic pressure*, the force exerted against artery walls when your heart beats and pushes blood out into your blood vessels. The second, lower number is the *diastolic pressure*, the force exerted between beats.

In 2019, the National Heart, Lung, and Blood Institute (NHLB) reported the results of four studies which compared the health benefits of DASH with the common American diet, plus a fifth, the Premier clinical trial funded by NHLB, all showing that DASH lowers blood pressure and reduces the blood level of "bad" LDK cholesterol.

Conquering the common cold

This section is not about chicken soup. That issue has been settled, and Dr. Mom was right. In the 1980s, Marvin Sackler of Mount Sinai Medical Center in Miami, Florida, published the first serious study showing that cold sufferers who got hot chicken soup felt better faster than those who got plain hot water, and dozens of studies since have said, man, he's right. Nobody really knows why chicken soup works, but who cares? It works.

So moving on to other foods that make you feel better when you have the sniffles — for example, sweet foods. Scientists do know why sweeteners — white sugar, brown sugar, honey, molasses — soothe a sore throat. All sugars are *demulcents,* substances that coat and soothe the irritated mucous membranes.

Lemons aren't sweet, and they have less vitamin C than orange juice, but their popularity in the form of *hot lemonade* (tea with lemon and sugar) and sour lemon drops is unmatched. Why? Because a lemon's sharp flavor cuts through to your taste buds and makes the sugary stuff more palatable. In addition, the sour taste makes saliva flow, which also soothes your throat.

Hot stuff — such as peppers, horseradish (freshly grated is definitely the most potent), and onions — contains mustard oils that irritate the membranes lining your nose and mouth and even make your eyes water. As a result, it's easier to blow your nose or cough up mucus.

Finally, there's coffee, a real boon to snifflers. When you're sick, your body piles up *cytokines,* chemicals that carry messages among immune system cells that fight infection. When cytokines pile up in brain tissue, you get sleepy, which may explain why you're so drowsy when you have a cold. True, rest can help to boost your immune system and fight off the cold, but once in a while you have to get up. Like to go to work.

The caffeine in even a single cup of regular coffee can make you more alert. Caffeine is also a mood elevator (see Chapters 24 and 30) and a *vasoconstrictor* (a chemical that helps shrink swollen, throbbing blood vessels in your head). That's why it may help relieve a headache. But nothing's perfect: Drinking coffee may intensify the side effects of OTC (over-the-counter) cold remedies containing decongestants and/or caffeine that make some people feel jittery.

FOOD AND SEX: WHAT DO THESE FOODS HAVE IN COMMON?

Oysters, celery, onions, asparagus, mushrooms, truffles, chocolate, honey, caviar, bird's nest soup, and alcohol beverages. No, that's not a menu for the very, very picky. It's a partial list of foods long reputed to be *aphrodisiacs,* substances that rev up the libido and improve sexual performance. Take a second look, and you'll see why each is on the list.

Two (celery, asparagus) are shaped something like a male sex organ. Three (oysters, mushrooms, and truffles) are said to arouse emotion because they resemble parts of the female anatomy. (Oysters are also high in zinc, the mineral that keeps the prostate gland healthy and ensures a steady production of the male hormone testosterone. A 3-ounce serving of Pacific oysters gives you 9 milligrams of zinc, about 82 percent of the 11 milligrams a day recommended for adult men.)

Caviar (fish eggs) and bird's nest soup are symbols of fertility. Onions — and *Spanish fly* (cantharides) — contain chemicals that produce a mild burning sensation when eliminated in urine; some people, masochists to be sure, may confuse this feeling with arousal. Honey is the quintessential sweetener: The Bible's Song of Solomon compares it to the lips of the beloved. Alcohol beverages relax the inhibitions (but overindulgence reduces sexual performance, especially in men). As for chocolate, well, it's a veritable lover's cocktail, with stimulants (caffeine, theobromine), a marijuanalike compound called anandamide, and phenylethylamine, a chemical produced in the bodies of people in love.

So do these foods actually make you feel sexy? Yes and no. An aphrodisiac food isn't one that sends you in search of a lover as soon as you eat it. No, it's one that makes you feel so good that you can follow through on your natural instincts, which is as fine a description as you're likely to get of oysters, celery, onions, asparagus, mushrooms, truffles, chocolate, honey, caviar, bird's nest soup, and wine.

WARNING

Check the label warnings and directions before using coffee with your cold medicine. Vasoconstrictors reduce the diameter of certain blood vessels and may restrict proper circulation. Check with your doctor, too, if you're taking meds for a chronic condition such as high blood pressure.

Eating for a Better Body (And Brain)

Citrus fruits are rich in vitamin C, an antioxidant vitamin that seems to slow the development of cataracts. Bran cereals provide fiber that can rev up your intestinal tract, countering the natural tendency of the contractions that move food through your gut to slow a bit as you grow older (which is why older people are more likely to be constipated). Getting enough calories to maintain a healthy weight helps protect against wrinkles. And although a diet with adequate amounts of fat doesn't totally prevent dry skin, it does give you a measure of protection. That's one reason virtually all sensible diet gurus, including the American Heart Association and the Dietary Guidelines, recommend some fat or oil every day.

And now for a word about memory. Actually, two words: Varied diet.

As long ago as 1983, a study of 250 healthy adults, age 60 to 94, at the University of New Mexico School of Medicine showed that the people who ate a wide range of nutritious foods performed best on memory and thinking tests. According to researcher Philip J. Garry, PhD, professor of pathology at New Mexico School of Medicine, overall good food habits seemed to be more important than any one food or vitamin. Maybe people with good memory are just more likely to remember that they need a good diet.

Or maybe it's really the food. No one knows for sure right now, but it may turn out that sticking with this same-old, same-old low-fat, high-fiber diet as you grow older may help you to remember to stick to the same-old low-fat, high-fiber diet — for years and years and years. (For much more on feeding your brain at any age, see Chapter 24.)

The Last Word on Food versus Medicine

Sometimes, a person with a life-threatening illness is frightened by the side effects or the lack of certainty in standard medical treatment. In desperation, she may turn down medicine and turn to diet therapy. Alas, this decision may be hazardous to her already-compromised health.

No reputable doctor denies the benefits of a healthful diet for any patient at any stage of any illness. Food not only sustains the body but also can lift the spirit, and some foods may enhance the effects of many common drugs. But there is no evidence that food alone is an adequate, effective substitute for (among other medicines)

» Antibiotics and other drugs used to fight infections.

» Vaccines or immunizations used to prevent communicable diseases. The emergence of an "antivax" movement has proven not that vaccines are hazardous but that avoiding them is. In the past few years, in parts of the

United States where parents have refused to vaccinate their children against childhood diseases, such as measles or whooping cough, the inevitable result has been epidemics of preventable illness.

>> Medicine used to treat cancer.

WARNING

If your doctor suggests altering your diet to make your treatment more effective, your brain will tell you, *Hey, that makes sense.* But if someone suggests chucking your doctor and tossing away your medicine in favor of food alone, heed the natural warning in your head. You know there's no free lunch and — as yet — no truly magical food, either.

THE HISTORY OF FOOD AND MEDICINE

Common wisdom to the contrary, doctors do have a sense of humor. Witness this "history of medicine" attributed to that famous author Anonymous and currently still making the rounds of medical meetings and blogs:

2000 B.C: "Here, eat this root."

A.D. 1000: "That root is heathen. Here, say this prayer."

A.D. 1850: "That prayer is superstition. Here, drink this potion."

A.D. 1940: "That potion is snake oil. Here, swallow this pill."

A.D. 1985: "That pill is ineffective. Here, take this antibiotic."

A.D. 2020: "That antibiotic doesn't work. Here, eat this root."

6

The Part of Tens

Chapter **27**

Ten Reliable Food and Nutrition Websites

The websites listed in this chapter give you accurate, balanced information complete with nutritional guidelines, medical news, and interactive features. But as terrific as they are, what's listed here is only a start. Had the *For Dummies* people chosen to call this part of the book "The Part of Hundreds" rather than "The Part of Tens," it would have been a cinch to fill it out.

This means, of course, that there's no good reason a curious reader like you can't dig up even more places that provide the news you need. Simply type *nutrition information* into your favorite search engine and — bingo! — up comes dozens of university and government sites plus commercial ones run by the food companies that really, really want you to try their nutritious yummies. After you check carefully to ensure that the site is reliable (the suffixes .gov, .edu, and .org are good signs), away you go.

WARNING

Beware of quackery! The internet is open to everyone and every opinion, some of which are miles away from real science. As we all know, if it sounds too good to be true, it usually is. So once again, look for those reliable three-letter identifiers at the end, which tell you what you're reading is from government, academic, or serious medical sources, including articles from medical journals whose final paragraphs ("conclusion") are more than likely understandable even to those of us without advanced degrees.

U.S. Department of Agriculture (USDA) Food Composition Website

Once upon a time, the USDA offered a single comprehensive database allowing anyone to look up any food at any time. Over the past few years, the agency has expanded and upgraded it offerings. Today, the USDA Food Composition website (www.nal.usda.gov/fnic/food-composition) is a multi-site site with nine specific subcategories covering everything anyone would ever want to know about food.

In descending order as they appear on your screen when you click on, the categories are:

Food Data Central: Expanded nutrient profiles plus links to related agricultural and experimental research from the USDA Nutrient Data Laboratory.

Nutrient Lists from Standard Reference Legacy (2018): This is essentially the old USDA Nutrient Database list, which allows you to pick a food, any food, and find out its exact nutrient values.

USDA Food Surveys Research Group: Up-to-date surveys on what Americans eat and drink.

Total Diet Study Analytical Results: Data on toxic elements such as industrial chemicals in specific foods.

Methods and Application of Food Composition Laboratory: A detailed explanation of the mission of the USDA Nutrient Data Laboratory.

Nutrient Information: A link to the American Society for Nutrition, which serves up facts about recent research and references for further information on vitamins and minerals, food sources, diet recommendations, and clinical information such as deficiencies and toxicity.

Food FYI: Links to other sites addressing foods, most often fruits and vegetables.

International Food Composition Resources: Databases, journals, conference proceedings, and websites across the world.

U.S. Food and Drug Administration (FDA)

Entering the U.S. FDA website at www.fda.gov is like opening the door to the world's biggest nutritional-information toy store. So much stuff is on the (virtual) shelves that you hardly know which item to grab first. Luckily, in this store, all the toys are free, and plenty of links to other helpful information means you can linger here happily for days, weeks, years, maybe forever.

The FDA's charter includes drugs as well as food, so at the top of the home page, you can click links to information on medicines for people and pets, poisons and side effects, medical devices (*think:* pacemakers), and products that give off radiation. But with a copy of *Nutrition For Dummies,* 7th Edition, in hand, the button to click is simply Food, which opens up a page with several links, from recalls and outbreaks to dietary supplements and packaging and labeling, plus tidbits about animals, vaccines and other meds.

As someone who writes about food and health, my favorite is Recalls, Outbreaks & Emergencies. I mean, who wouldn't want to know right away about the hazards lurking in the cupboard? After which you may need a soothing cup of really good, surprisingly healthful coffee (see Chapter 30).

Academy of Nutrition and Dietetics (AND)

The website for the Academy of Nutrition and Dietetics (www.eatright.org), formerly the American Dietetics Association, features nutrition recommendations, research, policy, and the world's largest membership group of nutritional professionals, primarily registered dietitians. (For a quick rundown on who's who in nutrition science and practice, see Chapter 1.)

The AND home page does serve up links to categories, such as Professional Development, that are clearly meant to appeal to association members. But the rest is tilted toward consumers with daily nutrition tips and nutrition position papers.

In other words, if you can bend your brain around the much-too-adorable net address ("eatright"? Give me a break!), this site, written and reviewed by nutrition professionals, is well worth a visit.

The American Heart Association (AHA)

The indisputable link between diet and the risk of heart disease, not to mention the AHA site's user-friendly approach, makes this site (www.heart.org) a must-stop on your nutritional tour of the web.

Starting at the home page, click Healthy Living at the top. When the next page arrives, click Healthy Eating. Then start with Eat Smart for facts about actual food and meals. Do not leave the site without checking into Heart-Check Foods, which describes what you find when you see the AHA "seal of approval" at the supermarket: Foods that have at least 10 percent of one or more important nutrients and are low enough in sodium and "bad" fats to meet AHGA standards. All in all, a thoroughly valuable series of clicks.

American Cancer Society (ACS)

Once upon a time, the American Cancer Society (www.cancer.org) was barely a blip on the screen of nutrition sources. Today, with a growing number of well-designed studies to demonstrate that some foods and diet regimens may reduce your risk of certain types of cancer while others may put you in harm's way, the ACS website offers solid reporting on this area of nutritional research.

Click the Stay Healthy link at the top of the ACS home page. Then scroll down to Stay Healthy Topics, then click on Eat Healthy and Stay Active for info about cancer and diet (plus exercise, of course).

Food Allergy Research & Education (FARE)

FARE (www.foodallergy.org), formerly the Food Allergy and Anaphylaxis Network, is a nonprofit membership organization whose participants include families, doctors, dietitians, nurses, support groups, and food manufacturers in the United States, Canada, and Europe. The group provides education about food allergies in addition to support and coping strategies for people who are allergic to specific foods.

From the home page, you can link to updates, daily tips, newsletter excerpts, and all the usual service-oriented goodies. The site's best feature is a no-charge email alert system. Scroll down to the site's best feature, a form you can fill out to connect to an early warning system with allergy-linked news and information about recalls of troublesome products, such as bags of cashews that may mistakenly contain peanuts.

Mayo Clinic

When you go to the Mayo Clinic web page at www.mayoclinic.org, type *nutrition* into the Search box. The day I reviewed the site for this edition of *Nutrition For Dummies,* that search pulled up nearly 2,000 entries, ranging from basics (what food labels mean) to the moderately exotic (Is yerba mate safe to drink?).

Of course, nutrition information isn't all this award-winning site has to offer. In fact, the virtue of a site created by one of America's premier medical centers is that it's packed with, well, medical links, many nutrition-related.

For example, when you're done with nutrients, return to the home page. and click Patient Care and Info to bring up an A–B–C box that enables you to check out any one of hundreds of diseases, medical conditions, symptoms, tests, and procedures. Is it any wonder that this site picks up awards every year or so?

Science Daily

Think of this one as your daily nutrition newspaper packed with reports and studies and snippets of strange and unusual but serious stuff gathered from across the entire world of healthful eating. Where else, for example, would you find on one day on one "page" an assortment of info ranging from how to fuel your walking and cycling with low-carbon foods to a protein that cleans up your muscles after a workout and the absolutely fascinating facts about how pickles can promote dental health? Nowhere, that's where, except for this exceptional, entertaining, and thoroughly professional site: `www.sciencedaily.com/news/health_medicine/nutrition/`

Enjoy!

WebMD

WebMD (`www.webmd.com`), the net's all-purpose medical information site, has scores of information on health and nutrition. To start, click Living Healthy from the home page. Here, you find lists of subjects too numerous to type in one simple entry here. As on all WebMD-related sites (Medscape, Medscape Reference, MedicineNet, eMedicineHealth, RxList, First Aid, WebMD Magazine, WebMD Health Record, and Physician Directory), the material is current, accessible, and sound.

Food Safety News

To prove that lawyers can be your nutrition friends, Seattle food-safety attorney Bill Marler created Food Safety News (`www.foodsafetynews.com`) in 2009 and assembled a staff to provide timely reporting on, well, food safety. The well-written, well-chosen, news-heavy reporting includes notices of recalls, safety measures, and legislation. The very best clickables are Find Your Health Department (a complete list of each state's agency) and Restaurant Inspections in Your Area (something not always readily available if your state, city, or town doesn't have the ABC ratings decals). You can find both of these links on the right-hand sidebar on the home page.

Chapter **28**

Ten Northern Nutrition Rules

I n January 2019, Health Canada, the Federal department responsible for helping Canadians maintain and improve their health, released the latest edition of its *Dietary Guidelines* along with a handy *Food Guide* offering ten sensible rules for healthful eating. The summaries are here, cross-referenced to their U.S. matches. For more complete info, click on `food-guide.canada.ca/en/healthy-food-choices/`

Be Mindful of Your Eating Habits

Rule number one is simple and straightforward: Eat when you're hungry, not when you're not. You can read more about how to tell the difference in Chapter 14, which explains how your hormones say "Eat Now!" and then "Stop! You've had enough."

Cook More Often

Doing your own meal prep increases your choice of fresh foods and requires you to plan ahead instead of just grabbing whatever's in the fridge, on the shelf, or in that nifty package from the people who send out nifty packages of prepared meals. Better yet, cooking can be a group experience: One person measures out ingredients, a second slices, a third stirs the pot, and so on. Best of all, this section of the complete *Guidelines* has recipes. For more about how cooking improves food, check out Chapter 20.

Enjoy Your Food

Who you are — meaning where your family come from — often determines what food and dishes are likely to grace your table. Celebrating your own cultural diet allows you to share your history with friends while sharing theirs as well. Of course, your own taste buds and experiences also count, so turn to Chapter 15 to find out why you like the foods you like.

Eat Meals with Others

Share the cooking, share the meal, share the experience. In short, make the dinner table a moment of togetherness among family and friends.

Eat Plenty of Vegetables and Fruits, Whole Grain Foods, and Protein Foods

The *Food Guide* strongly emphasizes plant foods, even urging you to choose your proteins from plant combos like the ones named in Chapter 6. The benefits? Getting vitamins and minerals the natural way and reducing consumption of those potentially artery-clogging animal saturated fats described in Chapter 7.

Limit Highly Processed Foods

If you absolutely totally cannot do without a hot dog now and then, compromise by keeping it to one that's been "improved" by modern food science as spelled out in the sidebar "Lemons, Limes, Oranges — and Bacon?" in Chapter 10. For no-nonsense definitions of food processing, including the often-maligned but useful preservatives, see Chapter 19.

Make Water Your Drink of Choice

No surprises here. Pass on the sugary drinks in favor of plain water, which hydrates without adding calories and other stuff. Chapter 12 makes that easy by listing and evaluating different kinds of water.

Use Food Labels

Proving that borders aren't impenetrable boundaries, citizens from both the U.S. and Canada agree on the new-and-improved label shown in Chapter 17.

Be Aware That Food Marketing Can Influence Your Choices

The pretty pictures of food on TV and in magazines all have one thing in common: The food has been cosmetically enhanced to make you want to reach right out and pluck it from the screen or page. Exercise restraint.

Check the Guidelines for Updates

Full disclosure: This one isn't actually listed in the *Guidelines* or *Food Guide*, but since the folks in Canada only wrote nine rules, it's added here to make a Dummies Ten. Makes sense, right?

Chapter **29**

Ten Superstar Foods

This chapter is by no means the complete A+ list of foods with extra special attributes. For example, I don't include chicken soup, because what more can anyone say about this universal panacea? How about this: These ten foods are super good enough.

Avocado

It starts with A, but the avocado is virtually an entire alphabet of nutrition goodness. According to the USDA National Nutrient Database, this pale green fruit with the thick and sometimes prickly skin is an excellent source of vitamins B-6, C, E, K, folate, niacin, pantothenic acid, and riboflavin, plus the minerals magnesium and potassium. The green fruit also delivers lutein, a carotenoid pigment that protects vision, and beta carotene, another carotenoid your body converts to a form of vitamin A. Finally, the creamy texture that hides a wealth of dietary fiber (6 to 7 grams per half fruit), comes from heart-healthy omega-3 fatty acids.

Just about the only drawback to the avocado is its calorie count, about 320 for one medium-size fruit. The good news is that you can cut that in half and maybe even spread the avocado on bread instead of butter or cheese for a luscious and calorie-conscious lunch.

Bananas

Looking for a good night's sleep? Peel a banana. Like turkey, bananas contain the essential amino acid tryptophan credited with making you sleepy after Thanksgiving dinner (although serious nutrition folks say it is actually all those calories common to this November feast that do the job). Add to that the muscle-relaxing minerals potassium and magnesium, plus B vitamins that help your body process tryptophan, and you can see why a 2017 report in the *Journal of Agriculture and Food Chemistry* showed eating one banana at bedtime produced a 180 percent jump in body levels of the sleep-inducing natural hormone melatonin. That's a sweet dream for the more than one-in-three Americans who suffer from insomnia at some point in their lives. (More on amino acids in Chapter 6.)

Beans

All beans are rich in soluble dietary fiber, the *gums* and *pectins* that mop up fats and cholesterol to prevent their being absorbed by your body. (Oats, which also are rich in gums, particularly gums called *beta glucans,* produce the same effect.)

Beans are also valuable for people with diabetes. Because they're digested very slowly, eating beans produces only a gradual increase in the level of sugar circulating in your blood. As a result, metabolizing beans requires less insulin than eating other types of high-carb foods, such as pasta and potatoes (see Chapter 8). In one now-classic study at the University of Kentucky, a diet rich in beans made it possible for people with Type 1 diabetes (their bodies produce virtually no insulin) to reduce their daily insulin intake by nearly 40 percent. Patients with Type 2 diabetes (their bodies produce some insulin) were able to reduce insulin intake by 98 percent.

Just about the only drawback to a diet rich in beans is gas resulting from the natural human inability to digest some dietary fiber and complex sugars such as *raffinose* and *stachyose,* which sit in your gut as fodder for the resident friendly bacteria that digest the carbs and then release carbon dioxide and smelly methane.

TIP

One way to reduce intestinal gas production is to reduce the complex sugar content of the beans before you eat them. Here's how: Bring a pot of water to a boil. Turn off the heat. Add the beans. Let them soak for several hours. The sugars leach out into the water, which means you can discard the sugars by draining the beans and adding fresh water to cook in. If that doesn't do the job, try two heat-and-soak sessions before cooking.

Celery

Hate kale? Loathe Lettuce? Can't stand spinach? Try celery. Like other leafy greens, this one boasts naturally occurring nitrate, which scientists at the Karolinska Institute in Sweden say reduces the buildup of fat in the livers of lab mice, thus preventing non-alcoholic liver damage, a major cause of chronic liver disease in humans.

TIP

Added bonus: Celery is crunchy, so it's a great low-calorie substitute for chips.

Cheese

For years, virtually every respected nutrition guru, organization, and report, including The Dietary Guidelines for Americans, have strongly advocated for low- or no-fat dairy products. But in 2018, researchers at the University of Texas Health Science Center (Houston) found zero "significant evidence" that dairy fats are linked to an increased risk of heart disease and stroke. In fact, having followed 3,000 adults age 65+ for 13 years from 1998 to 2011, the study's authors concluded that heptadecanoic fatty acid, one of the lipids in dairy food (including full-fat cheese), may actually lower the risk. Two years later, while prudently calling for more confirming studies, an article in the *Journal of the American Society for Nutrition* came to pretty much the same conclusion. Time to bring on the Brie and revel in the Roquefort — with whole-grain crackers, of course.

Chocolate

Westerners have been fools for chocolate ever since the Spanish conquistadors discovered it at Montezuma's Mexican court. And why not? The cocoa bean is a good source of energy, fiber, protein, carbohydrates, B vitamins, and minerals (1 ounce of dark sweet chocolate has 12 percent of the iron and 33 percent of the magnesium a healthy woman needs each day).

TECHNICAL STUFF

Chocolate is heart healthy. True, chocolate's fat, cocoa butter, is 59 percent saturated fatty acids, primarily stearic acid. But unlike other saturated fats, stearic acid neither increases LDLs ("bad cholesterol") nor lowers HDLs ("good cholesterol"). In addition, stearic acid makes blood platelets less likely to clump together into a blood clot, thus lowering the risk of heart attack or stroke. And, like other beans, cocoa beans contain gums and pectins that sop up fats before they reach your bloodstream (see the earlier section "Beans"). Finally, a study published in the *Proceedings of the National Academy of Sciences* in January 2006 credits the cocoa compound (−)epicatechin (translation: *minus epicatechin*) with the ability to help blood vessels relax — lowering blood pressure and once again reducing the risk of heart attack.

Chocolate is also rich in antioxidants, the naturally occurring compounds that inactivate free radicals (small particles that can damage cells). In 2007, when the U.S. Department of Agriculture created a scale to rank the antioxidant content of several hundred foods, red beans came in at #50 but unsweetened cocoa powder was #10; unsweetened baking chocolate, #16; and dark chocolate candy, #31.

Does all this mean chocolate is a bona fide component of a healthful diet? Yes. Especially because even though it is moderately high in calories, dark chocolate is a veritable happiness cocktail containing *caffeine* (a mood elevator and central nervous system stimulant), *theobromine* (a muscle stimulant), *phenylethylamine* (another mood elevator), and *anandamide,* a chemical that stimulates the same areas of the brain that marijuana does, although you'd have to consume 25 pounds or more unsweetened chocolate at one sitting to get even the smallest marijuana-like effect. (See Chapter 24 for more info.)

Nuts

Pass up the pretzels. Skip the chips. At snack time, reach for the almonds. Or the walnuts. Or whatever nut variety is currently in vogue among nutritionists. Although all nuts are technically a high-fat food, multiple studies, including several at California's Loma Linda University, say that adding moderate amounts of nuts to a cholesterol-lowering diet or substituting nuts for other high-fat foods, such as meats, may cut normal to moderately high levels of total cholesterol and LDLs ("bad cholesterol") by as much as 12 percent.

These guys should know. A while back, they made headlines with a walnut study in which volunteers were given one of two diets, both based on National Cholesterol Education Program (NCEP) recommendations. People on Diet #1 got 20 percent of their calories from fats in oils and fatty foods, such as meat. Folks on Diet #2 got 20 percent of their calories from high-fat nuts instead of meat, but both controlled-fat diets appeared to lower cholesterol levels.

The take-home message here is that although nuts are high in fat, their fats are polyunsaturated fatty acids and monounsaturated cholesterol busters (more about them in Chapter 7). And nuts also provide other heart-healthy nutrients such as arginine (an amino acid your body uses to make a clot-blocking compound called nitric oxide) and dietary fiber.

So feel free to go (sensibly) nuts for nuts, including the exception, peanuts — which are beans, not nuts, making peanut butter a protein-rich, low-saturated fat bean butter with its own heart-healthy benefits.

Sardines

True, a 3.5 ounce (100 grams) serving of canned tuna in water has a few less calories than an equal serving of canned sardines and a bit more protein. But the heart-healthy omega-3 fatty acid content is pretty much equal. The deciding point is the skin and bones in the sardines, which are packed with 240 milligrams of bone-protective calcium versus a measly 34 milligrams for the tuna. And there's this for environmentalists: Dolphins swimming alongside tuna are sometimes "accidentally" netted and killed, but not a single one ever went to his reward to make a sardine sandwich. *Caution:* The only fish bones considered safe to eat are the cooked and softened ones in canned sardines. All others, including the ones in fresh sardines, are hard, sharp, and hazardous to your health.

White Tea

Black and green? So 20th century. Since the turn of the 21st century, the hot new color in tea has been white. The leaves for all three teas come from one plant, *Camellia sinensis*. But those leaves meant for black and green teas are rolled and fermented before drying, while those destined for white teas — which actually brew up pale yellow-red — aren't. Nutritionally, this small change makes a big difference.

Flavonoids are natural chemicals credited with tea's ability to lower cholesterol, reduce the risk of some kinds of cancer, and protect your teeth from cavity-causing bacteria. Fresh tea leaves are rich in flavonoids called *catechins,* but processing the leaves to make black and green teas releases enzymes that enable individual catechins to hook up with others, forming new flavor and coloring agents called polyphenols (*poly* = many) that give flavor and color to black and green teas but lack the protective effect. Because white tea leaves are neither rolled nor fermented, fewer of their catechins marry into polyphenols. According to researchers at the Linus Pauling Institute (LPI) at Oregon State University, the plain catechin content of white tea is three times that of green tea. Black tea comes in a distant third.

Why should you care about this? Because all those catechins seem to be good for living bodies. For example, when LPI researchers tested white tea's ability to inhibit cell mutations in bacteria and slow down cell changes leading to colon cancer in rats, the white tea beat green tea, the former health champ. And when scientists at University Hospitals of Cleveland and Case Western Reserve University applied creams containing white-tea extract to human skin (on volunteers) and exposed the volunteers to artificial sunlight, the creamed skin developed fewer pre-cancerous changes. To be fair, green tea preparations were also protective, but white tea has less caffeine than either green or black tea, which makes it the perfect brew for a recovering caffeine fiend.

Whole Grains

Are you a man who plans to live forever? Then a team of nutrition scientists at Harvard/Brigham and Women's Hospital in Boston have three words for you: whole grain cereal. When the investigators took a look at the health stats for a one-year period in the lives of the 86,190 male doctors in the long-running Physicians' Health Study, they found 3,114 deaths among the study volunteers, including 1,381 deaths from heart attack and stroke. Then they looked a little closer and discovered that eating habits count. Men who ate at least one serving of whole grain cereal a day were 27 percent less likely to die than were men who ate refined grain products. The whole-grain group was also as much as 28 percent less likely to succumb to a heart attack, regardless of how much they weighed, whether they smoked or drank alcohol or took vitamins pills or had a history of high blood pressure and high cholesterol.

Nobody yet knows exactly why this should be so. But they do know that whole grains are a treasure-trove of dietary fiber, vitamins, minerals, and other phytochemicals (plant compounds such as antioxidants) that protect by lowering blood pressure and cholesterol while improving the body's ability to process nutrients, particularly carbohydrates.

The question is, how much cereal must you eat to benefit? The studies say more is better, but one serving a day is better than none at all. To find the right cereal, check the Nutrition Facts label. If whole grain is the first ingredient and each serving has at least 2 grams of dietary fiber, you've found breakfast. Hate cereal? Whole-grain bread is an acceptable alternative. And, yes, whole grains are an equal opportunity dish. Earlier studies suggest that women, too, may come out ahead by adding whole grain to their daily diets.

Chapter **30**

Ten Ways Coffee (and Tea) Make Life Better

Java, joe, mocha, mud — call it what you will, coffee is America's most popular drink. More than half of Americans drink it every day, an average of three cups per person, for a total national bill of about $40 billion each year. The good news is that coffee is actually a drink with benefits for virtually every part of the human body.

Start with the fact that coffee is nutritious. It's brewed from beans, so many of the nutrients that make them a powerhouse show up in your coffee cup. USDA numbers show that a single 6-ounce cup of plain coffee brewed from grounds delivers 12 percent of the magnesium and potassium and 16 percent of the calcium you'd get from a half cup of cooked kidney beans, all for a skinny 2 calories (versus 70 calories for the kidney beans). And while it's true that coffee has none of the protein, dietary fiber, and other nutrients you get with beans, there's more good coffee news from brain boost to good sex.

While tea gets less clinical study for its properties as a feel-good/be-healthy beverage, around the world it's the number one drink. Even in the coffee-loving United States, 23 percent of us have one cup a day. It, too, serves up caffeine (black tea more than green tea), but all teas have less caffeine than an equal amount of coffee. By the numbers, one 8-ounce cup of coffee has about 95 milligrams caffeine. The same cup of black tea has 48 milligrams, and green tea has a measly 29 milligrams. As you read through the benefits of the caffeine in coffee, think lesser but equally interesting benefits from tea. In short, coffee is a more powerful potion, but tea's a pleasant runner-up.

Coffee Lights Up Your Brain

Take a sip of coffee, and its caffeine zips from your mouth through your body to your brain where it blocks *adenosine,* a natural chemical that slows the transmission of messages from one brain cell to another. With adenosine sidetracked, two other natural brain chemicals, *norepinephrine* and *dopamine,* spring into action, firing up nerve cells that enable you to think faster. That's why caffeine makes you alert.

How much coffee a body needs to get this benefit depends on the body in question. In 2014, data from the Coffee and Caffeine Genetics Consortium published in *Molecule Psychiatry* suggested that genes related to caffeine metabolism make caffeine's effects more "rewarding" for some than for others.

As with all good things, a smart body knows its limits and "modulates" consumption to get the best possible effects. FDA suggests that, in general, "moderate" coffee drinking means about 400 milligrams of caffeine a day, what you might get from about four 8-ounce cups. FDA moderates that moderate advice by suggesting that women stick to no more than two 8-ounce cups a day. However, you know your own body best. If two cups of coffee make you jumpy or irritable, stick to one. If four cups simply make you mellow, enjoy.

WARNING
Not all coffees are caffeinated equally. For example, one very well-known coffee café chain packs that 400 milligrams into just 2.5 cups. Yikes!

Coffee Chases the Blues

Feeling down because it's raining or you just realized you have to lose 5 pounds to fit into your favorite jeans? One cup of coffee will definitely provide the temporary lift you need to make it through the afternoon.

WARNING
If you're feeling down for days or weeks, check in with your doctor. Although coffee can provide a short-lived lift, it isn't a substitute for effective antidepressant meds or therapy.

Coffee Powers Endurance Exercise

According to the American College of Sports medicine, more than 40 years' worth of studies shows that caffeine enhances your exercise endurance, probably by releasing adrenaline into your bloodstream. The adrenaline triggers the release of fatty acids that provide energy early in endurance exercises, such as a marathon, sparing glycogen (the muscle fuel) for later effort.

Laboratory studies with trained athletes who can actually run to exhaustion suggest that the effective dose is 3 milligrams of caffeine per 2.2 pounds of body weight. So, for a 150-pound marathon runner, that equals 204 milligrams of caffeine, about what you get from two 8-ounce cups (95 milligrams each) or three 6-ounce cups (71 milligrams each).

WARNING

This advice applies to coffee, not caffeinated "energy drinks," which may be loaded with several times the amount of caffeine in an equal serving of coffee. This caffeine overload is just jitter-making. Between 2000 and 2012, the U.S. Poison Control Center reported more than 500 calls documenting adverse effects from these liquids, ranging from gastrointestinal upset to kidney damage and psychiatric problems.

Coffee Is Cholesterol-Safe

You may have heard that drinking coffee raises your cholesterol. Not necessarily. The culprits are cafestol and kahweol, natural chemicals in coffee that may indeed raise your total cholesterol level by as much as 20 percent, increasing the level of LDLs (the bad" cholesterol) and triglycerides, a type of fat circulating in your blood. But running your coffee through a paper filter captures and removes them. Problem solved.

Coffee Lowers Your Risk of Stroke

In 2011, a report in the medical journal *Stroke* credited women coffee drinkers with a risk of stroke 25 percent lower than women who never lift a cup of java. Many similar studies followed, including one in 2013 in which researchers compared the "beverage habits" of more than 80,000 healthy men and women. This time, the coffee advantage was a 20 percent lower risk of stroke among those who drank at least one cup a day. Researchers credit the effect to caffeine's ability to expand blood vessels and reduce blood clotting.

TIP

Green tea has a similar but much less pronounced effect. To get the benefit provided by one daily cup of coffee, you'd have to slurp down four cups of green tea a day.

By 2015, the researchers had upped the protective effects of coffee and green tea, now asserting that one daily coffee (or two cups of green tea) is associated with a whopping 32 percent lower risk of stroke. In 2017, a confirming study showed that just a single cup a week reduced the risk by 7 percent.

Coffee Lowers Your Risk of Some Cancers

Absolutely no conclusive evidence shows that any one food guarantees protection against cancer, but consuming some foods — including coffee — does appear to be associated with a lower risk of some forms of the disease. In 2015, scientists at the European Prospective Investigation into Cancer and Nutrition Study (EPIC) found a 19 percent lower risk of endometrial cancer among women drinking three cups of coffee a day versus non-coffee drinkers. In the United States, the long-running Nurses' Health Study (NHS) showed an 18 percent lower risk among women drinking four cups a day compared with women who never drank coffee. Similar studies have shown a lower risk of colon cancer, liver cancer, and malignant melanoma among coffee drinkers.

Coffee May Ward Off Type 2 Diabetes

In 2014, researchers at the Nurses' Health Study (NHS) found a 20 percent lower risk of Type 2 diabetes among those drinking up to four cups of coffee a day compared with non-coffee drinkers. Add one more cup, and the risk is 30 percent lower.

While it is known that coffee maximizes insulin sensitivity, increasing our body's ability to metabolize sugars in a healthful manner, Frank Hu, the Harvard professor of nutrition and epidemiology who found these figures, still doesn't think there's enough info to say exactly how much coffee will keep Type 2 Diabetes at bay. But he definitely considers plain coffee (sorry, no cream or sugar) healthful.

Coffee Doesn't Keep Everyone Awake

The FDA says that it takes about four to six hours to metabolize half the caffeine you consume, which means that the wake-up power of caffeine lasts for about seven hours. So if drinking coffee makes it hard for you to get to sleep, have your last cup long before you normally head for bed. On the other hand, although nobody quite knows why, some people actually find a cup of coffee right at bedtime relaxing. Go figure.

Coffee Lowers a Man's Risk of ED

You knew I'd get around to this, right? So here it is: A 2015 report from The University of Texas Health Science Center in Houston shows that men who consume 190 to 285 milligrams caffeine a day — about what you get from two to three cups of regular coffee — reduce their risk of erectile dysfunction by 42 percent compared to non-coffee drinkers. As with other benefits from coffee, the mechanism appears to be relaxation of the blood vessels, increasing blood flow and a firm erection. (The only exceptions are men with diabetes.)

Coffee Drinkers Live Longer

Starting in 1995, the National Institutes of Health (NIH) tracked more than 500,000 American men and women for about 12 years. Their findings, published in *The New England Journal of Medicine* in 2013 showed a clear link between coffee-drinking (regular or decaffeinated) and healthy longevity.

According to Neal Freedman of the NIH National Cancer Institute, "The association was similar for men and women, and tended to get stronger as participants drank more coffee, though the result was very similar for those who drank two or three cups per day and those who drank more than that. The top category we had was six or more cups per day. And by cup, I mean a U.S. 8-ounce cup." Why? Freedman says no one yet knows exactly which of the hundreds of compounds in coffee may be responsible for the health benefits, but he's sure there will be more studies coming.

He was right. In 2015, a similar 30-year study at Harvard's T.H. Chan School of Public Health suggested that anti-inflammatory compounds in coffee might be beneficial, but like Freedman before them, the researchers called for more studies to finally pinpoint the protective element in the cup.

Chapter **31**

Ten Terrific Foods Starting with the Letter P

I f your first thought on seeing the title of this chapter is "Is this a joke?" think again. Count the listings in your favorite food book, and you're likely to discover that more foods have names beginning with *p* than any other letter of the alphabet. Choosing ten nutritious ones is a cinch.

Note for the curious: As is the case all through this book, the nutrient numbers in this chapter come from the USDA: www.nal.usda.gov/fnic/nutrient-lists-standard-reference-legacy-2018. (See Chapter 27 for more info.)

Papaya

The papaya, also known as the *paw-paw*, is a pear-shaped melon with versatile pale-yellow flesh that you can serve cooked when unripe or enjoy raw when ripe (look for an orange-y gold rind). Either way, one small ripe papaya provides about half an adult's daily value of vitamin A, more than a day's worth of vitamin C, and about 10 percent of the daily dietary fiber allotment. Note that cooking the papaya reduces the vitamin C content because vitamin C is heat liable.

Smart cooks should know that the leaves of the papaya plant are also useful in the kitchen. The leaves are packed with *papain*, the *proteolytic* (protein-breaking) enzyme found in commercial meat tenderizers. In Central America, where the papaya was born, wrapping meat in papaya leaves is the standard tenderizing technique. But papain can irritate the skin, so handle the leaves with care.

Pear

The pear is a botanical cousin of the apple, a late-summer early-fall fruit that grows most plentifully in the American northwest. (Washington State is the leading producer of both apples and pears.) Although the apple is more popular, the pear is a better bet, nutritionally speaking. True, a 5-ounce fresh pear has 9 more calories than a 5-ounce apple, but the pear has 25 percent more protein than the apple, 30 percent more dietary fiber, including soluble pectin in the flesh and the insoluble fibers hemicellulose in the peel and lignan in those tiny gritty particles that crunch when you chew the pear. The pear also has 40 percent more iron and 50 percent more *lutein* (a naturally occurring plant chemical that protects vision). So it's not surprising that, like people who eat an apple a day, those who substitute a pear are likely to need fewer prescription drugs.

TIP

Pears resent rough handling. Bruising or slicing one releases *polyphenoloxidase*, an enzyme that hastens the oxidation of *phenols* (alcohols) in the fruit, producing clumps of flesh-darkening brownish compounds. You can slow this natural reaction by dipping sliced pears in a protective acidic antioxidant solution, such as lemon juice or vinegar and water, a trick that also works for sliced apples, bananas, and potatoes.

Unfortunately, not every part of the pear is people-friendly. Like peach pits, apricot pits, and apple seeds, pear seeds contain *amygdalin*, a cyanide/sugar compound that breaks down into hydrogen cyanide in the stomach. An occasional seed isn't necessarily hazardous for an adult, but swallowing only a few may be lethal for a child.

Peas

Like other legumes (beans and peanuts), peas are high in dietary fiber (4.4 grams per half cup) and rich in protein (4.29 grams per half a cup). One-half cup of peas has 477 International Units, or IU, vitamin A (16 percent of the Recommended Dietary Allowance, or RDA, for a man, 21 percent for a woman), 11.36 milligrams vitamin C (19 percent of the RDA), and 1.24 milligrams iron (8 percent of the RDA for a woman of child-bearing age).

PICK A PECK OF PERFECT PEAS

Not all peas are the same. For example, *fresh peas* are garden peas, straight from the pod. *Petits pois* is French for "small peas," peas that are mature but not yet full size. *Dried peas* are whole peas minus the natural moisture, which means they must be soaked before cooking. *Split peas* are dried peas that have been boiled, skinned, and split in half; these dried peas can be cooked without soaking. Because dried peas are minus the natural water, you get more pea solids per ounce and thus more nutrients — including calories, of course. *Pea pods* are very early pods with only a hint of peas inside; the most tender are called *snow peas; sugar peas* are a variety of snow peas. And here's a bonus: When you eat the pods with the peas, you add dietary fiber to your diet.

Peas taste good, too. They start out high in sugar, but within hours after picking, nearly half the sugar turns to starch. The fresher you get them, the sweeter they taste. You can pop them raw, straight from the pod, into your mouth or your salad. If you cook them, better make it quick. Chlorophyll, the pigment that makes green peas green, is sensitive to acids. When green vegetables, including peas, are heated, the chlorophyll reacts with acids in the cooking water or in the pea itself, forming a brownish pigment called *pheophytin* that turns peas olive drab. Swift cooking avoids this curse of steamed table cuisine. A really good example to demonstrate this color difference is to compare canned and frozen peas.

Despite their virtues, peas aren't perfect. Legumes rank among the foods most likely to trigger allergic reactions. Some nutrition guides warn that dried peas may interact with the antidepressant drugs known as MAO (monoamineoxidase) inhibitors and send your blood pressure soaring. *Purines,* byproducts of protein metabolism, may worsen the pain of *gout* (a form of arthritis). Some nutritionists think that dried peas may have enough protein to produce this effect.

Pineapple

It's neither a pine tree nor an apple, but the pineapple is still a twofer in the kitchen. First, it's rich in dietary fiber (2.3 grams per cup) and vitamin C (79 milligrams per cup; 72 percent of the RDA for a woman, 60 percent for a man). Second, it contains a natural meat tenderizer, the proteolytic (protein dissolving) enzyme *bromelain,* which is similar to the papain in papaya (see earlier section in this chapter). Cover your beef, lamb, pork, or veal with chunks of fresh pineapple and let it set in the fridge overnight for a slightly sweeter, definitely tenderer meat.

Plantain

The plantain is a member of the banana family, but unlike its peel-and-eat cousin, the plantain is classified botanically as a vegetable. Another difference is that while the banana converts its starches to sugars as it ripens, the plantain doesn't so you have to cook the plantains before serving to make its starch granules swell and break open, softening the flesh. The "fried bananas" so popular in Latin American cuisine are usually fried plantains with lots of added sugar to sweeten the otherwise starchy food.

On the other hand, a serving of plantains has more than ten times as much vitamin A, twice the vitamin C, and one-third more potassium than an equal amount of bananas.

Like bananas, plantains are rich in serotonin, dopamine, and other naturally occurring *neurotransmitters* (chemicals that make it possible for brain cells to communicate) that act as mood elevators. And if the latest chocolate research is right, you might increase the bliss potential by dipping those plantains in melted dark chocolate (see Chapter 29).

Pork

Ounce for ounce, pork has fewer calories and less total fat, saturated fat, and cholesterol than lamb and beef. And as you read this book, a team of Canadian researchers at the Lacombe Research Centre in Alberta, the University of Alberta, and the Prairie Swine Centre in Saskatoon, Saskatchewan, is charging ahead with its attempts to pack pork with heart-healthy omega-3 fatty acids. Beginning in 2011, the scientists were feeding their test animals omega-3-rich flaxseed and canola oil to discover just how much they can enrich the pork while keeping it stable in storage and tasty on the plate.

Of course, some folks may say, why bother? If your goal is to consume omega-3s, why not just eat fish and seafood, the primary source of these good fats? But science marches on. Sooner or later, an omega-3 pork chop is sure to hit your table. Until then, Table 31-1 lists the comparable fat stats on pork, lamb, and beef.

TABLE 31-1 **Fat Content (100 g./3.5 oz. Roasted Loin)**

	Pork	Lamb	Beef
Calories	142	217	257
Total fat (g)	4.9	11.4	15.8
Saturated fat (g)	1.7	4.6	6.2
Cholesterol (mg)	53	90	83

Potato

Despite the myth that "potatoes make you fat," the humble potato is a filling food with indisputable nutrition virtues. One 7-ounce oven-baked potato, skin included, dishes up 220 calories, mostly starchy carbs, plus 4 grams dietary fiber, 5 grams protein, and practically no fat. True, the proteins are "incomplete," with limited amounts of some essential amino acids. But you can remedy that by serving potatoes the traditional way, boiled, with a little milk poured on. Or you could melt some (low-fat) cheese into a baked potato. (See Chapter 6 for more on the nature of proteins.)

Potatoes, which have lots of vitamin C, were once eaten raw to prevent *scurvy*, the vitamin C deficiency disease. The fresher the potato, the higher the vitamin C. For example, after three months' storage in a cold place, a potato loses about one-third of its vitamin C; after six months, about two-thirds. Long storage also turns the potato's starches to sugar, so it tastes sweeter and less potato-like. But the conversion of starch to sugar is temperature-related; if the potatoes are stored back at 70 to 75 degrees Fahrenheit, the sugars revert to starch.

The devastating mid-18th century Irish potato famine was caused by *Phytophthora infestans,* a fungus that rotted the crops, but potatoes can be pretty mean critters on their own. The potato is a member of the nightshade family that produces a nerve poison called *solanine* (hence the potato's scientific name, *solanum tuberosum*), which makes it hard for your cells to transmit messages back and forth. Solanine, found in the green parts of the plant (leaves, stem, green spots on the skin), doesn't dissolve in water and is unaffected by heat. Any solanine present in a raw potato will still be there after you cook it. Yes, an adult might have to eat about 3 pounds of potatoes or 2.4 pounds of potato skins at one sitting to develop solanine poisoning, but better safe than sorry: Toss any potato with sprouts or green spots.

Prawns

Americans and Britons both speak English, but sometimes the same word means one thing in the United States and another in the United Kingdom. Case in point: *prawns*. In the U.S., a prawn is a very big shrimp; in the U.K., it's any shrimp at all.

For a few years, prawns, like lobsters, crabs, oysters, clams, and mussels, were banned from a healthy diet due to their high cholesterol content. But as nutrition scientists zeroed in on the role played by various kinds of fatty acids, particularly the nefarious saturated fat (for more on that, check out Chapter 7), foods low in saturated fats were welcomed back onto the menu.

True, a 100-gram/3.5-ounce serving of prawns has about 195 milligrams cholesterol versus about 82 milligrams for a similar serving of 90 percent lean hamburger. But the burger has 4.2 grams saturated fat, 23 percent of the RDA, and 14 times the 0.3 grams saturated fat in the prawns. In addition, like other fish and seafood, prawns are a good source of heart-healthy omega-3 fatty acids plus minerals, such as magnesium and zinc, all wrapped in a diet-pleasing 99 calories per serving.

TIP

To get all this good stuff fast and easy, simply boil the prawns until they turn opaque and then enjoy with a dip.

Prune

If you call a prune a dried plum, do you love it more? In 2000, The California Prune Board convinced the Food and Drug Administration to approve renaming the fruit, which is why cartons of prunes are now labeled "dried plums."

Of course, no matter what you call it, the prune is a food jampacked with antioxidants, vitamin A, *nonheme iron* (the form of iron found in plants), and fiber. Lots of fiber: Ounce for ounce, the fruit has more dietary fiber than dry beans.

But who's kidding whom? The prune's true nutritional claim to fame is still its reliable ability to relieve constipation. Prunes contain *dihydrophenylisatin*, a naturally occurring chemical relative of *biscodyl*, the active ingredient in many over-the-counter laxatives. The dihydrophenylisatin is a stimulant that triggers intestinal contractions to move food along. As a result, if you eat too many prunes, you may experience diarrhea. But you'd expect that. What may take you by surprise is an allergic reaction to sulfites used to prevent the flesh of dried fruit, including prunes, from darkening. To reduce the risk of serious side effects, including potentially lethal *anaphylaxis* (a whole body reaction that can include respiratory problems), all dried fruit containing sulfites carries a prominent warning on the label. For more about food allergies, see Chapter 23.

Pumpkin

The pumpkin, a New World original now grown on every continent except Antarctica, is a member of the squash family with nary a smidgen of waste. Boiled pumpkin flowers and leaves are green veggies. Dried or roasted pumpkin seeds are high-protein, high-fiber snacks. Pumpkin meat is an extraordinarily good source of vitamins A and C.

The most nutritious pumpkins are the golden cylindrical varieties, such as the Dickenson pumpkins grown and processed by Libby, the leading marketer of canned pumpkin. In fact, canned pumpkin is one time when processed beats natural hands down: Ounce for ounce, plain canned pumpkin has up to 20 times as much vitamin A and up to 2.5 times as much calcium as boiled fresh pumpkin but less vitamin C.

With all this goodness, is it any wonder that farmers around the world compete to see who can bring in the biggest pumpkin of them all? The current American record holder is a 2,294-pound beauty grown by Connecticut's Alex Noel, but his giant is still outweighed by the world champion 2,626-pound pumpkin grown by Belgium's Mathias Willemijns in 2016. You can access a list of the world's biggest pumpkins along with ten tips on how to grow your own monster veggies at www.backyardgardener.com. Bet you can't look without saying, "Wow!"

Appendix

Glossary of Nutrition Terms

Like any science, nutrition has its own vocabulary, so throughout this book you will find many definitions of terms relating to the specific material in each chapter.

The Departments of Agriculture (USDA) and Health and Human Services (HHS) include a broader glossary in each new edition of *The Dietary Guidelines for Americans*. This Appendix includes the USDA/HHS definitions for the most recent Guidelines (2021- 2025).

Added sugars—Sugars that are added during the processing of foods (such as sucrose or dextrose), foods packaged as sweeteners (such as table sugar), sugars from syrups and honey, and sugars from concentrated fruit or vegetable juices. They do not include naturally occurring sugars that are found in milk, fruits, and vegetables.

All-cause mortality—The total number of deaths from any or all causes during a specific time period. This does not include cause-specific mortality (i.e., total number of deaths from a specific disease such as cardiovascular disease or cancer).

Body mass index (BMI)—A measure defining weight in kilograms (kg) divided by height in meters (m) squared. BMI is an indicator of deficient or excess body tissue, both fat and muscle. BMI status categories for individuals ages 2 years and older include underweight, normal weight, overweight, and obese. (Normal weight is often referred to as "healthy" weight.) Overweight and obese describe ranges of weight that are greater than what is considered healthy for a given height, while underweight describes a weight that is lower than what is considered healthy.

Calorie— A unit commonly used to measure energy content of foods and beverages as well as energy use (expenditure) by the body. A kilocalorie is equal to the amount of energy (heat) required to raise the temperature of 1 kilogram of water 1 degree centigrade. Energy is required to sustain the body's various functions, including metabolic processes and physical activity. Carbohydrates, fats, protein, and alcohol provide all of the energy supplied by foods and beverages. If not specified explicitly, references to "calories" refer to "kilocalories."

Carbohydrates—One type of macronutrient. Carbohydrates include sugars, starches, and fibers:

>> **Sugars**—A simple carbohydrate composed of one unit (a monosaccharide, such as glucose and fructose) or two joined units (a disaccharide, such as lactose and sucrose). Sugars include white and brown sugar, fruit sugar, corn syrup, molasses, and honey (see **Added sugars**).

>> **Starches**—Many glucose units linked together. Examples of foods containing starch include vegetables, dry beans and peas, and grains (e.g., rice, oats, wheat, barley, corn).

>> **Fiber**—Nondigestible carbohydrates and lignin that are intrinsic and intact in plants. Fiber consists of dietary fiber, the fiber naturally occurring in foods, and functional fiber, which are isolated, nondigestible carbohydrates that have beneficial physiological effects in humans.

Cardiovascular disease (CVD)—Heart disease as well as diseases of the blood vessel system (arteries, capillaries, veins) that can lead to heart attack, chest pain (angina), or stroke.

Cholesterol—A natural sterol present in all animal tissues. Free cholesterol is a component of cell membranes and serves as a precursor for steroid hormones (estrogen, testosterone, aldosterone), and for bile acids. Humans are able to synthesize sufficient cholesterol to meet biologic requirements, and there is no evidence for a dietary requirement for cholesterol.

Blood cholesterol—Cholesterol that travels in the serum of the blood as distinct particles containing both lipids and proteins (lipoproteins). Also referred to as serum cholesterol. Two kinds of lipoproteins are:

>> **High-density lipoprotein cholesterol (HDL-C)**—Blood cholesterol often called "good" cholesterol; carries cholesterol from tissues to the liver, which removes it from the body.

>> **Low-density lipoprotein cholesterol (LDL-C)**—Blood cholesterol often called "bad" cholesterol; carries cholesterol to arteries and tissues. A high LDL-C level in the blood leads to a buildup of cholesterol in arteries.

Dietary cholesterol—Cholesterol found in foods of animal origin, including meat, seafood, poultry, eggs, and dairy products. Plant foods, such as grains, vegetables, fruits, and oils, do not contain dietary cholesterol.

Complementary feeding— The process that starts when human milk or infant formula is complemented by other foods and beverages. The complementary feeding period typically continues to age 24 months as the young child transitions fully to family foods.

Complementary foods and beverages (CFB)—Foods and beverages (liquids, semi-solids, and solids) other than human milk or infant formula provided to an infant or young child to provide nutrients and energy.

Cup equivalent (cup eq)—The amount of a food product that is considered equal to 1 cup from the vegetable, fruit, or milk food group. A cup eq for some foods may differ from a measured cup in volume because: (1) the foods have been concentrated (such as raisins or tomato paste), (2) the foods are airy in their raw form and do not compress well into a cup (such as salad greens), or (3) the foods are measured in a different form (such as cheese).

Dietary pattern—The quantities, proportions, variety, or combination of different foods, drinks, and nutrients in diets, and the frequency with which they are habitually consumed.

Dietary Reference Intakes (DRIs)—Nutrient reference values developed by the National Academies of Sciences, Engineering, and Medicine that are specific on the basis of age, sex, and life stage and cover more than 40 nutrient substances. The DRIs provide reference values for vitamins, minerals, and other nutrients that: 1) indicate daily intake amounts that meet the needs of most healthy people, and 2) set intake levels not to exceed to avoid harm.

Acceptable Macronutrient Distribution Ranges (AMDR)—Range of intake for a particular energy source that is associated with reduced risk of chronic disease while providing intakes of essential nutrients. If an individual's intake is outside of the AMDR, there is a potential of increasing the risk of chronic diseases and/or insufficient intakes of essential nutrients.

Adequate Intakes (AI)—A recommended average daily nutrient intake level based on observed or experimentally determined approximations or estimates of mean nutrient intake by a group (or groups) of apparently healthy people. This is used when the Recommended Dietary Allowance cannot be determined.

Chronic Disease Risk Reduction Intakes (CDRR)—The lowest level of intake for which a sufficient strength of evidence exists to characterize a chronic disease risk reduction. This nutrient reference value is currently available only for sodium.

Estimated Average Requirements (EAR)—The average daily nutrient intake level estimated to meet the requirement of half the healthy individuals in a particular life stage and sex group.

Recommended Dietary Allowance (RDA)—The average dietary intake level that is sufficient to meet the nutrient requirement of nearly all (97 to 98 percent) healthy individuals in a particular life stage and sex group.

Tolerable Upper Intake Level (UL)—The highest average daily nutrient intake level likely to pose no risk of adverse health effects for nearly all individuals in a particular life stage and sex group. As intake increases above the UL, the potential risk of adverse health effects increases.

Dietary supplement—A product intended to supplement the diet that contains one or more dietary ingredients (including vitamins, minerals, herbs or other botanicals, amino acids, and other substances) intended to be taken by mouth as a pill, capsule, table, or liquid, and that is labeled on the front panel as being a dietary supplement.

Eating occasion—Ingestive event, including a meal, snack or beverage during which any caloric or non-caloric food or beverage is consumed (see **Frequency of eating**).

Essential calories—The energy associated with the foods and beverages ingested to meet nutritional goals through choices that align with the USDA Food Patterns in forms with the least amounts of saturated fat, added sugars, and sodium.

Exclusive human milk feeding—Feeding human milk alone and not in combination with infant formula and/or complementary foods and beverages (including water), except for medications or vitamin and mineral supplements.

Fats—One type of macronutrient (see **Solid fats** and **Oils**).

» **Monounsaturated fat**—Monounsaturated fats have one double bond. They are found in both animal and plant products. Plant sources that are rich in monounsaturated fat include nuts and vegetable oils that are liquid at room temperature (e.g., canola oil, olive oil, high oleic safflower and sunflower oils).

» **Polyunsaturated fat**—Polyunsaturated fats have two or more double bonds and may be of two types, based on the position of the first double bond. Polyunsaturated fats are found in many different plants and some fish sources.

>> **Omega-3 fatty acids**—The three main omega-3 fatty acids are alpha-linolenic acid (ALA), eicosapentaenoic acid (EPA), and docosahexaenoic acid (DHA). Alpha- linolenic acid is required because it cannot be synthesized by humans and, therefore, is considered essential in the diet. Primary sources include soybean oil, canola oil, walnuts, and flaxseed. EPA and DHA are very long chain omega-3 fatty acids that are found in fish and shellfish.

>> **Omega-6 fatty acids**— There are four main omega-6 fatty acids: linoleic acid (LA), arachidonic acid (ARA), gamma linoleic acid (GLA), and conjugated linoleic acid (CLA). Linoleic acid is required because it cannot be synthesized by humans and, therefore, is considered essential in the diet. Primary sources of LA are nuts and liquid vegetable oils, including soybean oil, corn oil, and safflower oil.

>> **Saturated fat**—Saturated fats have no double bonds. Major sources include animal products, such as meat and dairy products, and tropical oils such as coconut or palm oils. In general, fats high in saturated fatty acids are solid at room temperature.

>> **Trans fat**—Trans fats are unsaturated fatty acids that contain one or more isolated (i.e., nonconjugated) double bonds in a trans configuration. Trans fatty acids present in foods that come from ruminant animals (e.g., cattle and sheep). Such foods include dairy products, beef, and lamb.

Food categories—A method of grouping similar foods in their as-consumed forms, for descriptive purposes. The USDA/ARS has created 150 mutually exclusive food categories to account for each food or beverage item reported in What We Eat in America (WWEIA), the food intake survey component of the National Health and Nutrition Examination Survey (for more information, visit: http://sepr1. ars.usda.gov/Services/docs.htm?docid=23429). Examples of WWEIA Food Categories include soups, nachos, and yeast breads. When food items that contain multiple ingredients are assigned to food categories, they are not disaggregated into their component parts. For example, all pizzas are put into the pizza category (see **Food groups**).

Food components of public health concern—Nutrients and other dietary components that are overconsumed or underconsumed (compared to Dietary Reference Intake recommendations and to biological measures of the nutrient when available) and linked in the scientific literature to adverse health outcomes in the general population or in a subpopulation.

Food environments—Factors and conditions that influence food choices and food availability. These environments include settings such as home, child care (early care and education), school, after-school programs, worksites, food retail stores and restaurants, and other outlets where individuals and families make eating and drinking decisions. The food environment also includes macro-level factors and includes food marketing, food production and distribution systems, agricultural policies, Federal nutrition assistance programs, and economic price structures.

Food groups—A method of grouping similar foods for descriptive and guidance purposes. Food groups in the USDA Food Pattern are defined as fruits, vegetables, grains, dairy, and protein foods. Some of these groups are divided into subgroups, such as dark-green vegetables or whole grains, which may have intake goals or limits (for more information, see *Appendix E3.1 Table A1.* USDA Healthy U.S.-Style Food Patterns—Intake Amounts). When mixed dishes are assigned to food groups, they are disaggregated into their major component parts. For example, pizza may be disaggregated into the grain (crust), dairy (cheese), vegetable (sauce and toppings), and protein foods (toppings) food groups.

Food pattern modeling—The process of developing and adjusting daily intake amounts from food categories or groups to meet specific criteria, such as meeting nutrient intake goals, limiting nutrients or other food components, or varying proportions or amounts of specific food categories or groups.

Food security—A condition in which all people, now and in the future, have access to sufficient, safe, and nutritious food to maintain a healthy and active life.

Fortification—The deliberate addition of one or more essential nutrients to a food, whether or not it is normally contained in the food. Fortification may be used to prevent or correct a demonstrated deficiency in the population or specific population groups; restore naturally occurring nutrients lost during processing, storage, or handling; or to add a nutrient to a food at the level found in a comparable traditional food. When cereal grains are labeled as enriched, it is mandatory that they be fortified with folic acid.

Frequency of eating—The number of daily eating occasions (see **Eating occasion**).

Gestational diabetes—Diabetes occurring during pregnancy in women not previously diagnosed with diabetes.

Gestational weight gain—Weight a woman gains during pregnancy.

Health—A state of complete physical, mental, and social well-being and not merely the absence of disease or infirmity.

Human milk—A mother's own milk provided at the breast (i.e., nursing) or expressed and fed fresh or after refrigeration or freezing.

Human milk feeding—Feeding human milk alone or in combination with infant formula and/or complementary foods and beverages, such as cow milk.

Hypertensive disorders of pregnancy—Disorders occurring during pregnancy that include gestational hypertension, preeclampsia, and eclampsia.

Infant formula—A food that is represented for special dietary use solely as a food for infants by reason of its simulation of human milk or its suitability as a complete or partial substitute for human milk.

Isocaloric—Having the same energy values. For example, two dietary patterns that vary in macronutrient proportions but have the same energy content are isocaloric.

Lean meat—Any meat with less than 10 percent fat by weight, or less than 10 grams of fat per 100 grams, based on USDA and FDA definitions for food label use. Examples include 95 percent lean ground beef, cooked; broiled beef steak, lean only eaten; baked pork chop, lean only eaten; roasted chicken breast or leg, no skin eaten; and smoked/cured ham, lean only eaten.

Life stages—The age groups defined by the NHANES sampling weights or by the DRI age-sex groups.

>> Infants and toddlers (birth to less than 24 months)

>> Children and adolescents (ages 2 to 19 years)

>> Adults (ages 20 to 64 years)

>> Pregnant women (20 to 44 years)

>> Lactating women (20 to 44 years)

>> Older adults (ages 65 years and older)

Macronutrient—A dietary component that provides energy. Macronutrients include protein, fats, and carbohydrates.

Neurocognitive—Having to do with the ability to think and reason, including the ability to concentrate, remember things, process information, learn, speak, and understand.

Neurocognitive development—The maturation during infancy and childhood of the ability to think and reason. Domains include: cognitive development, language and communication development, movement and physical development, and social-emotional and behavioral development. Outcomes that affect, or can be affected by, neurocognitive development include academic performance, attention deficit disorder (ADD) or attention-deficit/hyperactivity disorder (ADHD), anxiety, depression, or autism spectrum disorder (ASD).

Nutrient-dense foods—Foods that are naturally rich in vitamins, minerals, and other substances and that may have positive health effects; that are lean or low in solid fats and do not have added solid fats, sugars, starches, or sodium; and that retain naturally-occurring components, such as fiber. All vegetables, fruits, whole grains, fish, eggs, and nuts prepared without added solid fats or sugars are considered nutrient-dense, as are lean or low-fat forms of fluid milk, meat, and poultry prepared without added solid fats or sugars. Nutrient-dense foods provide substantial amounts of vitamins and minerals (micronutrients) and relatively few calories compared to forms of the food that have solid fat and/or added sugars.

Nutrient-Dense Representative Foods—For the purpose of USDA's food pattern modeling, nutrient-dense representative foods are those within each item cluster in forms with the least amounts of added sugars, sodium, and solid fats.

Nutrition Evidence Systematic Review (NESR)—Formerly known as the Nutrition Evidence Library (NEL), NESR specializes in conducting food- and nutrition-related systematic reviews. NESR systematic reviews are research projects that answer important public health questions by using rigorous and transparent methods to search for, evaluate, analyze, and synthesize the body of scientific evidence on topics relevant to Federal policy and programs. For more information, visit: nesr.usda.gov.

Oils—Fats that are liquid at room temperature. Oils come from many different plants and some fish. Some common oils include canola, corn, olive, peanut, safflower, soybean, and sunflower oils. A number of foods are naturally high in oils, such as: nuts, olives, some fish, and avocados. Foods that are mainly made up of oil include mayonnaise, certain salad dressings, and soft (tub or squeeze) margarine with no *trans* fats. Oils are high in monounsaturated or polyunsaturated fats, and lower in saturated fats than solid fats. A few plant oils, termed tropical oils, including coconut oil, palm oil and palm kernel oil, are high in saturated fats and for nutritional purposes should be considered as solid fats. Partially-hydrogenated oils that contain *trans* fats should also be considered as solid fats for nutritional purposes (see **Fats**).

Ounce equivalent (oz eq)—The amount of a food product that is considered equal to one ounce from the grain or protein foods food group. An oz eq for some foods may be less than a measured ounce in weight if the food is concentrated or low in water content (nuts, peanut butter, dried meats, flour) or more than a measured ounce in weight if the food contains a large amount of water (tofu, cooked beans, cooked rice or pasta).

Portion size—The amount of a food served or consumed in one eating occasion (see **Eating occasion**).

Postpartum weight loss—Change in weight from baseline during the postpartum period to a later time point during the postpartum period.

Processed meat—Meat, poultry, or seafood products preserved by smoking, curing or salting, or addition of chemical preservatives. Processed meat includes bacon, sausage, hot dogs, sandwich meat, packaged ham, pepperoni, and salami.

Protein—One type of macronutrient. Protein is the major functional and structural component of every animal cell. Proteins are composed of amino acids, nine of which are indispensable, meaning they cannot be synthesized by humans and therefore must be obtained from the diet. The quality of dietary protein is determined by its amino acid profile relative to human requirements as determined by the body's requirements for growth, maintenance, and repair. Protein quality is determined by two factors: digestibility and amino acid composition.

> » **Animal protein**—Protein from meat, poultry, seafood, eggs, and milk and milk products.
>
> » **Vegetable protein**—Protein from plants such as dry beans, whole grains, fruit, nuts, and seeds.

Protocol—A plan used by the 2020 Dietary Guidelines Advisory Committee to conduct a systematic review of a scientific question.

Reference Amount Customarily Consumed (RACC)—The serving size listed on a Nutrition Facts Label, which is based on a reference amount of food or beverage that is commonly eaten at a single eating occasion, as determined by the Food and Drug Administration.

Refined grains—Grains and grain products missing the bran, germ, and/or endosperm; any grain product that is not a whole grain. Many refined grains are low in fiber but enriched with thiamin, riboflavin, niacin, and iron, and fortified with folic acid.

Sarcopenia—A progressive and generalized loss of skeletal muscle mass, alone or in conjunction with either or both low muscle strength and low muscle performance.

Seafood—Marine animals that live in the sea and in freshwater lakes and rivers. Seafood includes fish, such as salmon, tuna, trout, and tilapia, and shellfish, such as shrimp, crab, and oysters.

Socioeconomic status—An economic and sociologic measure defined by factors such as income in dollars, income as a percent of the poverty ratio, food security, eligibility for federal assistance programs, or level of education.

Solid fats—Fats that are usually solid at room temperature. Solid fats are found in animal foods except for seafood, and can be made from vegetable oils through hydrogenation. Some tropical oil plants, such as coconut and palm, are considered as solid fats due to their fatty acid composition. Solid fats contain more saturated fats and/or *trans* fats than liquid oils (e.g., soybean, canola, and corn oils), and lower amounts of monounsaturated or polyunsaturated fatty acids. Common fats considered to be solid fats include: butterfat, beef fat (tallow, suet), chicken fat, pork fat (lard), stick margarine, shortening, coconut oil, palm oil and palm kernel oil. Foods high in solid fats include: butter, full-fat cheeses, creams, whole milk, full-fat ice creams, marbled cuts of meats, regular ground beef, bacon, sausages, poultry skin, and many baked goods made using these products (such as cookies, crackers, doughnuts, pastries, and croissants). The fat component of milk and cream (butter) is solid at room temperature (see **Fats**).

Sugar-sweetened beverages—Liquids that are sweetened with various forms of added sugars. These beverages include, but are not limited to, soda (regular, not sugar-free), fruitades, sports drinks, energy drinks, sweetened waters, and coffee and tea beverages with added sugars. Also called calorically sweetened beverages.

Whole grains—Grains and grain products made from the entire grain seed, usually called the kernel, which consists of the bran, germ, and endosperm. If the kernel has been cracked, crushed, or flaked, it must retain the same relative proportions of bran, germ, and endosperm as the original grain in order to be called whole grain. Many, but not all, whole grains also are sources of dietary fiber.

Index

Symbols

A

Food Guide Pyramid, 222–224
Food Patterns, 226
food processing
  adding nutrients, 256–257
  air control, 254–255
  canning, 288
  chemical methods, 255
  chemistry
    food additives, 298–305
    genetically engineered foods, 306–307
    phytochemicals, 295–297
  chicken, 264
  cooking
    effect on food, 267–270
    food safety, 278–282
    methods, 266–267
    overview, 265
    pots and materials, 272–276
    protecting nutrients in cooked foods, 276–278
  drying
    effect on nutritional value, 289–290
    spray drying, 289
    sulfites, 290
  food substitutes
    fat replacers, 258–261
    overview, 257
    substitute sweeteners, 261–264
  freezing
    effect on food texture, 286–287
    overview, 283–286
    refreezing, 287
    thawing frozen food, 287
  intensifying flavor and aroma, 256
  irradiation, 255, 291–293
  moisture control (dehydration), 254

overview, 251–253
as protecting nutrients in food, 12
temperature control, 253–254
food safety
  microbes, 279–280
  overview, 278–279
  temperature, 280–282
Food Safety News, 365–366
food substitutes
  fat replacers
    carbohydrate-based, 258, 259
    evaluating, 258–259
    fat-based, 258, 260
    nutrition, 260–261
    protein-based, 258, 259
    side effects of, 261
    weight loss and, 260
  overview, 257
  substitute sweeteners
    Acesulfame-K, 263
    aspartame, 262
    compared to sugar, 263
    cyclamates, 262
    neotame, 263
    overview, 261–262
    polyols, 264
    saccharin, 262
    stevia, 263
    sucralose, 262–263
Fowler, James, 42
Framingham Heart Study, 35–36, 42
free radicals, 296
freezing food
  effect on food texture, 286–287
  freezer burn, 287
  overview, 283–286
  refreezing, 287
  thawing frozen food, 287

fruit
  bananas, 372
  dried fruit, 290
  fat in, 84
  papayas, 383–384
  pineapple, 385
Funk, Casimir, 122

G

gastric alcohol dehydrogenase (gADH) enzyme, 25, 113
gelatin, 72
gender differences
  calorie requirements, 57, 59, 61–62
  dietary recommendations, 33
generally recognized as safe (GRAS) list, 298. See also food additives
genetic code, 143
genetically engineered foods, 306–307
genetics, taste and, 200
genistein, 296
geography, taste and, 198–199, 203–204
German Federal Institute for Risk Assessment, 124
ghrelin, 184
GI (Glycemic Index), 96
glands, 58–59
glass pots, 274
glucobrassicin, 297
gluconapin, 297
gluconasturtin, 297
glucose, 79, 96–97, 334–335
glucose tolerance factor (GTF), 148
Glycemic Index (GI), 96
glycerol, 79
glycoproteins, 67
goiter, 149

Institute of Medicine.
    See IOM
insulin, 184
International Food Information
    Council (IFIC), 306
International Units (IUs), 125
intestinal alcohol
    dehydrogenase, 26
intestinal enzymes, 26
intolerance, 313
intracellular fluid, 156
intrauterine device (IUD), 152
iodine
    deficiency, 149
    iodized salt, 152
    megadose of, 150–151
    overview, 146
    RDA for, 39
IOM (Institute of Medicine),
    338–339
    choline and, 130
    views on calcium, 153
ions, 158
iron
    deficiency, 149
    iron overload, 150
    overview, 144
    RDA for, 38–39
    supplements, 145
iron pots, 275
irradiation, 255,
    291–293
ischemic stroke, 85, 115,
    379–380
isoascorbate, 127
IUD (intrauterine device), 152
IUs (International Units), 125

J

Jamestown Colony, 18
*Journal of the American Medical
    Association* (*JAMA*), 171,
    176, 311

K

keratin, 65
Keshan disease, 146
ketogenic diets, 56–57, 79
ketosis, 79
kilocalories, 53–54. *See also*
    calories
kumiss (drink), 110

L

lactic acid, 115
lactobacilli (bacteria), 110
lactoferrin, 142
lard, 84
large intestine, role in digestive
    system, 27–28
Latin American Diet Pyramid
    and Plate, 225
LDLs (low-density lipoproteins),
    88, 89, 90
Lenhoff, Alex, 245
leptin, 185
limiting protein, 71
lingual lipases, 25
linoleic acid, 80
lipases, 78–79
lipids, 77. *See also* fat (dietary)
lipoproteins, 66–67, 79,
    88–90, 113
Lithuanian University of
    Health Sciences Medical
    Academy, 124
liver
    cholesterol production by, 89,
        90, 91
    role in digestive system, 27
longevity, coffee and, 381
long-term memory, 325
losing weight
    gaining muscle vs., 60
    later in life, 46
    realistic rules enabling,
        50–52

low-density lipoproteins (LDLs),
    88, 89, 90
low-protein diet, 351
low-quality proteins, 69–71

M

macrominerals, 141–144
macronutrients, 9–10
macular degeneration, 123
magnesium
    megadose of, 150
    overview, 143–144
    RDA for, 38–39
major minerals, 141–144
malnutrition, 13, 55
manganese, 39, 147
MAO inhibitors (monoamine
    oxidase inhibitors), 330
margarine, 82
mast cells, 312–313
Mayo Clinic, 364–365
mcg (micrograms), 36
meat
    beef, 387
    cholesterol in, 91, 92
    fat in, 84
    lamb, 387
    pork, 386–387
    protein, 10
mechanical digestion, 22
medication. *See also* food and
    drug interactions
    alcohol affecting, 118
    colchicine, 164
    as diuretics, 164
    vitamins and, 135
    water and, 164
medicine, food as, 14
    disease prevention, 351–356
    extra-potassium diet, 351
    high-fiber diet, 350–351
    history of, 358

N

NAD (nicotinamide adenine dinucleotide) coenzyme, 113

National Cancer Institute, 115, 130

National Cholesterol Education Program (NCEP), 89–90

National Heart, Lung, and Blood Institute, 89–90

National Institute of Health, 47

National Institute on Drug Abuse, 117

National Institutes of Health, 160

National Research Council, 131, 135

National Resource Defense Council, 161

Natural and Non-prescription Health Products Directorate (NNHPD), 168

NCEP (National Cholesterol Education Program), 89–90

NDRI (norepinephrine and dopamine reuptake inhibitor), 330, 331

neoglucobrassicin, 297

neomycin, 164

neotame, 263

Neuhouser, Marian L., 171

neurotransmitters, 67, 330, 386

neutral spirits, 110–111

niacin, 38, 128

nibbling, 185–186

nicotinamide adenine dinucleotide (NAD) coenzyme, 113

nitrates/nitrites, 304

nitrogen (amino) group, 65

nitrosamines, 304

NNHPD (Natural and Non-prescription Health Products Directorate), 168

nonessential amino acids, 68–69

non-heme iron, 144

nonstick pots, 275

norepinephrine and dopamine reuptake inhibitor (NDRI), 330, 331

nose, role in digestive system, 23

nucleic acids, 66

nucleoproteins, 66, 67

nutraceuticals, 167

nutrients

AI of nutrients, 31, 34, 37–39

in alcohol, 111

defined, 9

Dietary Guidelines for Americans, 214

Dietary Reference Intake, 31, 35–36, 39

digestion of, 24, 25, 26

essential, 10–12

food additives, 298

food processing and, 256–257

from food vs. supplements, 178

groups of, 9–10

protecting in cooked foods

minerals, 277

overview, 276–277

vitamins, 277–278

protecting in food, 12

Recommended Dietary Allowances, 31–33, 37–39

terms used to describe recommendations, 36

units of measurement for, 37

nutrition

basic principles of, 8–9

overview, 1–4, 7–8

reliable information about, finding, 14–17

Nutrition Facts Label, 227–235

health claims, 230–231

ingredients, 235

Nutrition Facts Panel

amount per serving, 229

DRV, 230

Percent Daily Value, 229–230

RDI, 229–230

serving sizes, 228–229

organic, 233–234

overview, 227

science-based definitions, 232–233

nutrition reporters and writers, 15

nutrition scientists and researchers, 15

nutritional status, 13–14

nutritionists, 15

nuts, 374–375

O

obesity, 189–190

across cities and states, 42–44

as epidemic, 42

overview, 41

obesogenic environment, 44

ocular arteries and veins, 87

oils, 77, 84. *See also* fat (dietary)

avoiding when eating out, 240

fatty acids in, 83

Oldways pyramids

African Heritage Diet Pyramid and Plate, 225

Asian Diet Pyramid and Plate, 224

Latin American Diet Pyramid and Plate, 225

Mediterranean Diet Pyramid and Plate, 225

Vegetarian Diet Pyramid and Plate, 225

omega-3 fatty acids, 86, 323

online resources

ACS website, 364

AHA website, 363–364

FARE website, 364

FDA website, 362–363

Food Safety News, 365–366

pumpkins, 389

PURE (Prospective Urban Rural Epidemiology) survey, 162

pyridoxine, 128–129

PYY (peptide tyrosine-tyrosine), 185

Q

Quetelet, Lambert Adolphe Jacques, 47

Quetelet Index, 46

R

radioallergosorbent test (RAST), 313

radiolytic products (RPs), 291

RAST (radioallergosorbent test), 313

RDAs (Recommended Dietary Allowances)

defined, 35

for micronutrients, 10

minerals, 38–39, 148–151

overview, 31–33

terms used to describe recommendations, 36

vitamins, 37–38

vitamins and, 121–123, 131–134

RDI (Reference Daily Intakes), 229–230

RDs (registered dietitians), 15

reactions to food

brain food

adult brain, 325–329

developing brain, 321–324

emotional brain, 329–336

injured brain, 336–339

food allergies

coping with, 315–319

delayed reactions, 314

diagnosing, 311–314

identifying, 314

immediate reactions, 314

metabolic reaction, 319

mood and behavior changes, 320

physical reaction, 319

psychological reaction, 320

Reasonableness Test, 15, 17

Recommended Dietary Allowances. *See* RDAs

red blood cells

protein deficiency affecting, 74

protein in, 66

red meat, 92

REE (resting energy expenditure), 57–59

Reference Daily Intakes (RDI), 229–230

refreezing food, 287

registered dietitians (RDs), 15

rejection reactions, 23

resting energy expenditure (REE), 57–59

retinoids (chemicals), 123

retinol, 36

retrograde amnesia, 325

retrospective studies, 17

ribitol, 127

riboflavin (vitamin B2), 38, 127–128, 136

RNA (ribonucleic acid), 66

RPs (radiolytic products), 291

S

saccharin, 262

salicylates, 317

saliva, role in digestion, 24–25

salt/sodium

overview, 162

recommended daily intake, 209

sodium pump, 159

sodium-restricted diet, 351

water weight, 212

sardines, 374–375

satiety, 79

saturated fat, 82, 83

saturated fatty acids (SFA), 81–83

Science Daily, 365

scleroproteins, 65–66

sedentary persons, calorie requirements for, 61–62

selective serotonin reuptake inhibitors (SSRIs), 331

selective serotonin-norepinephrine reuptake inhibitors (SNRIs), 331

selenium, 39, 146, 151

semipermeable membrane, 158

Semi-Vegetarian Indulgence Pyramid, 226

serotonin, 330

serving sizes

Nutrition Facts Panel, 228–229

when eating out, 238

sex glands, 59

SFA (saturated fatty acids), 81–83

SGSD (sulforaphane glucosinolate), 297

short-term memory, 325

simple carbohydrates, 94

sinigrin, 297

sleep

bananas and, 372

body weight and, 52

small intestine

alcohol in, 113

role in digestive system, 25–27

smell, sense of, 196

smokers, 135

SNRIs (selective serotonin-norepinephrine reuptake inhibitors), 331

sodium ascorbate, 127

soft water, 166

solanine, 387

soy isoflavones, 296

soybeans, 69, 70

sparkling water, 166

About the Author

Carol Ann Rinzler is a former nutrition columnist for the *New York Daily News* and the author of more than 30 health-related books, including *Controlling Cholesterol For Dummies*, *The New Complete Book of Food*, the award-winning *Estrogen and Breast Cancer: A Warning for Women*, and *Leonardo's Foot*, which the American Association for the Advancement of Science described as "some of the best writing about science for the non-scientist encountered in recent years."

Author's Acknowledgments

First, my thanks to the skilled and pleasant professionals at Wiley. Acquisitions editors Tracy Boggier and Elizabeth Stillwell shepherded the project from idea to completion. Project editor Christina Guthrie kept things moving smoothly even through the inevitable crises. And technical editor Rachel Nix made the content even stronger with her comments and suggestions.

As with previous editions of *Nutrition For Dummies*, I am indebted to those who took time to share with me their knowledge and expertise. Stephanie Miceli and Dana Korsen with the National Academies of Sciences, Engineering, and Medicine provided valuable insight into the science behind the *Dietary Guidelines for Americans*. Akiva Cohen of the University of Pennsylvania School of Medicine and the Children's Hospital, Philadelphia; Roger Härtl of Weill Cornell Medical College; Kalman Rubinson; and Donald Wilson of NYU Langone Medical Center-NYU School of Medicine read and commented on parts of the manuscript. Mel Rosenfeld of the NYU Robert Grossman School of Medicine generously opened for me the door to the extraordinary world of neuroscience, and Jim Mandler of NYU Langone Medical Center was always ready with an expert to offer a quote.

William Eakins shared his encyclopedic knowledge of historical fact. Between book chapters, Alexis Gelber prevented nutrition overload by assigning articles on the COVID-19 pandemic. David Handlin solved my math problems, such as the number of zeros in 108. William Hicks kept me up to date on medical ethics. Dane Neilson explained the wondrous thermodynamic concept that there is no cold, only the absence of heat. Peter Sass was simply and seriously logical. Shahzaib Shaikh showed me the importance of right angles. Minna Elias and Ed Morrissey's balanced politics at opposite ends of the spectrum kept the chaos of the 2020 election in perspective. Rosemary Cardillo, Louise Dankberg, and Ruth Edenbaum patiently heard my complaints on days when the writing was hard. Each of these people made this a better book.

Publisher's Acknowledgments

Senior Acquisitions Editor: Tracy Boggier

Senior Editorial Assistant: Elizabeth Stillwell

Editorial Project Manager and Development Editor: Christina N. Guthrie

Managing Editor: Michelle Hacker

Technical Editor: Rachel Nix, RD

Production Editor: Mohammed Zafar Ali

Cover Photo: ©udra11/Shutterstock